STUTTERING:
SCIENCE, THERAPY & PRACTICE

The Most Complete Book About Stuttering

Thomas David Kehoe

THE COVER PHOTO is of the author (center) in 1972 (age ten) and his Cub Scout den (photo by Thomas F. Kehoe). The background pattern is from *Kodai Moshiki Zuko* (Picture Album Of Traditional Patterns), reproduced as *Japanese Border Designs*, edited by Theodore Menten (New York: Dover, 1975). The chapter "Zen and Stuttering" suggests that words should slip from your tongue as easily as snow slips from a bamboo leaf.

Printed on recycled paper

Stuttering: Science, Therapy & Practice

ISBN 0-9657181-0-7 SAN 299-2566

Casa Futura Technologies
P.O. Box 7551
Boulder, CO 80306-7551

(303) 417-9752
FAX: (303) 413-0853
kehoe@casafuturatech.com

Warning — Disclaimer

This book is designed to provide information in regard to the subject matter covered. It is sold with the understanding that the publisher and author are not engaged in rendering medical or legal services. If medical or other expert assistance is required, the services of a competent professional should be sought.

It is not the purpose of this book to reprint all the information that is otherwise available to the author and/or publisher, but to complement, amplify and supplement other texts. You are urged to read all available material, learn as much as possible about the subject matter, and to tailor the information to your individual needs. For more information, see the many references provided.

Stuttering cannot be cured quickly. Any stutterer who decides to improve his or her speech must expect to invest considerable time and effort.

Every effort has been made to make this book as complete and as accurate as possible. However, there **may be mistakes** both typographical and in content. Therefore, this text should be used only as a general guide and not as the ultimate source of stuttering information. Furthermore, this book contains information on stuttering only up to the printing date. If you find mistakes, notify the publisher immediately and every effort will be made to correct the problem.

The purpose of this book is to educate and entertain. The author and publisher shall have neither liability nor responsibility to any person or entity with respect to any loss or damage caused, or alleged to be caused, directly or indirectly by the information contained in this book.

If you do not wish to be bound by the above, you may return this book to the publisher for a full refund.

Reviews of *Stuttering: Science, Therapy & Practice*

The Speak Easy Newsletter:

a meticulously-fashioned masterpiece...On the cover page, under the book's title, Mr. Kehoe calls it, "The Most Complete Book About Stuttering." If it isn't, it certainly comes close to it.

Journal of Fluency Disorders:

Ambitious yet eminently practical...a wealth of information...

Insights into the world of people stutter as well as the world stutterers have to contend with...

The dominant theme of the book is that people who stutter should take command of their lives, their stuttering, and the treatment of their stuttering...

This book belongs on the bookshelf of every speech-language pathologist.

ADVANCE For Speech-Language Pathologists:

The therapy section is...a standout...People who stutter will find this particularly useful...This book is an excellent presentation that is worthwhile reading for a wide variety of readers.

ASHA Leader:

Speech pathologists, educators, stutterers, and families of stutterers will be enlightened by this text...From a speech therapist's viewpoint I was encouraged that readable information was available to our clients with fluency disorders...I found the book heartwarming, encouraging, and challenging.

William Perkins, Professor Emeritus, University of Southern California:

A breath of fresh air; you've produced more new sources of information than I've found anywhere else.

CONTENTS

INTRODUCTION

SCIENCE

PRACTICE

INTRODUCTION

What's So Great About Stuttering?

Stuttering is a remarkable disorder. It's the easiest disease to treat, and the hardest to cure. On occasion, stutterers can talk fluently, when they're alone, by changing their manner of speaking, thinking differently, using an electronic device, or even seeing their speech therapist walk into the room.

But stutterers can go right back to stuttering, even after months of the best therapy. Temporary "cures" are a dime a dozen, but a universal, permanent cure has never been found.

Stuttering occurs when we want most to speak well, such as job interviews, public speaking, or speaking to authority figures. Stuttering is characterized by overtense speech-production muscles. We try too hard, tense, stutter, try harder, stutter more, and get more stuck in a vicious cycle. The most frustrating aspect of stuttering is that it gets worse when we try not to do it.

Some stutterers have extreme physical symptoms, such as head jerks and facial grimaces. Other stutterers hide their stuttering by substituting or avoiding words. The latter can be more disabling, because the stutterer is afraid that people will discover that he stutters. The stutterer may refuse promotions that require talking, or avoid social interaction.

Despite the disabling effects of stuttering, the greatest orators have been stutterers. Demosthenes was the greatest orator of ancient Greece. Aesop was master storyteller of Babylon. Winston Churchill and Aneurin Bevan were the best orators in the British Parliament in the 1930s. Today, James Earl Jones is the most in-demand voice in Hollywood.

These stutterers found ways to speak fluently, and developed these techniques into strengths.

Demosthenes improved his articulation by speaking with pebbles in his mouth, improved his volume by shouting over the ocean waves, and took lessons from an actor to speak with his emotions.

Bevan also found fluency when expressing his emotions, and as leader of the Labor Party during the Depression made passionate speeches about the plight of the working class.

Churchill was fluent when he prepared and rehearsed his remarks in advance — so he devoted long hours to mastering every political issue and having an answer ready for every objection.

Jones recited Shakespeare and developed his acting talent along with his fluency.

Men find their strengths only after finding their limitations (Bly, 1990). For other men, the age of 35 may be when the dreams of their youth crash down. But for stutterers this is often the age at which they overcome stuttering, and find that they can achieve the goals they never thought possible.

Stutterers are both hyperaware and unaware of stuttering. Before talking to a stranger, we have fear and anxiety that we will stutter. But when we stutter, we lose awareness of what our speech-production muscles are doing. Our minds seem to go "someplace else." We lose awareness of time.

You can't overcome stuttering until you admit that you stutter. Ironically, admitting that you stutter gets easier as you improve your fluency. People who stutter severely can be the least willing to talk about or do anything about their stuttering.

But after you make progress on your speech, you happily talk about stuttering. You attend support groups and stuttering conventions. You want to tell everyone what you did to overcome stuttering.

Stuttering is one of few disabilities that get better over time. Most children outgrow it. Even adults who stutter severely in their 20s usually learn to manage their stuttering in their 30s. People with almost any other disease face a lifetime of worsening symptoms. But your most severe stuttering is probably behind you.

Stuttering is difficult to treat because it involves all aspects of your life — muscle control, emotions and anxieties, cognitive awareness, and social interaction. But by working on the different aspects of stuttering, your reward is not just fluent speech, but improvements in all areas of your life.

Glenn Doman wrote (1974):

> In no area is man more vulnerable to misunderstanding, criticism and downright abuse from his fellow man than if he should fail to develop speech, or having gained it, should lose it — for when man loses the ability to express himself by speech he is suspect...of having lost, also the [faculties to arrive] at the conclusions which he would express in speech. The world feels...that if he can't say his name...he doesn't know his name.

About the Author

I stuttered severely until I was about thirty years old.

I had blocks lasting five minutes or more. When I was 22, a speech pathologist measured my most fluent speech (reading out loud alone) as averaging two seconds per syllable, or ten times slower than normal speech.

I took five or ten minutes to say what a non-stutterer could say in thirty seconds. I had the full range of facial grimaces and head jerks.

I added starter sounds, for example, adding a /k/ sound in front of words starting with /l/, so that I introduced my friend "Lou" as "Clue." I had to change these starter sounds every few weeks, as their effectiveness wore off.

People couldn't understand what I said, so they nodded and guessed, and guessed wrong. I thought people were stupid because I'd tell them how to fix something, and they'd go on with the broken thing. I didn't realize that they couldn't understand me.

My mother recalls me, at the ages of 4 and 5, being less than fluent, but not stuttering. I was probably "borderline stuttering." I liked my kindergarten teacher, and recall this as a happy year.

When I was six, my family moved from Nebraska to Wisconsin. My first-grade teacher was a cold, uncaring older woman, and I remember coming home in tears. My brother remembers this as a stressful period for the family, possibly due to both parents starting new jobs. My mother recalls stress from a housekeeper who didn't work out.

Whatever the problems, this was a stressful period, and I started stuttering. One traumatic experience stands out. I had learned to read in kindergarten in Nebraska, but in Wisconsin children learn to read in first grade. Because I could read, the teacher had me go to the front of the room and read stories to the class, while the other children drew pictures of me. Somehow the drawings terrified me, and I associate this with the beginning of stuttering.

After a few months we moved to another neighborhood. I started in a new school with a new teacher. My stuttering went away.

But I started stuttering again in second grade (even though I liked my teacher). My parents consulted psychologists, who evaluated the family and found nothing wrong.

In third grade I was treated by a speech pathologist at the nearby university. I recall working on articulation exercises, not stuttering, and a year of therapy had some, but not great effect. This was 1971, and stuttering therapies were not as advanced as today.

My parents consulted with a speech pathologist at another

university, who recommended some reading materials. My parents concluded that no cause or treatment for stuttering was known. This conclusion was confirmed because the Ph.D. speech pathologist (who has since written several textbooks on stuttering) stuttered severely. If he couldn't help himself, there must not be a treatment. This ended my stuttering therapy for ten years.

As a child I had the usual circle of friends, and enjoyed Cub Scouts and other group activities. But as a teenager I became withdrawn, developing an introverted shell. This was due a combination of family patterns and stuttering. I was depressed through my teenage years. The only activities I liked as a teenager were long-distance bicycling and solo backpacking. In college, I liked photography and became yearbook editor and darkroom manager. This allowed me to spend long hours alone in the darkroom. I majored in philosophy, which I never enjoyed, but fit my introspective shell. I spent all my time sitting in the library reading.

These activities didn't help me improve my speech or develop social skills. My extroverted true nature always managed to come through, conflicting with the introverted shell. I've always talked a lot, and enjoyed writing. But I tended to express anger or insult people. This satisfied my extroverted need for attention, and maintained the strong shell that kept people away.

As an adult, I was unaware of how severely I stuttered. I didn't know that my speech was all but incomprehensible. I didn't know that my speech was painful to watch, or that listeners barely had the patience to wait for me to finish a sentence.

People are surprised when I say that I was barely aware of my stuttering. But no one told me that I stuttered. Family and friends never talked to me about my speech. Teachers, supervisors, guidance counselors — no one suggested I should improve my speech, or where I could begin. Again, my protective shell kept away anyone from getting close enough to have a personal conversation with me.

By 1981, when I was 19, I tried a new stuttering therapy, Precision Fluency Shaping Program (PFSP). This therapy had no effect on my speech.

When I was 22, I completed a PFSP refresher course. The speech pathologist videotaped me at the start of the therapy program. Again the therapy had no effect on my speech. Then at the end of the program, I saw the videotape — the first time I'd seen myself on video. I was shocked by how severely I stuttered. I had never known that I talked, or looked, like that.

I instantly was able to talk fluently outside the clinic for the first time in my life. I used the slow fluency shaping speech, but I was fluent.

This fluency lasted three days. My stuttering then came back. The speech pathologist hadn't told me to expect relapse. He'd given me the impression that the therapy program was over, I was talking fluently, and I was cured. I was too embarrassed to call and tell him that I'd somehow failed.

I'd graduated from Reed College, but had difficulty getting a job. For a few years, my friends got me jobs (I never made it past the first interview with people that didn't know me). When I was 26 I was managing the data processing department at a market research firm, supervising a half-dozen employees. I was only paid $6.50/hour, after 3 years with the company, and the executives avoided me, although they were satisfied with my department's work. I went to the local speech clinic again.

Again I learned fluency shaping techniques. After three months of therapy, my speech became comprehensible (a great advance), and the president of my company gave me a promotion. I continued in therapy a few more months. I'd gotten completely fluent in the speech clinic, but was making no progress on my speech outside the clinic. Eventually the speech pathologist said there was nothing more she could do. We discontinued the therapy, and my stuttering returned.

When I was 28 I went to graduate school, studying for an MBA at the University of Chicago. By now I knew that improving my speech was paramount, and I began stuttering therapy at the university's hospital.

I saw two speech therapists at the university hospital. The first taught me the Benjamin Bogue arm-waving technique, which went out of favor about 1935. He knew little about stuttering. When the hospital hired a new Ph.D. speech pathologist that had written her dissertation on stuttering, I started seeing her.

Each week, the Ph.D. speech pathologist asked me what my speech goals were. My extroverted true self came out when I envisioned myself not stuttering. I said that I wanted to be a great public speaker.

Demosthenes had gone from severe stuttering to become the greatest orator of ancient Greece. James Earl Jones had gone from being mute from stuttering to being the most in-demand voice in Hollywood. For three days after the PFSP program I'd experienced the pleasure of relaxed, clear, confident fluent speech. I knew that if I could control of my speech, I could speak better than anyone else. I wanted so badly to talk that I was hyperaware of how poorly many non-stutterers speak. They had the gift I wanted, and they squandered it by rambling off topics, mumbling, ignoring listeners, etc. If only I could talk fluently, I would never make those mistakes. I would speak better than anyone!

Each week, the speech pathologist told me that adults who stutter severely could never hope to talk fluently. I wouldn't be able to make any progress until I lowered my goals and admitted to myself that I would always stutter. She wasn't going to teach me any techniques to talk fluently.

After a few months of this lecturing, I stopped seeing her. I found a speech pathologist in private practice. The new speech pathologist taught me Van Riper techniques for modifying my stuttering — cancellations, pull-outs, bouncing. I didn't like voluntary stuttering or bouncing, and my poor awareness of my stuttering made the stuttering modification techniques ineffective.

The speech pathologist also helped me work on slow, relaxed speech. I made slow but steady progress. My speech moved from incomprehensible to comprehensible, severe stuttering.

I read Malcolm Fraser's *Self-Therapy for the Stutterer*, the first book I'd found about stuttering, but I lacked the vocal control to do the exercises. I tape-recorded my job interviews. Each time I was sure I'd been almost fluent, but I'd listen to the tape and find that I'd stuttered on almost every word. I kept thinking I was making progress, but the tapes showed that I wasn't.

During a summer internship in California, I saw another speech pathologist. She had a high-tech operation: she videotaped each session, and we used a delayed auditory feedback (DAF) device. The DAF device seemed pointless, because I was fluent in her office. I continued to stutter outside, but it never occurred to me to borrow the DAF device.

I graduated with my MBA when I was 30. Despite more than 50 job interviews, no one hired me. This was before the Americans with Disabilities Act, and interviewers discriminated against me.

I did some temp work. Three weeks later, a telephone I was using at a job malfunctioned, and I heard an echo of my voice, delayed enough to slow my speech and make me talk fluently. I recognized this was DAF, and I wanted a telephone to do this all the time!

I talked to a telephone company engineer, who said that such a telephone would be easy to make, but they wouldn't make one. I quit my temp job and figured out how to build DAF telephones.

To talk fluently, I had to set the delay extremely slow, so that I sounded like a robot. But I was fluent, and even this speech was faster than my stuttering. My friends were amazed (although a few asked if I was working on an improved version, which would run faster!). I sold a few DAF telephones to other stutterers, while looking for a permanent job.

After a few months, I was able to talk fluently with the DAF set to a "slow-normal" speed. I used the DAF telephone for an hour a day or so, but it wasn't really usable off the telephone.

My speech without the device was getting better. I still stuttered, but I'd lost the head jerks and facial grimaces, and conversations didn't take forever.

For the first time in my life, I could talk without stuttering. OK, it was just on the telephone, but that changed my entire outlook on life. My extroverted self happily my telephone calls at every opportunity. The anger and bitterness I'd experienced all my life dissolved away in those first six months. I no longer tried to treat people badly, or take out my frustrations on people. I felt like all my life I'd been in prison, and now I was free.

Now I wanted to help other stutterers talk fluently. I'd learned that stuttering wasn't just a speech disorder. Stuttering was pain, frustration, menial jobs, accomplishments that were ignored, disrespect from strangers, people that wouldn't return my calls, friends that never asked me to go out with them.

I stopped looking for a job. I worked full-time developing electronic devices for stuttering. I was elected president of our local National Stuttering Project (NSP) self-help group.

I joined the American Speech-Language Hearing Association (ASHA). I read speech pathology textbooks and journals. I attended the ASHA and NSP conventions. I met hundreds of stutterers and speech pathologists.

I then developed biofeedback devices for stuttering, training me to talk with relaxed speech-production muscles. Two years after building my first DAF telephone, I had a portable device that produced consistent carryover fluency. If I used the device for a few hours, I was fluent the rest of the day. If I used the device for a few days, I was fluent for a week. Afterwards my stuttering would return, but always less severely.

I've spent another three years improving the anti-stuttering biofeedback devices. I'm now 35, and my speech is fluent or I stutter mildly. The mild stuttering doesn't bother me.

I've learned a lot about stuttering. Now I hope to share what I've learned. Perhaps the most frustrating aspect of stuttering was not knowing anything about it. Ten or twenty years ago, if someone had handed me a book about stuttering, or taken me to a self-help group meeting, or told me about an effective stuttering therapy, my life would have been different. Perhaps only silence is worse than stuttering.

Overcoming stuttering is a long road. I hope this book and the resources it points you to will help you along the road.

About This Book

This book is divided into three main sections: Science, Therapy, and Practice. Each section is independent, so you can skip sections that don't interest you.

Much scientific research has been published about stuttering. This book provides an overview of the major points, and then refers you to books and journals.

Much less is published about stuttering therapies. This book goes into more depth in this section. This section is intended to help you choose an appropriate therapy program for your needs.

The "Practice" section is also in-depth, because little has been published about practical issues. This section also points to other resources, including organizations, books, and Internet resources. The goal is to overwhelm you with ideas to try.

This book includes stutterers' personal stories. Many stutterers have written about their personal experiences, for example in the book *To Say What Is Ours*. However, this book keeps to personal stories that illustrate scientific or therapy points, or how the person overcame stuttering.

A survey of the *Journal of Fluency Disorders* found that over 90% of the studies were "science," mostly stuttering etiology (the nature and causes of stuttering). Less than 10% of the studies were about therapy. No articles were about practical issues.

Stutterers need the opposite. We need to know our rights under disability laws, whether a military career is possible, and how to improve communication in a relationship. Stutterers need to know enough to choose the most appropriate therapy. We don't need to know the percentage of phonological errors 3-year-olds make, or other scientific minutiae.

SLAUGHTERING THE SACRED COWS

This book presents the "conventional wisdom" of stuttering. Then scientific research is presented which slaughters these sacred cows. Lastly, I present original theories, which conform to the scientific data.

This thesis—antithesis—synthesis model may seem contradictory or confusing at times. For example, the chapter on childhood therapy suggests that parents should speak slower. Then there is research finding that changing parents' speech does not reduce children's stuttering. Because stuttering varies between individuals, a therapy technique that doesn't help 95% of stutterers could work for you. Maybe you are one of the 5%. When there is no clear answer or solution, this book gives you lots of ideas, and you can see what works. Doing *something* about your speech is better than doing nothing.

Stutterers say that "someone," maybe *Consumer Reports*, should do a study comparing stuttering therapies. This shows poor understanding of stuttering therapy. Many aspects of stuttering therapies can't be measured, such as fear and avoidances. Some therapies aim to improve your life, without directly altering your speech. A scientific study that pools many stutterers to get an "average" number is meaningless, because no two stutterers are alike. It's better to find out what kind of stutterer you are, and what approaches to therapy are available, and then you choose the most appropriate therapy for your needs. That is the aim of this book.

This book presents stuttering in the context of motor learning theory. No other book does this. Some reviewers objected to this, saying that this was "misleading, inaccurate and, indeed, absurd" (Venkatagiri, 1998). This ignorance about motor learning theory among speech pathologists is one reason I wrote this book.

All legal issues discussed in this book refer to United States laws. Laws in other countries may vary.

THE STUTTERING SCIENCE & THERAPY WEBSITE

The Stuttering Science & Therapy Website (http://www.casafuturatech.com) has a variety of resources:

- The Casa Futura Technologies catalog of electronic stuttering therapy devices.
- The Stuttering Penpals webpage — hundreds of men and women who stutter, parents of children who stutter, speech pathology students. All ages (18 or older), professions, and geographic areas are represented.
- The "Stuttering FAQ" file, which is a short version of this book (about 1/15th of the length).
- Links to other stuttering websites.

SCIENCE

Many scientific books and journals about stuttering are available. If you want to know more, several books and journals are recommended in the chapter "Books And Journals About Stuttering."

Definition of Stuttering

A widely-quoted definition of stuttering is (Wingate, 1964):

I. (a) disruption in the fluency of verbal expression, which is
(b) characterized by involuntary, audible, or silent repetitions or prolongations in the utterance of short speech elements, namely: sounds, syllables, and words of one syllable. These disruptions
(c) usually occur frequently or are marked in character and
(d) are not readily controllable.

II. Sometimes the disruptions are (e) accompanied by accessory activities involving the speech apparatus, related or unrelated body structures, or stereotyped speech utterances. These activities give the appearance of being speech-related struggle.

III. Also, there not infrequently are (f) indications or reports of the presence of an emotional state, ranging from a general condition of "excitement" or "tension" to more specific emotions of a negative nature such as fear, embarrassment, irritation, or the like.

(g) The immediate source of stuttering is some incoordination expressed in the peripheral speech mechanism; the ultimate cause is presently unknown and may be complex or compound.

The World Health Organization adds that stutterers know what they wish to say — they just can't say it.

Wingate's definition is from the point of view of the listener, who hears what the stutterer can say. The stutterer, on the other hand, is aware of what he can't say. To the stutterer, a repetition is a word he can say — it's the next sound or syllable that he can't produce.

My definition of stuttering is talking while using your speech-production muscles in a way that makes speech difficult or impossible.

Woodruff Starkweather believes that "stuttering is the elevated activity in the muscles that are involved in speech production" (Starkweather, 1995). In other words, stutterers tense their speech-production muscles (breathing, vocal folds, jaw, lips, and tongue) too much, and hold the tension too long.

Starkweather defines fluency in four parameters (Starkweather, 1987):

- Smoothness, or lack of interruptions.
- Speaking rate.
- Prosody, or emotional intonation.
- Mental effort.

Stuttering also includes avoidance and substitution techniques. Many stutterers talk 100% fluently — but substitute words, avoid answering the telephone, refuse jobs that require speaking to strangers, or just avoid talking, to hide their stuttering.

Stammering is the British word for stuttering.

EXAMPLES OF STUTTERING

Wendell Johnson, one of the most influential speech pathologists, arrived at the University of Iowa in 1926 and soon met Lee Edward Travis:

> A few days after I arrived, Dr. Travis asked me to come with him to one of his classes. He explained that he wanted the students to observe my speech. I sat in a chair beside his desk at the front of the room. There were thirty or forty students looking at me. Dr. Travis told them who I was and that I was from a small town in Kansas and then he handed me a book and asked me to read aloud to the students. I read for five minutes — and got out four words.
>
> After class I went with him to his car and we got in and started for the other end of campus. When we had gone about a block he stopped to give one of his staff members a ride and as she got in the car he introduced us. Then he started the car again and we drove down a long curving hill and crossed a river…Altogether we had gone about a mile when all of a sudden I finally managed to blurt out, "Puleased to meet you!" They were startled, and so was I, and I wished I hadn't said it, only I would have been more embarrassed if I hadn't said anything at all. (Johnson, 1961)

The internal, invisible effects of stuttering are as important as the stumbling speech that listeners hear. One stutterer sent me the following e-mail:

> I'm a 25 year old male. I'm not the typical stutterer in that no one guesses that I have a problem. Even my family and friends don't believe me when I tell them. What they don't realize is that for my

whole life I've been constantly struggling to get my words out fluently. When I speak, I substitute words. I completely avoid certain words, situations and people. However, when I'm comfortable, I LOVE to talk. I've made flawless speeches at a Toastmasters club and many people have told me that I am an excellent communicator.

When I speak, people don't actually hear me stutter. When a difficult word comes, I either avoid it completely or I struggle very hard to say it (silently though). I guess this is what is called a 'silent block.' The people I am talking to think that I am pausing to think (or hesitating).

I suppose you could say that my dysfluency rate is 0.5% but this is very misleading. You must take into consideration the avoidances, substitutions, mental stress etc. to achieve this rate. My stuttering behavior is avoidance.

I started taking therapy when I was a child but I can not remember how it was. When I was in high school and college I avoided people completely except for people I knew I was fluent with. I was (and still am) very much a loner. When I completed University, I enrolled in the late Dr. Boberg's program at the Institute for Stuttering Treatment and Research (ISTAR) in Edmonton [Canada] (1995). This was an excellent program. Due to this program, I slowly increased the amount of speaking situations I went into. I enrolled in a Toastmasters club and I volunteered as a teacher for several places. In February 1996, I went to Korea to teach English for a year! I came back just a few days ago.

Even though I've made improvements, I'm still very frustrated. The ISTAR program (though it has done wonders for me) has been difficult for me to maintain and I have a strong desire to speak at whatever rate that I want. It's also difficult for me to freely admit to everyone that I stutter. The ISTAR program brought me up to a level that enabled me to accomplish many of my hopes. Now that I've reached that level, I want to go further.

There are some words that I consistently have problems with but sometimes I do not know I will have problems with a word until just before I try to say it. My biggest worry is when I have to say a word that there is no substitute for. I'll have no choice but to try to say the word out loud. In this case I will stutter loudly and the people I'm talking to will notice. I've been very lucky that I've been able to avoid situations like that in most cases.

I do remember a time where I had to say my name. This was during a time when I feared to say my name. It took me 20 seconds of continuous loud stuttering to get it out. I was devastated.

When I went to Korea I was worried that I would have problems saying the city I came from. Luckily I either lied about the city or said my province's name. A few times though, I was able to say my city fluently.

WHAT CAUSES STUTTERING?

As you will see in this book, there are many hypotheses about what causes stuttering. But the question "What causes stuttering?" is really two questions — one easy to answer, one hard to answer.

The easy question is "What causes stuttering in adults?" The answer is that they stuttered when they were children. The speech patterns we learn as children — accent, grammar, language, etc. — become "hard-wired" as our brains grow. An adult stutterer can learn to talk fluently about as easily as an adult non-stutterer can learn to speak Chinese.

Because stuttering develops as a child's speech and language develops, this disorder is called *developmental stuttering*. Developmental stuttering is distinguished from *neurogenic stuttering* (caused by strokes and head injuries) and *psychogenic stuttering* (caused by psychological trauma). These types of stuttering are presented in the chapter "Other Fluency Disorders."

The hard question is "What causes stuttering in children?" Paradoxically, childhood stuttering looks simple compared to the complex behaviors of adult stuttering. But while the cause of adult stuttering is simple, the cause of childhood stuttering is an enigma.

How Speech Is Produced

Speech uses many organs and muscles. While no single organ has developed primarily for speech, many human organs have evolved to be suited for speech.

For example, the larynx is lower in humans than other mammals, creating a space for sound to resonate and be manipulated. Babies are born with their larynx higher (allowing babies to breathe and swallow at the same time), but by age two the larynx has descended to produce speech.

Children also learn a new way to breathe in their second year. In addition to steady, relaxed, diaphragmatic breathing, children develop speech breathing, using their upper chests. Speech breathing draws in more air, with fast inhalation, and releases the air slowly, enabling the child to cry longer and louder. This breathing also prepares the child for speech.

Speech begins with breathing. Your lungs fill with air, more air than you would inhale if you weren't talking. You expand your upper chest, as well as your diaphragm, to get all this air in. Your lung pressure and respiration muscle tension increases.

Next, you release air through your throat, past your vocal folds (also called vocal cords or chords). Your vocal folds are a pair of small muscular folds in your larynx. If you tense these muscles slightly, and release a little air, your vocal folds vibrate. This is called phonation. If you place your fingers or palm across the front of your throat, and hum or talk, you can feel your vocal folds vibrating.

Men vibrate their vocal folds about 125 Hz, or 125 times per second. Women vibrate their vocal folds about 250 Hz. This is too fast for your brain to control. Vocal fold vibration is the only muscle activity that your brain doesn't directly control. Phonation results from the coordination of respiration muscles with slight tensing of your vocal fold muscles.

If you tense your vocal folds too much, you block off your throat and prevent any air from escaping your lungs. This is a good thing to do when you are lifting heavy weights. By blocking your larynx and tensing your respiration muscles, you increase lung pressure, which strengthens your chest and you can lift more weight. Similarly, a tire inflated to a high pressure can carry a heavier car. But this is what stutterers do when they talk, and this is not a good idea.

The space above the larynx is called the pharynx. Here your vocal fold vibrations resonate.

Above this are your oral and nasal cavities. More vocal resonation is produced in the nasal cavity. Your jaw and lips and tongue (your articulation muscles) modify your voice into intelligible speech.

Vowels are produced by your vocal folds, and modified by your articulation muscles. Some voiced consonants, such as /b/ and /d/, are also produced with vocal fold vibration, and modified by your jaw, lips and tongue. Other consonants are voiceless, such as /p/ and /t/, and are produced by your articulation muscles modifying airflow, without your vocal folds vibrating.

When you whisper, you don't vibrate your vocal folds. You just modify the airflow with your articulation muscles.

Your ears are essential but overlooked speech-production organs. You can't speak correctly if you can't hear — deaf persons can't articulate certain sounds quite right. The role of hearing in stuttering is not well-known. Some theorists have proposed that stutterers have defective hearing in some way. Despite over 40 years of research, no such defect has ever been found. Stutterers appear to have normal hearing.

Speech requires coordination of over 100 muscles and many organs. The average person speaks about 150 words per minute. Each word requires a different configuration of most of those 100 muscles. Speech is our most complex, balanced neuromuscular activity. Learning to talk takes many years. There are a lot of mistakes you can make!

Symptoms of Stuttering

Studies in this chapter are referenced in *A Handbook On Stuttering* (Bloodstein, 1995), except as otherwise noted.

LARYNGEAL DISORDERS

Laryngeal dysfunction is widely-believed to be the core stuttering behavior. The vocal folds have been the focus of research since the nineteenth century. However, laryngeal dysfunction in stuttering is not simple.

There are many muscles in the larynx. Different stutterers tense different muscles. Some people stutter without laryngeal dysfunctions. Some people have stuttering-type laryngeal muscle activity when they're not talking (called "internal stuttering").

The typical laryngeal dysfunctions are:

- High levels of laryngeal muscle activity (too much muscle tension).
- Poor muscle timing, such as starting phonation too late, or holding tension too long.
- Poor coordination of muscles, e.g., incompatible contractions of opposing muscles.

Frances Freeman used electromyography to measure muscle activity during stuttering. She found that stutterers tense their vocal folds too much, and that antagonistic muscles were poorly coordinated.

Conture, McCall, and Brewer (1985) concluded that stutterers do not "simply 'squeeze' their vocal folds together in all instances of stuttering."

Smith, *et al.* (1996) concluded that

> Compared to periods of fluent speech, intervals of disfluent speech are not typically characterized by higher levels of activity in [laryngeal] muscles; and...normally fluent adults show robust and sometimes near maximal recruitment during conversational speech. The adults who stutter had a lower operating range for these muscles during conversational speech, and their disfluencies did not produce relatively high activation levels. In summary, the present data require us to reject the claim that adults with a history of chronic stuttering routinely produce excessive levels of intrinsic laryngeal muscle activity.

On the other hand, Martin Schwartz felt this study overgeneralized (Schwartz, 1996):

> The article looked as two muscles and generalized to all the intrinsic muscles. The crico-thyroid is innervated by the superior laryngeal branch of the vagus nerve — that's different from all the other intrinsics. And they did not look at pre-speech tensions, which I believe are the critical ones. And the two most important intrinsic muscles — the posterior crico-aryntenoid and the lateral crico-aryntenoid — were not examined.

Regardless of whether stutterers use our vocal folds in a abnormal way, changing how you use your vocal folds is one of the most effective ways to improve fluency. The section on stuttering therapies discusses this at length.

OTHER PHYSIOLOGICAL DISORDERS

Stuttering is associated with other physiological disorders. Generally, speech-production muscles are tensed too much, and the tension is maintained too long:

1) Breathing disorders. Many studies associate stuttering with disordered respiration. Breathing disorders include antagonism between abdominal (belly) and thoracic (upper chest) respiratory muscles; complete cessation of breathing, and interrupting exhalation with inhalation.

2) Articulation disorders. Many studies have found dysfunctions of the lips, jaw, and tongue in stuttering. As with the laryngeal dysfunctions, these unusual muscle activities occur in only some persons who stutter. Some articulation dysfunctions occur when the stutterer is talking fluently, or even when not talking. Unlike other speech disorders, in which people place their articulators in the wrong positions,

> stutterers place their articulators in virtually the same position for a particular sound as non-stutterers; however, the inability to precisely time the movement from that position to the position for the subsequent sound is a distinctive characteristic of stuttering. (Caruso, 1994)

Low-frequency tremors are seen in the neck, jaw, and lip muscles of adult stutterers. These are found to a lessor extent in older children, and not found in young children who stutter. (Kelly, 1995)

3) Aerodynamic studies found abnormalities in the airflow of stutterers. These studies show that stutterers try to speak through a constricted airway.

THE STUTTERING MOMENT

Bloodstein (1995) presents three general concepts of the stuttering moment:

1) *Repressed need.* A variety of psychological hypotheses have proposed that stuttering is the repression of an psychological need or desire. Stutterers seem to start to do one thing, then stop it, then try again, stop again, and so on. Stuttering appears (to certain psychologists) to be the conflict of opposing desires:

• Psychoanalytic oral erotic and anal erotic models are described in the subsection on psychological studies in the chapter "Physical Constitution and Personality of Stutterers."

• Stuttering is a covert expression of hostility or aggression, which the stutterer fears to express openly.

• Stuttering is an unconscious desire to suppress speech.

These psychological views are no longer widely-regarded.

2) *Anticipatory struggle.* Oliver Bloodstein describes this concept as, "stutterers interfere in some manner with the way they are talking because of their belief in the difficulty of speech...stutterers have difficulty whenever they expect to stutter and...speak fluently when not 'thinking' about their speech." (Bloodstein, 1995) He added, "if a stutterer were to forget that he was a stutterer, he would have no further difficulty with his speech." (Bloodstein, 1996)

One variation of the "anticipatory struggle" is that stutterers try to consciously control automatic speech processes, like the imaginary centipede who couldn't walk after he thought about which leg to move first. Another variation is that "stuttering is what the speaker does while trying not to stutter."

Scientific research has cast doubt on the anticipatory struggle hypothesis (see the subsection "The Placebo Effect" in the chapter "Belief: Anticipation, Distraction, Stress, and Placebos").

3) *Breakdown under stress.* Stuttering is seen as a physical breakdown caused by emotional stress. Oliver Bloodstein writes that this concept presumes "a momentary failure of the complicated coordinations involved in speech. In the context of such theories, the words *breakdown*, *disorganization*, *disintegration*, and *disruption* are often used." (Bloodstein, 1995)

Usually this breakdown is viewed as discoordination of respiration, phonation, and articulation (i.e., your breathing, vocal folds, and jaw, lips and tongue don't work together). Or this breakdown is believed to be in the brain, perhaps due to left/right hemisphere dominance breakdown.

Another view is that stutterers have a threshold of speech-production muscle control, and talking in certain ways pushes you over the threshold and your brain can no longer coordinate these muscles. Zimmerman suggests this involves brainstem reflexes (Bloodstein, 1995). Martin Schwartz believes that stutterers have a lower threshold for laryngeal tension, and that by "subtracting" laryngeal tension prior to speaking, stutterers can talk fluently below their threshold for vocal fold locking.

The problem with the "breakdown" hypothesis is that stuttering is not the absence or failure of a speech process. The stutterer doesn't not hear something, or fail to remember a word (aphasia), or is unable to produce certain speech sounds (disarthria), or is unable to move certain muscles (strokes). The stutterer's speech functions work.

There is no lack of coordination in stuttering — stutterers are quite coordinated in their production of prolongations, blocks, repetitions, and secondary behaviors. Anyone who has seen speech pathology students or other non-stutterers trying to imitate stuttering can see that considerable coordination is needed to stutter. Non-stutterers are able to tense their upper chest respiration muscles, *or* lock their vocal folds, *or* force their lips, jaws, and tongues into fixed positions, but not all at the same time. Stuttering is a complex, coordinated speech behavior.

Stuttering is not a lack of control over certain muscles, such as their vocal folds. Stutterers' vocal folds do not lock up without reason. Stutterers lock their vocal folds in response to specific cues — e.g., trying to speak to an authority figure, or leaving a message on an answering machine. Stutterers lack *conscious* control, but do not lack control.

4) I propose a fourth alternative to Bloodstein's three descriptions of the stuttering moment — stuttering is a *developmental maladaptive motor skill.* Stuttering is the retrieval of the memory of how to stutter, in response to an environmental cue. Stuttering is a behavior learned in childhood and stored as a one of many ways of speaking. Stutterers also learn when to use this form of speech, and when to use other, fluent forms of speech.

This is analogous to a person growing up in Texas, and then moving to Minnesota. When she is in Minnesota and hears the Minnesota accent, her brain retrieves the memory of how to speak with a Minnesota accent. But when she returns to Texas and hears Texas accents, her brain retrieves the memory of how to speak with a Texas accent.

Similarly, stutterers retrieve stuttering or fluent speech motor plans from memory depending on the situation they are in.

SECONDARY BEHAVIORS

Most stutterers have stuttering symptoms unrelated to speech production:

• Physical movements such as eye-blinking, wrinkling of the forehead, sudden exhaustion of breath, frowning, and quivering of the nostrils. There may be jerky movements of the head, arms, legs, etc.

• Interjected words, such as "um," "er," "you know," "in other words."

• Vocal abnormalities, such as changes in speaking rate, vocal pitch, odd inflections, or monotone speech.

• Looking away from the listener, and not maintaining eye contact.

• Articulating an unrelated sound (e.g., forming a /t/ sound when trying to say /s/).

Some stutterers have few secondary behaviors. Others have many secondary behaviors. Extensive studies have failed to find any secondary behavior patterns common to all stutterers.

Secondary symptoms are believed to begin as a way to relieve speech-production muscle tension. For example, if your vocal folds are uncontrollably locked, slapping your thigh might relax your vocal folds.

But the secondary symptoms soon lose their effectiveness, and are retained out of habit.

Charles Van Riper suggested five classifications for secondary behaviors:

1) Avoidance of feared words, such as substitution of another word.

2) Postponement of the feared word, with pauses or filler words.

3) Starting tricks, such as an "uh" before the feared word.

4) Escape tricks, such as head jerks, exhausting one's breath and speaking on residual air, "backing up and getting a running start," etc.

5) "Anti-expectancy" speech behaviors to prevent stuttering such as speaking in a rapid monotone, or affecting an accent.

Many studies have found unusual physical behaviors associated with stuttering, such as eye movements, changes in heart rate and blood distribution, and hand tremors. Abnormal brain waves have been found. However, no consistent patterns or commonalties are clear.

WHAT STUTTERING FEELS LIKE

Stutterers report three types of sensations:

1) A sense of being frustrated in the attempt to talk. Stutterers know the word they are trying to say, but the word is stuck. The advice, "Think about what you are going to say before you say it" does not help stutterers.

Stuttering can be almost visual. You see the person waiting for the word. You visualize the word stuck in your mouth. You wonder, if I'm expending so much mental effort on this word, why can't the word telepathically jump from me to the listener and save me all this struggling?

2) A feeling of muscle tension, usually in the speech-production muscles (breathing, throat, jaw, lips, and tongue). Sometimes this tension is felt in the arms or legs or shoulders.

3) Emotions and anxiety may be felt before, during, or after stuttering.

Prior to stuttering, stutterers often feel apprehension or anticipation, even panic.

POOR AWARENESS OF STUTTERING

During stuttering, stutterers usually feel a mental "blankness." Our minds go "someplace else."

Several studies have found that stutterers lose their ability to use their hands during stuttering. Other studies have found that stutterers lose sense of time during stuttering.

Stutterers are unaware of what they do during stuttering. Because they don't perceive what they are doing, they can't alter their behavior. This is why stuttering is involuntary. When stutterers are not stuttering, they may be capable of any behavior anyone asks them to do, such as altering breathing, relaxing certain muscles, making eye contact, etc. But during stuttering they lose awareness and control of their speech activities.

Stutterers may be hyperaware that they are going to stutter before talking to a stranger. They may experience great anxiety during stuttering. But during stuttering, they have little awareness of how long their blocks are, how many times repetitions they did, secondary symptoms, etc.

Stutterers are often surprised when they hear tape recordings of their speech. This suggests that they feel anxiety during stuttering, but don't hear repetitions, prolongations, feel head jerks, etc.

After stuttering, stutterers feel embarrassment, shame, and guilt. They feel especially shameful if they have completed a speech therapy program and know that they can talk fluently.

Recent brain scan research has found changes in cerebral activity that may explain why stutterers often have poor physical awareness of what they do during stuttering (see the chapter below on "Neurology of Stuttering").

One stutterer wrote, "When I would stutter, my mind would come to a kind of blankness for a second, a kind of pause. Then all the 'shame' and 'pain' would rush in. I [overcame stuttering when I] taught myself to focus in on that 'pause'" instead of focusing on the shame and pain. (Glenn, 1996)

To listeners, stuttering is heard, and seen as muscle jerks or spasms. The listener doesn't experience the stutterer's anxieties. Listeners should realize that stuttering has a large emotional aspect. But more importantly, stutterers should improve their physical awareness of stuttering. See the chapter on "Psychological Self-Therapy" for a variety of techniques to do this.

Some non-stutterers report similar lack of awareness during public speaking. Afterwards, they can't remember what they said. If a brain scan could be done of a non-stutterer performing public speaking, we might see a pattern similar to stuttering, with abnormally-high right-brain emotions and anxiety, and abnormally-low left-brain central auditory processing.

ATTITUDES AND EMOTIONS

There are stutterers who believe that:

1) Stuttering is shameful and embarrassing. Many stutterers won't even read a book or watch a television program about stuttering. Some stutterers avoid other stutterers, and won't go to self-help groups. Some stutterers insist they don't stutter, but maybe "have trouble getting words out."

2) Speech is threatening and difficult. Certain words or sounds are believed to be especially difficult. Stutterers often substitute words. Stutterers avoid certain words or speaking situations, for example, by driving to a store instead of calling first, or not asking a salesperson for help finding something.

3) Stuttering occurs for no apparent reason, and can't be controlled. Dean Williams referred to stutterers' magical belief in a "something" inside that prevents them from speaking. Even experts

on stuttering believe there must be a physiological or neurological cause for stuttering, though decades of research have failed to find such an abnormality. (Research has found physical correlations, not causes of stuttering.)

4) Non-stutterers are believed to never experience speech hesitancy, anxiety, or fears. Stutterers may believe that non-stutterers' speech is perfect.

5) Stutterers may try to overcompensate or gain approval by working extra hours, doing favors for people, or excelling at non-speaking activities such as music or sports.

6) Stutterers fear using telephones. On telephone calls, listeners can't see the stutterer struggle, and think there's a "bad connection." Also, telephone conversations have more time pressure. You are expected to reply immediately. In face-to-face conversations, a pause in replying is acceptable.

7) When stutterers listen to non-stutterers, they tend to not do the smiling and nodding that non-stutterers do when listening. Stutterers' faces tend to be immobile. Conversations between stutterers and non-stutterers tend to lack simultaneous utterances, and there are fewer turn-taking switches. Conversations tend to be less spontaneous.

8) Listeners are perceived as critical, impatient, pitying, or amused. In reality, when non-stutterers talk to stutterers, they tend to nod their heads more, engage in "compulsive" smiling, and express less anger. But stutterers don't realize this.

9) Schoolchildren who stutter may say "I don't know" or even give a wrong answer, to avoid stuttering when called on in class.

10) In spite of all this, many stutterers, especially children, seem unconcerned about their stuttering. Franklin Silverman asked 62 children who stutter (grades 2 to 5) to make three wishes. Only four children made wishes related to speech, and one of these children wished he could go to speech class forever! This study was repeated in 1985 with 12 children who stutter, and only one wish out of 72 was related to speech (Culatta, 1985). Younger children don't view themselves as inferior to their classmates. This belief develops as the child grows up.

Adults can also be unconcerned about stuttering. Stutterers' minds "go someplace else" during stuttering. Listeners tend to be polite and pretend to not notice stuttering. Stutterers avoid thinking about stuttering. Friends and family don't discuss stuttering. Stutterers can be unconcerned and oblivious to their speech problems.

READING OUT LOUD

Some stutterers are more fluent reading out loud than in conversations. Others are the opposite. This has never been explored scientifically, but several reasons may be hypothesized:

1) The fluent-when-reading stutterers pretend to be robot readers, and switch off higher brain functions: not forming complex sentences in our minds; not forming complex thoughts; and not getting emotionally involved in the message.

2) The fluent-in-conversation stutterers substitute words in conversations to appear fluent. When reading, they can no longer substitute words, and saying feared words and sounds causes anxiety. They scan ahead in the text looking for feared words. Reading ahead with your mind while reading something else out loud demands high brain activity, leading to stuttering.

AND JUST TO CONFUSE YOU...

The American Speech-Language Hearing Association (ASHA) says that stuttering is not a medical condition or disease. The United States Food and Drug Administration (FDA) says that stuttering is a disease. California's Department of Equalization says that stuttering is not a disease.

The issue is whether speech is a bodily function, like breathing, versus whether speech is a learned behavior, like playing tennis. Not being able to play tennis is not a disease (although diseases and physical disabilities can effect your ability to play tennis). Choosing not to speak is not a disease, e.g., if you're a Trappist monk. Not being able to breathe is another story.

This may seem like a purely philosophical debate, but it effects whether health insurance providers pay for your speech therapy, whether schools provide stuttering therapy to children, and whether you pay sales tax for an anti-stuttering device.

THE FLUENT SPEECH OF STUTTERERS

The "average" stutterer is disfluent on 10% on words. Stated conversely, stutterers are fluent on 90% of words. Is stutterers' fluent speech normal? Or are there abnormalities even in stutterers' fluent speech?

Some studies found that listeners could differentiate the fluent speech of stutterers from that of normal speakers. Other studies found that listeners could not hear a difference.

Some studies have found abnormal laryngeal activity in the fluent speech of stutterers. Other studies found no abnormalities.

Spectrographic analysis did not find abnormal pitches in stutterers' fluent speech. But electromyographic and aerodynamic studies found abnormalities in stutterers' fluent speech.

The problem may be that in what each research team considered to be fluent speech. Some studies used mild stutterers, other studies used severe stutterers. Some stutterers may have used therapy techniques resulting in abnormal muscle activity in order to sound fluent.

DO STUTTERERS TALK TOO FAST?

Stutterers will tell you that they talk too fast, and this results in stuttering. Stutterers may appear to talk faster than fluent speakers. Internally, stutterers feel like their minds can produce sentences faster than their speech-production muscles can move, so they stumble over their words.

Children who stutter do not talk faster than non-stuttering children. Children who stutter do not talk faster on utterances in which they stutter, compared to utterances in which they are fluent. One study found that children who stutter talk slower than non-stuttering children (Yaruss, 1997).

Several studies found that altered auditory feedback (DAF and FAF) enabled stutterers not only to talk fluently, but to talk extremely fast (averaging 6.5 words per second), while reading out loud (Kalinowski, 1993, 1994, 1995).

Martin Schwartz suggests that a fast start on a sentence increases vocal fold tension before the first word of a phrase, which then leads to stuttering. He believes, however, that speaking fast on the rest of the sentence has less effect on stuttering.

Stutterers' fluent speech is speech is slower than non-stutterers' speech. Early studies measured overall speaking rate of fluent speech (not counting disfluencies), and found that stutterers talk slower.

One study found that stutterers have shorter vowel-to-consonant transitions, and hold vowels longer.

Another study found "articulatory slowness" in stutterers. But a similar study found deviations in the order of articulation movements, not slowness.

Many other studies have found various results, sometimes faster, sometimes slower. Stutterers seem to do some speech movements faster, and other speech movements slower, which result in an overall slower speaking rate.

Variance in these studies may also be due to some stutterers having learned compensation techniques (from therapy or on their own) to produce fluent speech. Many such techniques involve slowing down aspects of speech production. Or the slowness in stutterers' speech may be due to apprehension and excessive caution learned over years of stuttering.

Stutterers sometimes shorten the syllable before a disfluency, as if they anticipate stuttering on a certain word, and rush up to it to get a "running start." If stutterers keep all syllables about equal in length, they don't stutter.

Physiology and Personality of Stutterers

Studies in this chapter are referenced in *A Handbook On Stuttering* (Bloodstein, 1995), except as otherwise noted.

PHYSICAL STUDIES

Researchers found that stutterers have normal breathing (when not talking); heart rate, blood pressure, and basal metabolic rate; alveolar carbon dioxide and salivary pH; blood calcium, phosphorus, potassium, and blood sugar; electrical potentials of the left and right masseter muscles; oculocardiac and solar plexus reflexes; stretch reflexes of jaw closing muscles; biceps muscle tension; manual strength, and regularity and accuracy of reproducing rhythmical patterns.

Stutterers have normal hearing, including auditory threshold, phase disparities, sound localization, binaural loudness balance, and discrimination of speech distorted by frequency filtering, early latency potentials, and middle ear muscle activity. Stutterers have normal vision, reading achievement, and oral sensory and perceptual abilities.

A 1941 study found stutterers to be slightly less capable of carrying a full glass of water. Next time you spill something, you have an excuse!

Various studies of complex, difficult manual tasks, requiring organizing sequential motor activities, have sometimes found stutterers to be less proficient than non-stutterers. Other studies found stutterers to be normal. Examples of these tasks include transcribing sequences of letters faster than people can write; or tapping four fingers in various sequences, while pressing a foot pedal. This might sound bizarre, but many of these tests were designed to create interference between the left and right brain hemispheres.

Stutterers are slower to vocalize in response to a signal. These studies failed to show whether stuttering is caused by vocal folds that react slowly, or whether the subjects initiated vocal fold vibration slowly because they stutter.

Six studies found that stutterers are slower at pressing a button with their fingers in response to a signal. Six studies found that stutterers are normal.

Studies found that stutterers had normal births, diseases, injuries, allergies, and surgical operations.

PSYCHOLOGICAL STUDIES

Sigmund Freud wrote, "Whatever the source of stuttering is, it is not amenable to the treatments I have developed. I therefore refuse to deal with it further." (Schwartz, 1991)

Two of Freud's followers failed to follow the great psychologist's advice. In 1928, Isador H. Coriat advanced a theory that stuttering was an attempt to satisfy unresolved oral-erotic needs. (If this were true, there would stuttering phone sex lines. Imagine looking through the back of *Penthouse* magazine and seeing ads with scantily-dressed women saying, "Call me! I stutter!")

Otto Fenichel wrote a chapter about stuttering in his 1945 book, *The Psychoanalytic Theory of Neurosis.* He attributed stuttering mainly to fixation on the anal-sadistic level.

A 1939 study using the Bernreuter Personality Inventory found that stutterers were more neurotic, more introverted, less dominant, less self-confident, and less sociable than non-stutterers. Examination of the personality test found sixteen speech-related questions, including "If you are dining out do you prefer someone else to order dinner for you?" The psychologists had interpreted stutterers' reluctance to order in restaurants as evidence of neuroses, rather than as difficulty talking. This would be like concluding that paraplegics are anti-social because they don't like to participate in softball games.

Studies using the Minnesota Multiphasic Personality Inventory (MMPI) found that stutterers are slightly less well-adjusted than non-stutterers, but within the normal range.

Rorschach tests (finding images in inkblots) found little or no differences between stutterers and non-stutterers. A similar type of study, the Thematic Apperception Test, found no significant differences between stutterers and non-stutterers.

A 1954 study involving cartoons depicting events of psychosexual interest in the life of a dog named Blacky found that stutterers significantly exceeded non-stutterers in scores indicative of anal fixation. For example, one question in this category asked, "What was Blacky's main reason for defecating there?" (Blacky was defecating between Mama and Papa's doghouses.) The psychologists concluded that stutterers show "evidence of disturbance in such Blacky dimensions as oral eroticism, oral sadism, castration anxiety, and penis envy."

A 1946 study found differences in obsessive-compulsive character traits between stutterers and non-stutterers. Current thinking, however, is that there may a subset of stutterers with obsessive-compulsive disorder, possibly linked to Tourette's Syndrome.

A 1952 study of hostility and aggression found stutterers more likely to turn hostility inward. A 1953 study found the opposite, that stutterers are more likely to direct aggression outwardly at people that bother them.

A 1951 study found that stutterers' self-concept was no different from non-stutterers. A 1976 study found no difference in levels of aspiration. A 1967 study found no differences in drawings of body images. A 1974 study found no differences on the Sarbin-Hardyck Role Perception Test. A 1941 study of handwriting found no differences. A 1967 study found no difference on the Vineland Social Maturity Scale. The birth order of stutterers is normal (although one study found that only children are more likely to stutter).

Some studies have not found abnormal behavioral symptoms, such as exaggerated fears, sleep disturbances, hyperactivity, temper tantrums, excessive thumb sucking or nail biting, etc. Some studies have found somewhat more symptoms of maladjustment in stutterers.

"Locus of control" refers to whether you think things happen to you and are out of your control, or whether you are in control of satisfying your basic needs. Stutterers generally don't differ from non-stutterers. A recent study found that locus of control could not predict success in stuttering therapy or fluency two years after therapy. (De Nil, 1995)

Finally, a recent study found that stutterers are not more anxious or depressed than non-stutterers. (Miller, 1992) This study did find that stutterers have "poor communication attitudes," but this is a rational response to stuttering.

LANGUAGE STUDIES

There is evidence that children who stutter start talking later or are slow in developing language skills. This has not been conclusively proven.

By school age, stutterers have caught up with other children in language ability. In some tests, such as grammar, children who stutter did better than non-stutterers.

Some studies have found stutterers to be poor in auditory processing of language. Other studies have found no differences. A recent study compared 32 young children in three groups: children who stuttered briefly and then recovered; children who stuttered for a longer period before recovery; and children who continued to stutter. No differences in language development was found, but the children who stuttered longer had greater variability of language development (Watkins, 1997).

A study of 94 children who stutter found no cognitive or linguistic deficits (Häge, 1997).

Some studies have found that stutterers have problems with phonetic perception. For example, stutterers have difficulty figuring out that the word "caught" backwards produces the word "talk." (Stutterers may be immune to hidden, reversed Satanic messages in rock music!)

Many studies have shown that children who stutter also have articulation disorders, such as lisping, indistinct speech, or difficulty saying the sound /r/. Stuttering and articulation disorders appear to be related.

A recent study found that adults who stutter do not differ from non-stutterers in "speed of word identification" when reading, but stutterers "retrieve semantic information more slowly" (Bosshardt, 1996). The subjects were asked to read sentences and find a certain word, or a word that rhymes, or a word fitting a definition, in normal sentences, nonsense sentences with correct grammar, and random strings of words.

Stutterers had more difficulty than non-stutterers switching stress from the second syllable to the first syllable of the word "tatatas" (Jäncke, 1997).

Another study found substantial differences between stutterers and non-stutterers in learning "novel pseudowords." 7 controls and 5 stutterers were taught the nonsense words "abisthwoychleet" (abîs†wøîtßlit) and "eepashfwujbok" (ipæßfwudΩbok). In 11 trials, the controls averaged getting the words about 80% right. The stutterers averaged about 55% right. By the end of the 11 trials, the controls had learned the words about 90%, but the stutterers were still down in the 60% range.

Among the five stutterers, the severity of their stuttering inversely correlated with their ability to learn the words (the severe stutterers had poorer learning).

None of the stutterers had language-processing deficits. The study concluded that stutterers have an inefficient speech/language production system, and, in particular, "the interconnections between the input-output speech system and semantic and cognitive processing seem less efficient in those who stutter." (Ludlow, 1997)

MOTOR PROGRAM PRODUCTION

Several recent studies tested whether stutterers have trouble assembling abstract motor plans in their minds before speaking (van Lieshout, 1996a). The hypothesis was that speech is produced by first producing a phonological abstract motor plan, or plan of the sounds you are going to say, and storing this in short-term memory; then each phoneme's motor plan is retrieved from long-term memory (you remember which muscles produce a sound); then these units are "unpacked," i.e., you remember the individual muscle commands for the sound; and finally you execute the muscle commands.

To test whether stutterers have problems assembling abstract motor plans, the researchers conducted *reaction time* studies. When non-stutterers are asked to say a word quickly after seeing a word or a picture, they quickly say a short word, but take longer to say a multi-syllable words or multi-word phrase. The hypothesis was that stutterers take even longer to say the multi-syllable words or multi-word phrase. This would indicate that stutterers can't "assemble abstract motor plans" as well as non-stutterers.

Reaction times to say short words, long words, symbols, pictures, and choices of words were studied. Both audible reaction time and muscle (electromyographic) reaction time were measured.

The studies found that stutterers had longer speech reaction times than non-stutterers for both simple and complex responses, as you would expect. However, the number of syllables in the word did not make a difference. The researchers concluded that stutterers "do not...have problems in assembling motor plans for speech production or in building and retrieving memory representations of symbol-word combinations." (van Lieshout, 1996b)

INTELLIGENCE

Studies seem to indicate that children who stutter score about five IQ points lower than children who don't stutter. Five IQ points isn't much, and many of these studies had problems, such as lacking a control group.

Other studies found that college students who stutter are more intelligent than their peers. However, any person with a disability has to be especially intelligent and motivated to attempt college work, so this doesn't mean that stutterers are more intelligent in general.

Stuttering among mentally-retarded individuals appears to be far higher than the general population. In Down Syndrome, prevalences from 21% to 45% have been reported. This may be because mentally deficient children (and adults) are less able to overcome stuttering. Stuttering therapies require a great deal of intelligence and mental effort, and are only effective for about 70-75% of stutterers. We would expect mentally deficient stutterers to be more likely to fail at therapy. They would also be less likely to overcome stuttering by themselves.

It's also possible that these children are not stuttering, but have speech and language disabilities (such as speech interruptions) that sound like stuttering. See the chapter "Stuttering Therapies For Mentally-Retarded Individuals."

PARENTAL ATTITUDES AND BEHAVIORS

Several studies suggest that

> Compared with non-stuttering children, stuttering children are more likely to be raised
>
> (1) in less harmonious families [i.e., the parents do not have a happy marriage],
>
> (2) in less sociable and less close families [e.g., the parents don't belong to organizations, or aren't friendly to their neighbors], and
>
> (3) by parents having less formal education and/or lower intelligence…
>
> such home environments may exacerbate conditions that lead to speech difficulties and withdrawal tendencies…[it's also possible that] parents who stutter, especially fathers…personal inhibitions led them to…maintain more isolated social lives, and obtain lower levels of education… (Yairi, 1996)

American studies of socioeconomic status found that children who stutter tend to belong to more upper-class families. British studies have found the opposite. All studies found these trends to be weak.

Psychological studies of parents' personalities (e.g., hostility, anxiety) on balance have shown negative results. In other words, parents of stutterers seem to have normal personality traits.

Many studies have examined parental attitudes and behaviors, such as acceptance and expectations regarding intelligence or school performance; child-rearing behavior regarding food, health, toilet training, etc.; and social-communication interaction such as number of verbal interactions initiated, or number of negative statements made. On balance the results have been negative. The only exception is that parents of children who stutter tend to be overprotective and overanxious.

A 1961 study found that mothers were superficially accepting of their children who stuttered, but seemed to reject their children in subtle, hidden ways. It wasn't clear if this subtle rejection had caused stuttering or was caused by stuttering, or whether mothers of other disabled children had similar mixed feelings. Other studies have found that parents tend to hold unfavorable images of a stuttering child.

Several studies have investigated whether children who stutter have "ambivalent sex-role identification," distance anxiety, inadequate or punishing fathers, lack of acceptance, etc. Again, different studies found different results.

Many studies have investigated parental reactions to stuttering, and often found that parents have negative reactions to their child's disfluencies. However, the studies tend to be inconsistent.

Studies of parents' speech patterns have not found anything unusual.

Generally, studies done in the 1950s found positive results, and studies done recently have found negative results. This could be because scientific methods have improved, or because families today are more supportive of children who stutter. References for this chapter are Yairi (1996) and Bloodstein (1995).

Incidence and Prevalence of Stuttering

Preschool. The typical age for stuttering to begin is 3 or 4. One study found that three-quarters of stutterers begin by age 6, and all before the age of twelve. Recent research moves these ages earlier: the average age for stuttering to begin is 2.5 years old (30 months); and 75% of risk of stuttering has passed by age 3.5 (Yairi, 1992).

Schoolchildren. Oliver Bloodstein (1995) reviewed 37 studies of stuttering prevalence among schoolchildren (mostly grades 1-8, about half American studies and half foreign studies), from 1893 to 1981. Samples sizes ranged from 3,000 to 200,000 children. He concluded that, "the data in general are quite consistent. They point to a prevalence of stuttering of approximately 1 percent." In other words, 1% of school-age children stutter.

The lifetime incidence of stuttering about 5%, in other words, 5% of people recall stuttering at some point in childhood. The incidence surveys are less reliable then the prevalence surveys.

Even less reliable are the surveys of spontaneous recovery without therapy, but a figure of 80% is usually quoted.

The prevalence of stuttering is constant at 1% from grade 1 through grade 8. This seems strange — as a cohort of children grows up, many of the stutterers should recover, and few should start stuttering. The prevalence should diminish as children grow up. Bloodstein explains these "puzzling" statistics by saying that stuttering is "passed about" among schoolchildren, "new cases arising to take the place of those that disappear." As children grow up, fewer and fewer start stuttering, but fewer and fewer recover from stuttering.

These studies were done before the federal government mandated that schools provide speech therapy. If most young children who stutter are now being treated successfully, hopefully fewer than 1% of older children now stutter.

Adults. No surveys of stuttering in adults have been done. Bloodstein references two longitudinal studies from 1st through 12th grade. One found that stuttering diminished from 1% in 8th grade to 0.5% in 12th grade. The other study found that stuttering diminished from 1% in 8th grade to almost zero in 12th grade. These trends can't be reliably projected beyond 12th grade, but it would seem likely that the prevalence of stuttering beyond 12th grade is between zero and 0.5%, and probably closer to 0.1% by age 30.

The two biggest stuttering treatment programs — Hollins College and the National Center for Stuttering — have each treated 4,000-

5,000 teenagers and adults. All other programs and speech clinics have probably treated an equal number of individuals, so about 20,000 adults have received stuttering treatment. There are only a few hundred speech pathologists who are members of ASHA's Special Interest Division on Fluency Disorders. If each has treated 50 stutterers, then about 20,000 stutterers have been treated. This suggests that about 0.01% of Americans have been treated for stuttering.

Many adult stutterers do not seek treatment. Many are able to hide their stuttering. Assuming that 90% of adult stutterers do not seek treatment, then about 0.1% of adults stutter.

SEX RATIO OF STUTTERING

80% of adult stutterers are men. 93% of speech pathologists are women. This book refers to stutterers as "he" and speech pathologists as "she."

Of two- and three-year-olds, equal numbers of boys and girls stutter (Yairi, 1983). The sex ratio becomes 3:1 by the first grade, and 5:1 by the fifth grade, the same ratio as adults.

Girls begin stuttering earlier, but are more likely to outgrow it. Boys start stuttering later, and are less likely to outgrow it.

A theory that testosterone causes stuttering is unlikely because 3-year-old boys have little testosterone. When boys develop greater testosterone at puberty, their stuttering doesn't dramatically change.

The preferred theory is that the earlier development of language in girls enables them to cope with stuttering better (Andrews, 1983). Additionally, boys' interactive styles are more stressful:

> Boys in [all-boy] groups are more likely than girls in all-girl groups to interrupt one another; use commands, threats, or boasts of authority; refuse to comply with another child's demand; give information; heckle a speaker; tell jokes or suspenseful stories; or call another child names. Girls in all-[girl] groups, on the other hand, are more likely than boys to express agreement with what another speaker has just said, pause to give another girl a chance to speak, or when starting a speaking turn, acknowledge a point previously make by another speaker. This account indicates that among boys, speech serves largely egoistic functions and is used to establish and protect an individual's turf. Among girls, conversation is a more socially binding process. (Maccoby, 1990)

A boy who stutters will be frustrated when trying to assert himself, leading to a vicious cycle of increased effort and increased frustration reinforcing stuttering. A girl who stutters will not be frustrated by her peers because they try to be “nice” to sustain their social relationship.

I will speculatively add that girls’ brains also mature earlier than boys’ brains in terms of social skills. The combination of better social skills and better language skills enable girls to speak calmly and fluently in situations that over-excite a six-year-old boy and trigger his stuttering.

For example, I taught five six-year-olds to make a slinky walk down stairs. The three girls sat together at the top of stairs, took turns, and encouraged each other. One girl was good at the task, one was OK, and the third girl was completely inept. But all three girls sat still and cooperated. Learning this motor skill required social skills, including turn-taking, co-operation, and not distracting each other. Similarly, learning to speak fluently requires not only learning respiration control, vocal fold control, etc., but also listening skills, conversational turn-taking, etc.

The two six-year-old boys couldn’t stop wrestling on the stairs. They lacked attention span, ability to follow instructions, and self-discipline. But they had plenty of energy. I suspect that a neurochemical development, possibly related to adrenaline, enables six-year-old girls to calmly handle the new demands of school and social situations. Six-year-old boys lack this neurochemical maturity, and respond to increased social demands by getting excited (e.g., running around chasing each other), so the increased social pressure of schools makes it difficult for them to outgrow stuttering.

Genetics of Stuttering

DNA STUDIES

A study of 225 persons with Tourette's Syndrome examined three genes associated with the neurotransmitter dopamine. The study found that "each gene individually showed a significant correlation with various behavioral variables" including stuttering. More importantly, subjects who had loading on all three genes were more likely to have various behaviors, including stuttering.

This suggests that Tourette's Syndrome has a genetic origin, in these three genes. The study also suggests that among Touretters, stuttering has a genetic origin. The study does prove that stuttering has a genetic origin among people that don't have Tourette's Syndrome. The study found that attention deficit hyperactivity disorder (ADHD) had the highest association with these three genes. Other associated symptoms included tics, obsessive-compulsive disorder, mania, alcohol abuse, and anxiety attacks. If you don't have these other symptoms, your stuttering probably isn't caused by these three genes (Comings, 1996).

Also, speech pathologists did not verify that subjects stuttered — the subjects were simply asked, "Have you ever had problems with stuttering?" Self-reports for stuttering are not considered to be 100% reliable.

Some stutterers have a genetic predisposition to stutter, and other stutterers don't. If you have other dopamine-related disorders, such as ADHD, your stuttering is likely to be genetic.

British researchers recently found a gene that causes a rare speech/language disorder resulting in poor articulation, speech that is "very difficult to understand," rudimentary language skills, and "impaired coordination of the orofacial musculature affecting non-speech movements" (Porterfield, 1998). While this discovery has no direct connection to stuttering, it shows that genes influence the develop of speech and language.

FAMILIAL INCIDENCE

Studies of the families of stutterers failed to find simple Mendelian types of inheritance, such as sex-linked, autosomal dominant, or recessive.

Stutterers are more likely than non-stutterers to have relatives who stutter. At least 25 studies have been done, but the results vary widely. Somewhere between 20% and 74% of stutterers say they have a relative who stutters. Control studies found that 1% to 42% of non-stutterers said they have a relative who stutters (Yairi, 1996). One study found that if you stutter, you are about three times more likely to have a close relative who stutters (Andrews, 1983).

A study of children aged 2 to 6 found that more than two-thirds of stuttering children have relatives who stutter. This study found that male and female children were equally likely to have relatives who stutter. This study also found that stuttering was more likely in first-degree relatives than in second- or third-degree relations. (Ambrose & Yairi, 1993)

An informal study of 13 adopted stutterers found that 4 had adopted relatives who stuttered. This suggests against genetic transmission of stuttering. (Bloodstein, 1993)

TWIN STUDIES

A half-dozen studies of twins have found that concordance for stuttering (both twins either stutter or don't stutter, rather than one twin stuttering and the other not stuttering) is much more likely in identical twins than in fraternal twins. The exact numbers vary between studies, in part because some studies only looked at same sex twins (a male and female fraternal twin pair is unlikely to both stutter because males are more likely to stutter than females) (Yairi, 1996).

On the other hand, a study of 95 pairs of identical twins reared apart found 5 stutterers (2% of the subjects, the expected prevalence). None of their twins stuttered. This is in spite of finding similarities in talkativeness, pitch, and hoarseness, as well as tastes in clothing, books, etc. This suggests that stuttering is not genetic. (Bloodstein, 1995)

Twins are more susceptible to all disorders, so the results from twin studies may not extrapolate to singletons (non-twins). It's possible that if one twin has any disorder, the other is more likely than other siblings to pick it up environmentally.

AGGREGATION

Several studies have found that female stutterers are more likely than males to have relatives who stutter. This suggested that the few females who stutter might have a stronger genetic component in their families. (Analogously, men are more likely to be tall than women, but tall women are more likely to have tall relatives.) (Yairi, 1996)

However, a recent study of adult stutterers "did not find that relatives of female [stutterers] were more likely to stutter than relatives of the male [stutterers]." (Janssen, 1996).

SUBGROUPS

Studies of the family incidence of stuttering have compared left-handed stutterers to right-handed stutterers, speech motor skills, anxiety, and reading ability. Familial differences were found only for speech motor skills.

Two studies of birth or developmental trauma had contradictory results. A study of adults suggested that there are two causes of stuttering: genetic, and trauma or illness. A similar study of children who stutter reached the opposite conclusion.

Two studies found that severe stutterers were no more likely than mild stutterers to have relatives who stutter. Two more studies found no familial differences between recovered and persistent stutterers. (Yairi, 1996)

GENETICS VS. ENVIRONMENT

It's possible that stuttering is socially conditioned, not genetic. However, imitation has been ruled out for a variety of reasons. Some related persons stutter, without the child having met the relative. Also, beginning stuttering is associated with different behaviors than adult stuttering.

A more likely possibility is that families have a common environment that is conducive to stuttering. For examples, some families have a "climate of anxiety," while others are "laid-back." Highly-educated families may place more language demands on children than do less-educated families.

A researcher in 1940 studied five generations of an Iowa family, with stuttering in all generations. In the third generation, three of four children in one family stuttered. The children grew up, and three moved to Kansas and lost contact with the sibling remaining in Iowa. Of the descendants of the woman remaining in Iowa, 40% stuttered. Of the descendants of the Kansas siblings, only 6% stuttered.

The researcher concluded that the Iowa family had a "tone" that was conducive to stuttering. These relatives were sure that stuttering was genetic, and they anxiously watched their children looking for signs of stuttering. This fear of stuttering in the parents may have caused the stuttering in the children.

Twenty years later, another researcher studied the next generation. Only 2% of these children stuttered, and the researcher reported that there had been a change in the familial assumptions and attitudes about stuttering. (Bloodstein, 1995)

Another speech pathologist then looked at the original study, and concluded that, “genetic transmission has been judged to provide an equally viable explanation for the data.” (Wingate, 1986)

Conditions That Increase or Decrease Stuttering

Studies in this chapter are referenced in *A Handbook On Stuttering* (Bloodstein, 1995), except as otherwise noted.

CHARACTERISTICS OF STUTTERED WORDS

Stuttering is most likely to occur on:

• The initial sound or syllable of a word (90% of stuttering). Initial consonants are more difficult than initial vowels.

• The first word of a sentence.

• Accented syllables of words.

• Content words (nouns, verbs, adjectives, and adverbs) rather than function words ("and," "but," "he").

• Longer words, more than shorter words.

• Less-frequently-used words.

• Transitions from voiceless to voiced sounds (i.e., when switching on your vocal fold vibration.)

If listeners are given a sentence word by word, they can easily guess the next word, in certain phrases, but are unlikely to guess other words. Stuttering occurs more often on words that can't be easily guessed (which is why listeners fill in our sentences wrong!).

Children are more likely to stutter on longer utterances, vowel-consonant transitions, and in the middle of sentences and words (Rommel, 1997).

No conclusive evidence has been found that stuttering occurs in waves, cycles, or clusters, when reading out loud. For some stutterers, a disfluency is followed by other disfluencies. For others, a stutter is followed by a period of fluency. Some stutterers start speaking relatively fluently, and disfluencies increase the longer they talk (Ingham, 1997).

CONDITIONS THAT INCREASE STUTTERING

• Syntactic complexity. Young children stutter more on complicated sentences, and stutter less on simple sentences. This phenomenon seems to disappear by adolescence (Silverman, 1997). Normal disfluencies and errors continue to be more likely in complex sentences. Children stutter more on sentences with more clauses (Logan, 1997).

• Speaking on the telephone. In telephone conversations, pauses are less acceptable. You are expected to continuously keep the conversation going. Also, you are unable to use non-verbal communication.

• Saying one's name.

• Telling jokes. Timing is critical to jokes, so there is more anxiety about saying a punchline fast.

• Saying something important or meaningful. Stuttering is less likely when, for example, reading a list of numbers or nonsense words (Ludlow, 1997).

• Time pressure.

• If you believe a listener is hard to talk to or critical. You are likely to stutter less with someone you perceive as easy-going or understanding.

• Speaking to an audience.

• Talking to an authority figure or a person with higher status.

• Talking to a person of the opposite sex (who is the appropriate age for romantic interest). However, one woman told me that she is fluent on dates. Perhaps dating is more stressful for male stutterers, who are expected to make the first call and initiate conversations and activities, and less stressful for female stutterers, who can talk a more passive role.

• Talking to strangers. Many stutterers are shy about talking to strangers. Of course, many non-stutterers are shy about this too.

• Talking to friends and co-workers. This may sound surprising, but stutterers are most embarrassed about their speech when talking to people they've known for years. In stuttering therapy, stutterers are more willing to use therapy techniques (e.g., a slower speaking rate) when speaking to strangers, than when speaking to friends and co-workers. One stutterer went through fluency shaping stuttering therapy, but refused to use the therapy techniques at work. "I've been working with these people for 20 years, " he said, "what would they think if I came to work talking like that?"

CONDITIONS THAT DECREASE STUTTERING

• Whispering reduces stuttering about 60%. Whispering does not use phonation (vibration of the vocal folds). "Lipping" or silently moving one's lips, jaws, and tongue almost eliminates stuttering. This suggests that "stuttering is a function of complexity of phonatory coordinations with articulatory and respiratory processes" (Perkins, 1976). In other words, stutterers can articulate, or breathe, or phonate, but trying to do all three at the same time results in stuttering.

• Saying a phrase repeatedly, or reading something out loud several times, reduces stuttering. This is called *adaptation*. "...the decrease in stuttering frequency during adaptation readings is an effect of *practice* of speech movements and may be considered a result of *motor learning*." The adaptation effect does not result from "silent rehearsal without oral movements" and the effect is reduced with "silently performed speech movements or when whispered speech is used" (Caruso & Max, 1997).

• Speaking in chorus (unison) with another person. If you have a phrase you say often, but stutter on (such as answering the telephone at work), buy a micro digital tape recorder (Radio Shack #63-945, $15), and record yourself saying the phrase fluently. When you need to say the phrase, push the button and speak in chorus with your fluent recording. Combined with the adaptation effect, eventually you should be able to say the phrase fluently without the microrecorder.

• Some people can reduce stuttering by trying to stutter, saying that they stutter, or not hiding their stuttering. Some of us, on the other hand, succeed whenever we try to stutter.

• When speaking alone or to animals, many stutterers are fluent.

• Many stutterers can read out loud fluently, especially if they don't feel emotionally connected to the book. However, other people only stutter when reading out loud, because they can't substitute words.

• Many electronic technologies reduce stuttering. See the chapter "Computers and Electronic Devices for Stuttering Therapy."

• Talking a lower status person. Adult stutterers stutter less when talking to children (although children are more likely to laugh or ask "What's wrong with you?"). Military officers who stutter are able to give commands to subordinates fluently.

• Stutterers can sing fluently. Singers who stutter include: Mel Tillis (country), Carly Simon (pop), Robert Merrill (opera), "Scatman" John Larkin (jazz), and John Melendez (rock). Singing uses continuous phonation and diaphragmatic breathing, like stuttering therapy. Singing doesn't require forming new sentences (the words are written for you).

• Lowering your vocal pitch reduces stuttering 75-85%. This is due to relaxing your vocal folds and reducing subglottal pressure (Ramig, 1981).

• Acting and speaking with a different accent increase fluency. No research has investigated why this works.

• Various studies have increased or decreased stuttering through punishment and reward (operant responses). Electric shocks contingent on stuttering reduce or eliminate stuttering. Stuttering returns when the electrodes are removed. (In 1810, Dr. Joseph Frank suggested "regular beatings" as the preferred treatment for stuttering in his book *Practice of Medicine*.)

• A study found that a speech pathologist saying "right," "wrong," or "tree" all decreased stuttering equally. It didn't matter if the word was said after fluent words or disfluencies.

• A 1935 study found that stutterers could talk fluently while walking on all fours. This may sound ridiculous, but crawling apparently aids neurological growth in infants. One physical therapist developed crawling therapy for brain-injured children and adults. (Doman, 1974)

• Most stutterers can swear fluently!

DOES ALTERED VOCALIZATION REDUCE STUTTERING?

Does altering your speaking rate, vocal volume, or vocal pitch improve fluency?

• Speaking rate. Wingate (1976) believed that slowing down your speaking rate was the most important variable in improving fluency. Recent research (Kalinowski 1993, 1994, 1995; Glover, 1996) has shown that slowing down is not essential for reducing stuttering. Several fluency-enhancing conditions enabled stutterers to increase speaking rate. These include singing and electronic devices, such as delayed auditory feedback (DAF) and frequency-shifted auditory feedback (FAF) (see the section "Computers and Electronic Devices For Treating Stuttering").

• Vocal volume. Stager (1997) found that reduced vocal volume (talking quietly) reduced stuttering, but only in combination with other aerodynamic changes, including reduced air pressure and reduced air flow, and increased vowel duration. In other words, relaxing you breathing and relaxing your vocal folds tends to reduce vocal volume, and improve fluency. But talking quieter without relaxed breathing and vocal folds won't improve fluency. Yelling loudly forces diaphragmatic breathing, and improves fluency. Again, increasing volume without using diaphragmatic breathing won't improve fluency. Altering vocal volume alone doesn't alter fluency.

• Vocal pitch. Ramig and Adams (1981) studied the effect of altered vocal pitch on stuttering. They studied 18 adults and 18 children, half stutterers and half non-stutterers. They found that, for the children, an increased vocal pitch (speaking in a high voice) cut stuttering in half. Decreasing vocal pitch (speaking in a deep voice) cut stuttering by three-quarters.

The effect on the adults was even greater — the high pitch reduced stuttering 70% and the low pitch reduced stuttering 85%. Note that with both children and adults, the low pitch had half the stuttering of the high pitch.

The researchers explained the dramatic effect of the lower pitch noting that

> …at lower-than-normal pitches, the vocal folds are thick and lax…there is more subglottic pressure values that can initiate vocal fold vibration when the folds are lax. This is important because lax folds should then enhance fluency by means of making it easier to start and sustain voicing. Thus, lax vocal folds may be viewed as a physiological state that would add to or support fluency.

Ramig and Adams add that speaking at a lower vocal pitch reduces your vocal range. This "simplifies the speech act," and simpler speech muscle movements are a fluency-enhancing condition.

This latter aspect explains why a lower vocal pitch is not widely-practiced in stuttering therapy programs. With less vocal range, you are less able to express a wide range of emotions.

However, the emotions you express at lower vocal pitches are relaxation, confidence, and authority. Speaking at a lower vocal pitch can be seen as not limiting your emotional range, but enhancing your ability to emote relaxation and confidence.

A similar strategy of altering vocal resonance has been developed by Don Campbell as part of music therapy to treat a variety of physical and mental disorders (not stuttering specifically). Campbell has written several books about this, including *The Mozart Effect.*

Ramig and Adams found that speaking at a higher vocal pitch produced twice the disfluencies of the lower pitch, but still much less than speaking at your normal pitch. They found that the subjects increased their vocal volume when speaking at the higher pitch (vocal volume at low and normal vocal pitches were similar). The researchers believe that the increased volume was due to increased subglottic pressure (air pressure below your vocal folds), so there was a greater drop in air pressure across the glottis, "…thus making the onset and continuity of vocalization easier to achieve."

There was also a small decrease in speaking rate with both the lower and higher pitches. Speaking rates slowed 10% with the higher pitch, and 20% with the lower pitch. This also contributed to increased fluency.

GOOD DAYS AND BAD DAYS?

Any stutterer can tell you that he has “good days” — with less stuttering — and “bad days” — when he can’t get a word out without stuttering. On “bad days,” he finds that his therapy techniques, electronic devices, or other fluency enhancers don’t help.

The “good days/bad days” syndrome may be due to varying levels of dopamine in the brain. The neurotransmitter is affected by several factors, including diet. Foods that increase dopamine levels — e.g., low-fat fish — appear to increase stuttering, although no research has been done. See the chapter “Neurology and Drug Treatments” for more about dopamine.

A recent study tested whether “daily stress” increases stuttering (Blood, 1997). First, stutterers and non-stutterers completed the “Social Readjustment Rating Scale” to see how stressful each person’s life was. No difference was found between the stutterers and non-stutterers.

Next, each stutterer made a tape of their speech and filled out a “Daily Stress Inventory” each evening. The questionnaire had 58 questions about events that day. The 58 questions were grouped into five types of stress: interpersonal (e.g. arguments), personal competency (e.g., late for an appointment), cognitive (e.g., heard bad news), environmental (e.g., sleep loss), and “varied” (e.g., a rude waiter).

The stutterers had more interpersonal problems than the non-stutterers, but fewer of the other four types of stress. The “interpersonal” category had more items related to speaking situations.

The researchers found that stuttering increased 50% on “high stress” days as compared to “low stress” days (“average stress” days were ignored). The researchers did not analyze the data to discover if certain categories of stress had a greater impact on stuttering.

Belief — Anticipation, Distraction, Stress, and Placebos

Studies in this chapter are referenced in *A Handbook On Stuttering* (Bloodstein, 1995), except as otherwise noted.

ADAPTATION AND ANTICIPATION

In 1937, Wendell Johnson conducted a series of tests of *adaptation* and *anticipation*, in which stutterers repeatedly read a passage out loud:

1) Johnson marked the stuttered words in the first reading. In the second reading, of an unmarked copy, the stutterer was asked to read only words on which he did not expect to stutter. This eliminated 98% of stuttering. The 2% of stuttering was on words which were stuttered in the first reading. In most cases, the stutterer afterwards said knew he would stutter on the word, but failed to follow the instructions not to read it.

2) The stutterer marked the words in the text on which he expected to stutter. He then read the passage out loud 15 minutes later, and a second time the next day. In both cases stuttering occurred on about 50% of the marked words, and on about 10% of the unmarked words. In 1975, Wingate repeated this experiment but altered the sequence of the words, and found little relationship between anticipated and stuttered words.

3) Johnson noted the stuttered words as each stutterer read a passage ten times repeatedly. Most subjects stuttered on the same words in each reading. This showed that developmental stutterers stutter on certain words, and say other words fluently. In contrast, some forms of neurogenic stuttering may have random stuttering on any word. Later researchers tried to make the subjects forget which words they'd stuttered on, by reading other material, or by waiting several weeks between readings. Stutterers continued to stutter on the same words.

4) Johnson increased stuttering by having the person read to an audience or by other means. Later, the person read out loud to one person. Stuttering increased on passages with cues associated with the audience reading, such a colored border on the page or a similar subject matter. Johnson theorized that the colored border reminded the person of previous stuttering.

5) Johnson blacked out the stuttered words in heavy pencil, and the stutterer skipped those words. For some subjects, this elimi-

nated stuttering, but most subjects then stuttered on new words. These new stuttered words were adjacent to the blacked-out words.

6) Johnson had stutterers silently read a passage twice, several weeks apart, and mark words they expected to stutter on. Stutterers marked the same words each time.

Johnson theorized that stutterers associate a word with past stuttering or failure (a cue). These studies show that certain words are stuttering cues for individual stutterers, just as certain speaking situations can cue an individual to stutter.

In 1971, Rappaport and Bloodstein repeated Johnson's fifth experiment, but divided subjects into two groups, and added a second test. In the second test, random words had been blacked out. The subjects who did Johnson's test first and then read the random test stuttered on the words adjacent to the blacked-out words. The subjects who read the random test first did not stutter on adjacent words. The stutterers were trained to stutter to a new cue — blacked-out words.

DOES DISTRACTION REDUCE STUTTERING?

According to some speech pathologists, "Distraction methods can be used to eliminate stuttering temporarily" (Kuehn, 1994). But if distraction worked, stutterers would work a Rubik's cube or play a pocket video game whenever they wanted to talk fluently. Distraction does not reduce stuttering:

• Distraction from speech-production muscle tension. This is believed to be the origin of secondary symptoms. Tensing non-speech muscles (e.g., eye blinking, foot-stamping) distracts attention from vocal tension. The stutterer may relax his speech muscles momentarily and the word pops out. But he will soon block again, and if he continues to do the secondary behavior it will become habitual. It will also become ineffective. *Distraction from vocal tension is ineffective.*

• Distraction from anticipation of stuttering. Wendell Johnson showed that stutterers know which words they will stutter on. If this anticipation could be distracted, maybe the person wouldn't stutter on those words? A 1982 study had stutterers step on and off a 10-inch platform while reading out loud (step aerobics stuttering therapy!). A 1985 study had stutterers manually track an irregular line on a rotating drum while speaking. Neither distraction was able to reduce stuttering. Another study (James, 1981) had nine adult stutterers take a 10-second "time-out" after disfluencies, while a control group of nine stutterers got random 10-second "time-outs." "Time-outs" after disfluencies reduced stuttering 46%. Random "time-outs" had no effect on stuttering, proving that "time-outs" do not reduce stuttering via "distraction." These three studies show that *distraction from anticipation is ineffective.*

• Distraction from the fear of stuttering. There are many stories of a stutterer being "too scared" to stutter (see the section below "Does Stress Increase Stuttering?"). This is a real and fascinating phenomenon, but has no practical value as a therapy for stuttering. For example, we could train a Rottweiler to attack you whenever you stutter. If you brought the dog with you everywhere you went, this might cure you of stuttering, but it would be a cure worse than the disorder.

• Increasing attention to one aspect of speech may reduce attention to other aspects of speech. For example, speaking in a foreign accent requires careful attention to your articulation. Other examples of increased attention may be to relaxed breathing or to speaking slower. These techniques can be effective, but the effectiveness is from increased attention to a fluency-enhancing aspect of speech, not due to distraction or decreased attention to fluency-inhibiting aspects of speech.

• Distraction causes stuttering, when stutterers use therapy techniques. When learning to use a new motor skill, the inhibition of other neuronal linkages is as important as the development of the target neural linkage: "Each motor engram is a pathway of excitation surrounded by a wall of inhibition" (Kottke, 1978). A golfer must keep her eye on the ball. Tennis pros are infamous for demanding silence from fans. Stutterers often say that they can use therapy skills in a clinical environment, but the distractions of normal conversations make fluent speech difficult.

DOES STRESS INCREASE STUTTERING?

A stutterer asked: "If stress is supposedly a catalyst for stuttering, or if stuttering is some sort of response to stress, then why is it that I seem to stutter much more in situations which *should* be non-stressful?"

"Stress" is defined as "a state…resulting from factors that tend to alter an existent equilibrium" (Merriam-Webster, 1996). "Stress" is a broad term that can refer to many different physical and mental states:

• Physiological stimulation, such as elevated heart rate or blood pressure. Physical activities such as running or bicycling are physiologically stimulating, but have little or no effect on stuttering. No one has studied whether sleep deprivation, the flu, etc., effects stuttering.

• Emotional stimulation. Aneurin Bevan, the British labor leader and member of Parliament, developed great public speaking skills by getting emotionally involved in his subject.

• Fear or anxiety. Fear is anxiety directed at an object. Anxiety is more general, such when taking an exam. Fear and anxiety are emotions, but are distinguished from other types of emotional stimulation.

• Time pressure is a form of stress, and increases stuttering.

• Cognitive stress is hearing or seeing several contradictory things at once. For example, talking to someone who is watching television is cognitively stressful. This increases stuttering.

One study had stutterers state the color that the name of a different color was written in (Caruso, 1994). For example, the word "red" was written in yellow on a computer monitor. The subjects had to say "yellow," not "red." This was cognitive stress.

The researchers also added time pressure. Heart rate and blood pressure were monitored, as well as disfluencies, speech rate, response time, and acoustic content of the words.

The hypothesis was that increased speed, cognitive stress, and heart rate and blood pressure would cause subjects to stutter more and take longer to respond. This was hypothesized for both stutterers and non-stutterers.

The study found that cognitive stress and increased speed caused or increased disfluencies for both stutterers and non-stutterers. These results were dramatic: stutterers went from 1% stuttered words, to 3% with time pressure, to 9% with speed and cognitive stress. Non-stutterers went from 0%, to 2% disfluencies with time pressure, to 4% with speed and cognitive stress. Neither group made many errors in naming the colors. Increased cardiovascular measures did not correlate with increased disfluencies in stutterers.

The first two types of stress above — physiological and emotional arousal — do not increase stuttering, and may decrease stuttering. The last two types of stress — cognitive stress and time pressure — increase stuttering.

The third type of stress — fear and anxiety — increases or decreases stuttering depending on whether the fear is speech-related. Speech-related fear and anxiety, such as public speaking, increases stuttering.

Non-speech-related fear and anxiety do not correlate with

stuttering (Miller, 1992). Non-speech-related fear and anxiety may even reduce stuttering in some cases. For example, one night someone threatened me physically for several hours. I experienced anxiety and emotional stimulation, which caused a "fight or flight" response and physiological stimulation. I have never been so fluent in my life! My voice was calm and relaxed to get the person to calm down. But I didn't feel calm or relaxed!

Oliver Bloodstein describes a World War Two stutterer who could talk fluently for mortar communication in combat — again, physiological and emotional arousal, but cognitively focused on one task. Bloodstein adds (Bloodstein, 1995):

> stutterers who tell of speaking fluently under conditions of acute fear or emotional stress sometimes report more stuttering "after it was all over." One subject who had no stuttering immediately after an automobile accident said, "And then when I got home I was shot. I could hardly say one word without having a bad block."

There may be a neurochemical explanation for these phenomena. Noradrenaline and adrenaline compete with dopamine for the binding sites on D4 receptors, and when bound, acts as an agonist. At the same time, through feedback inhibition, norepinephrine inhibits tyrosine hydroxylase, which in turn inhibits the production of dopamine. Because dopamine in the striatal system increases stuttering (see the section "Neurology and Drug Treatments for Stuttering"), and adrenaline blocks dopamine, "fight or flight" situations that increase adrenaline may reduce stuttering (Newman-Tancredi, 1997).

Pharmacist Richard Harkness adds (Harkness, 1996):

> Stress, I think, is given far too much weight. Stress certainly can be an aggravating factor in stuttering just as it can be in diabetes and high blood pressure, but it certainly doesn't cause any of those conditions. PWS stutter whether they're under stress or not. I think the element of stress is one of those simplistic things that we want to "find" to explain stuttering. For example, if we can stop the stress, we can stop the stutter. Would be great if it were true!

Another stutterer wrote:

> I am person who stutters (mild to moderate), also a speech-language pathologist, and last week my grandfather passed away. I was alone with him when this occurred. Immediately after I went home and wrote

a few pages about him. My family requested that it be read/presented at the service but they suggested my older brother (business exec). I strongly stated that I wanted to do this and so I did.

I spoke at the pulpit in front of a crowded church for about 6 minutes without a single disfluency, the last 20 seconds was fairly emotionally charged but I completed my task. I rate this experience as my greatest ever public speaking activity. In terms of my speaking behavior, it was slow, proper phrasing and very effective. The material was typed on pages but it was also memorized, having practiced approximately 10 times while alone in my car driving varying places.

So I guess what my question is, Why was I so fluent? I had thought previously about it several times and always with my concern on not crying, stuttering was never a issue, if I stuttered so what. It was the content I cared about not necessarily the delivery.

Almost every person at some point commented to me on the quality of the eulogy, many were strangers, even my brother was impressed. The minister later while having coffee suggested to me that I should "Praise the Lord" for successful speaking. I believe I expected fluent speech, separated the emotion from behavior and utilized standard techniques such as slow rate, continuous airflow, phrasing and easy onsets.

STUTTERING REDUCES STRESS

A study by Perkins and Dabul (1973) found that stuttering reduced stress. 16 adult male stutterers were subjected to "uncomfortable" electric shock to their right arms. This caused an average 3% increase in systolic blood pressure. The subjects then received 5 "treatments" to reduce stress:

• Stuttering, while reading a list of "least-used English words designed to encourage stuttering." The "mean frequency" of stuttering was 23.7.

• Fluent speech, reading a poem "shadowing" the speech of an examiner. The "mean frequency" of stuttering was 1.7.

• Chewing gum "vigorously."

• Finger tapping.

• Sitting quietly for three minutes.

The results were dramatic. All treatments resulted in a 2% reduction in blood pressure, except finger tapping, which resulted in almost no change in blood pressure, and stuttering, which reduced blood pressure over 10%. Maybe cardiologists should teach people with high blood pressure to stutter?

THE PLACEBO EFFECT

A placebo is a pill without a drug in it. Placebos are used to compare people taking a drug to control groups of people, who take a pill without the drug.

More generally, a placebo is an inactive, nonspecific medical treatment, which achieves its effect via altering the beliefs of the patient. A placebo does not have to be a pill. One study found that the physician telling the patient that he or she had no serious disease and would soon be well improved the health of the patients more than the physician saying that the cause of their ailment was unclear (Brown, 1998).

Placebos are effective treatments for almost every disease and symptom:

> Study after study showed that, for virtually any disease, a substantial portion of symptoms — roughly one-third, by most estimates — would improve when patients were given a placebo treatment with no pharmacological activity. Patients simply believed that the treatment would help them, and somehow, it did. (Goleman, 1993)

> …for a wide range of afflictions, including pain, high blood pressure, asthma and cough, roughly 30 to 40 percent of patients experience relief after taking a placebo…placebos seem to be most reliably effective for afflictions in which stress directly affects the symptoms…pain, asthma and moderate high blood pressure can become worse when the patient is upset…placebos may work in part by lessening the apprehension associated with the disease [because] the immune system falters under stressful conditions. (Brown, 1998)

In other words, placebos are effective for diseases that are made worse by getting upset, or by a weakened immune system. Stutterers are often fluent when they get upset. The immune system does not affect stuttering. Because stress can increase, decrease, or have no effect on stuttering, placebos should not effect on stuttering.

Placebos change the beliefs of the patient. An Internet support group member expressed the view that stuttering can be reduced via the placebo effect:

> My personal experience [is]…That our beliefs about stuttering seem to be one of the main factors in stuttering severity. (Neiders, 1997)

Oliver Bloodstein wrote, under the heading "The Influence of

Beliefs," (Bloodstein, 1997)

> ...if a stutterer were to forget that he was a stutterer, he would have no further difficulty with his speech.

No study has changed the attitudes and beliefs of a group of stutterers, then compared changes in their fluency to a control group. Bloodstein provides only anecdotal accounts to support his view, such as a student who stopped stuttering when she became a Christian Scientist. He refers to a 1946 hypnosis study which found that 8 out of 40 stutterers had self-reported "easy and relaxed" speech for two or three days after the hypnosis sessions — which doesn't prove much either way. Bloodstein and Rappoport's 1971 study (described in the first section of this chapter) supports his theory, but wasn't a strong enough change in belief to be conclusive proof.

A double-blind crossover study of haloperidol and placebos found no reduction in stuttering with the placebo (Prins, 1980).

A study of clomipramine, desipramine, and placebos found that placebos had no effect on stuttering (Stager, 1995). But placebos had the greatest side effects. The average placebo subject reported three side effects — including constipation, sexual dysfunction, dizziness, sweating, tremors, etc. The placebo was 50% more powerful than clomipramine, and six times more powerful than desipramine, in producing side effects. The placebo was the most powerful drug in the study — but not for reducing stuttering!

These placebo studies prove that belief that you will or won't stutter has no effect on fluency. Stutterers can't be "psyched" into fluency. The placebo studies show that stuttering is less psychological than heart disease, asthma, etc. — the opposite of the long-held belief that stuttering is a psychological problem.

Motor Learning Theory

Our muscle movements, or *motor skills*, are paradoxical. One the one hand, we execute complex, precise movements when we speak, walk, dance, play a guitar, etc. These activities are difficult to learn, requiring years of practice.

On the other hand, once we learn these skills, we perform them without cognitive effort, without even thinking about them. In fact, many of these skills can only be performed when we don't think about them. Our performance degrades when we exert conscious control. Some stutterers even suggest that this is the cause of their stuttering — trying to control speech, instead of letting automatic processes produce speech.

How do we learn new motor skills? How do we unlearn undesired or *maladaptive* motor skills? What is the role of *cognition* (mental attention) in motor learning? How should practice sessions be structured to maximize motor learning and retention? These questions are studied by physical and occupational therapists, athletes and coaches, psychologists and human factors engineers. This field is called *motor learning and control*. (Except as noted, this chapter references the textbook *Motor Learning and Control*, by Charles Shea, Wayne Shebilske, and Stephen Worchel, 1993.)

Few stuttering therapies incorporate the principles of motor learning theory. Few speech pathologists have addressed the questions of how fluent speech motor skills are learned, and whether stuttering is an undesirable motor skill, which can be unlearned. Research in this area could revolutionize stuttering therapy.

STIMULUS AND RESPONSE

To *behaviorists* such as B. F. Skinner, motor control is an environmental *stimulus* followed by a resulting *response*. Psychologists have broken down stimulus-response into its components:

1) *Sensation*, or neural transmission from sensory receptors in your eyes, ears, etc., to your brain.

2) *Perception*, which retrieves long-term memory to organize, classify, and interpret your sensations. In other words, perception changes sensation data into perceived information or meaning.

3) *Response selection.* You use current perception and past experiences to formulate a course or action. For example, in baseball, a batter watches the pitcher and decides whether to swing

at a pitch, hit or bunt, hit to left field or right, etc. Psychologists differentiate conscious *decisions* from unconscious *translations*, or relating a particular stimulus to a particular response.

4) *Response execution* of an action plan — a step-by-step sequence of events that make up the planned movement. In these events, motor neurons carry signals from the brain or spinal cord.

The stimulation or *afferent* processes take about 15 milliseconds. Sensation takes about 45 milliseconds. Response selection takes about 75 milliseconds. Response execution takes about 45 milliseconds, and the *efferent* or motor neuron processes take about 15 milliseconds. The total time for a stimulus and response is about 200 milliseconds.

CLOSED-LOOP VS. OPEN-LOOP CONTROL

You can see a problem here — what if events occur faster than 200 milliseconds? Specifically, what if the response selection time or response execution time is reduced? A gymnast's double-back somersault requires muscle movements lasting only tens of milliseconds. Many speech elements last less than 50 milliseconds.

In *closed-loop control*, you continually adjust your movements according to your perceptions. You can't perform closed-loop control quickly. For example, in threading a needle, you move slowly, with each adjustment taking about 200 milliseconds. Psychologists have found that proprioceptive feedback (sensation of your body movements) takes 160 milliseconds to process, and exteroceptive feedback (sensation of your environment) takes about 190 milliseconds to process. The advantages of closed-loop control include accuracy, movement flexibility, and the ability to produce unpracticed movements. The disadvantages are increased attention demands, and increased time for executing corrections.

When stutterers slow their speech to about 200 milliseconds per syllable, they become almost 100% fluent. See the subsection about delayed auditory feedback in the chapter "Computers and Electronic Devices for Stuttering Therapy."

Reduced response selection time is a problem in sports. For example, the 100-mph fastball requires the batter to make a decision in 200 milliseconds or less. He can either make a decision based on incomplete information, or he can anticipate based on previous experience. The performance may occur in a closed environment, such as a video game, or in an open environment, with continually-changing conditions, such as a football game. In football, if the offensive team varies its plays to create uncertainty in their opponents, the defensive team will rely more on incomplete information. If the offensive team plays predictably, the defensive team will rely more on anticipation based on past experience.

In speech, reduced response execution time is a more important problem than reduced response selection time. Normal speaking rates are about 1200 phonemes or sounds per minute, or about 50 milliseconds per sound. Some sounds are longer, and others are shorter. A gymnast's complex movements are performed at similar speed.

Psychologists refer to this as an *open-loop control* system. All information processing is done before the movement begins. The movements must be preprogrammed, stored in long-term memory along with their sequence and timing. This memory is called a *motor program*, and is defined as a "set of muscle commands that are structured before a movement sequence begins, and that allows the sequence to be carried out uninfluenced by peripheral feedback."

After winning the gold medal in gymnastics at the 1984 Olympics, Mary Lou Retton said that coach

> Bela [Karolyi] can really teach, I've learned so much from him. Many long hours were spent in the gymnasium…repetition, feedback, repetition, and experimentation. Somehow, after a lot of bumps and bruises, it got easier, as if I could float.

Karolyi added,

> Someone should be able to sneak up and drag you out at midnight and push you out on some strange floor, and you should be able to do your entire routine sound asleep in your pajamas. Without a mistake. That's the secret. It's got to be a natural reaction.

Open-loop control has the advantages of producing rapid movements, without feedback; and little or no attention is required. The disadvantage is that there's no error regulation — if your speech motor programs contain errors that produce stuttering, you'll continue stuttering rather than correcting your speech. Also, open-loop control may be ineffective in changing environments, or when precision is needed.

SCHEMATA THEORY

Schemata theory suggests that you learn certain *invariable characteristics* of a motor skill, and you learn certain execution rules or *parameterization schema*. You then combine the invariable elements with the rules to produce a motor plan.

For example, a waitress from Oklahoma asked me if I wanted *ah-iss*. When I figured out that she was asking about *ice*, I affirmatively answered *yay-iss*. I knew the invariable characteristics of "yes," and when I'd learned the rules of an Oklahoma accent — e.g., break monosyllabic words into two syllables— I was able to say words I'd never heard.

Fluent speech is open-loop, preprogrammed motor programs. You don't listen to your speech, or feel your muscle movements, and correct your speech as you go along (except when speaking very slowly in a speech clinic). Many of these motor programs and schemata rules are stored during childhood. For example, your accent is hardwired into your brain in childhood. Stuttering develops and becomes permanent at this time, suggesting that stuttering is a stored motor program.

We usually think of motor skills and motor programs as desirable — the ability to serve a tennis ball, or to touch-type. But motor skills and motor programs can also be undesirable or *suboptimal*. Coaches can tell you of bad habits their athletes have. I type with two fingers, at 45 words per minute. These suboptimal motor skills are like stuttering in that you can play tennis or type or talk, but you don't do it as well as you should be able to.

Stuttering is an undesirable parameterization schema learned during childhood. A stutterer combines the invariable characteristics of words with stuttering parameters, and produces stuttered speech. For example, one stuttering rule may be, "When you perceive time pressure, tense your vocal folds."

RESPONSE SELECTION

Response selection is critical for speech. You choose between many words, as well as ways to execute each word. For example, if someone asks your name, you can say, "My name is Ernest Wingnut," or "Ernie," or "I'm Ernie Wingnut," or hand out your business card. You can say a word with a different accent. You can say a word quickly or slowly. You can stutter or say the word fluently.

You can either make a conscious *decision*, or an unconscious *translation* of stimulus to response. When speaking, you mostly make unconscious translations. For example, if the person asks you a question quickly, you respond by answering quickly. If the environment is relaxed, you may respond with relaxed, fluent speech.

This suggests that stutterers store several motor programs. You have the invariable characteristics of “yes” stored, and you have various schemata for creating a motor program to say “yes.” The schemata include accent, speaking rate, quiet or loud volume, emotional inflection, and whether you say the word fluently or disfluently. According to psychological cues, your brain sometimes retrieves the fluent schemata, and sometimes retrieves the stuttering schemata. For example, when you perceive time pressure, you retrieve the motor program for fast, tense speech, and when you perceive a relaxed listener, your brain retrieves the motor program for relaxed, fluent speech.

According to this model, stuttering is partly the motor programs you stored as a child, and partly your response selection for various psychological cues. You can change your fluency by changing either your motor programs or your response selection. To oversimplify, fluency shaping therapy focuses on changing motor programs, and stuttering modification therapy focuses on changing response selection.

For an exercise in stuttering therapy, write down all the psychological cues that affect your speech. Note your response to each stimulus (e.g., a fast talker makes you respond fast). Then note which stimulus-response cues increase your stuttering, and which decrease your stuttering.

Now think of a stimulus cue, and imagine yourself responding in a way that decreases stuttering. For example, someone speaks quickly to you. Instead of responding quickly, you pause, and then answer slowly. You can do this as role-playing games in a support group. Work through every stimulus-response cue on your list. This is explained in more detail below in the section on *personal construct therapy* in the chapter “Stuttering Therapy Programs.”

THREE STAGES OF MOTOR LEARNING

In 1964, psychologist Paul Fitts proposed three stages of motor learning:

1) In the *cognitive stage*, a teacher introduces you to the motor task. You learn the objective of the skill. You learn the relational and psychological cues that control and regulate the movements.

For example, a speech pathologist may teach you the “gentle onset” fluency skill. She explains to you that the purpose is to improve vocal fold control. She demonstrates gentle onset for you, and you hear and see what she is doing. She explains the cues such as taking a relaxed breath, letting out a little air, starting to produce sound softly, and then gradually increasing volume.

This stage of motor learning places high demands on sensation and perception. You learn stimuli and meaning. You make conscious decisions about response selection. You do little with response execution.

2) In the *associative stage*, you learn to perform and refine the motor skill. You move from response selection to response execution. You replace conscious decisions about response selection with unconscious translations from stimulus to response. You focus on timing your movements better, becoming more efficient. For some motor skills you work on executing your response more quickly.

One process in this stage is the *chunking* of memory. In short-term memory, most people can remember only seven things, or chunks of memory. For example, if someone tells you a 7-digit telephone number, you'll probably be able to repeat it, at least for the 30 seconds or so that short-term memory works. But add an unfamiliar area code and you won't remember the 10-digit number.

In learning, you chunk several items together in memory. For example, a familiar area code is one chunk, but an unfamiliar area code is three chunks. If you regularly call people in New York City, you recognize 212 as the New York City area code, and you're able to remember a new telephone number with that area code. In a well-known study, expert and novice chess players were equally able to remember chess pieces when placed randomly on a chessboard. When the pieces were arranged according to the rules of the game, the experts could recall the positions almost perfectly, while the novices' memory did not improve. The chess experts used the game rules to chunk pieces together, e.g., a knight attacking two pieces is chunked into a "knight hook."

Stuttering therapy starts to work when you begin "chunking" therapy techniques. At first, fluency shaping therapy is hard, with a six or seven different fluency skills to remember, with each fluency skill having several components. You can't possible remember all those things! But with practice, you "chunk" relaxing your breathing with relaxing your vocal folds, and then with slowing your speaking rate, and the fluent speech becomes easy. Chunking reduces information processing demands, allowing you to feel less rushed, and enabling you to respond to other stimuli.

3) In the *autonomous stage*, the motor skill becomes automatic. You can walk and perform other cognitive tasks at the same time.

In the autonomous stage, your conscious decisions are entirely replaced with unconscious translations of stimuli into responses. For example, when someone asks your name, you unconsciously take a relaxed breath, let out a little air, gently increase vocal fold tension, and fluently say your name.

If you've completed a stuttering therapy program, you probably completed the cognitive stage (learning the principles of the program) relatively quickly, in a few hours or days. The associative stage (learning to speak fluently in the speech clinic) took longer, probably weeks or months. The autonomous stage probably is still causing you trouble. You have spontaneous fluency at times, but at times you have to consciously control your speech. Perhaps you're one of the estimated 25-30% of stutterers who never reached the autonomous stage, and you continue to stutter outside the speech clinic.

How you move from the associative stage to the autonomous stage is the big question in motor learning theory. The rest of this chapter will explore this area.

INFORMATION FEEDBACK

"Most of the researchers in motor learning consider information feedback to be a very important, if not the most important, variable affecting performance and learning." (Shea, 1993, p.209) Psychologists classify information feedback into two categories: *knowledge of results* (KR) and *knowledge of performance* (KP).

Knowledge of results concerns whether you accomplished your intended goal. For example, if your task was to kick a football between goal posts, you'd want to know if the football went between the goal posts.

Knowledge of performance concerns whether you moved as you intended. In athletics, coaches often have you improve your "form," or how you kick, throw, hold a racket, etc. For the moment you ignore the goal of the sport.

Early theorizing about KR explored rewards and punishment. However, research has shown that *error information* is more important than rewards or punishment.

Error information is essential for motor learning. "The data from KR research suggest that subjects tend to change their behavior when they are provided error information. When this information is not presented, they tend to repeat their original behavior...When large errors result, subjects tend to make larger changes in their behavior than when smaller errors are observed." (Shea, 1993, p.210)

This suggests that because stutterers repeat their speech errors, stutterers may not be aware that they are making errors. Stutterers may be aware that their speech is "bad," and experience punishment, but stutterers may not be aware of what they are doing wrong (e.g., breathing abnormalities, incorrect vocal fold tension). Stuttering therapy sometimes consists of a speech pathologist saying when you do exercises right or wrong, but not providing useful error information. In comparison, the Computer-Aided Fluency Establishment & Trainer (CAFET) stuttering biofeedback computer system, which is probably the most effective stuttering treatment available (described in the chapter "Computers and Electronic Devices for Stuttering Therapy"), provides detailed and immediate error information.

While KR improves motor learning, too much KR may have a detrimental effect on retention. You can become dependent on KR, using it to guide your performance. You may ignore other sources of information. The ideal is to do some trials with KR and some without. You'll retain your new motor skills better. For example, one study compared 100% KR (results presented for every trail) with 33% KR (results shown only for every third trial). The 100% KR group performed better during the trials, but two days later the 33% KR group performed better, indicating better retention of the motor skill. (Shea, 1993, p.214)

Psychologists spend much time figuring out the optimum plan for KR. Usually you have a *fading schedule*: lots of KR for the first trials, and as your performance improves you do trials without KR. For example, the CAFET biofeedback system at first provides visual feedback of your breathing and vocal volume on the computer monitor, and error messages across the bottom of the screen. After you successfully complete each performance task a number of times (usually 20 correct trials in a row), the visual display switches off, and you see only the error messages, in real-time as you talk. After 20 more correct trials, the error messages are held until after you finish a trial. The goal is to complete 20 trials without KR and without errors.

Psychologists also suggest using a *bandwidth of KR* schedule, in which large errors are displayed, but small errors are not displayed. This prevents a tendency for you to overcorrect small, inconsequential errors, leading to larger errors on the next trial. This is called *maladaptive short-term corrections*.

In most sports, KR is immediate — you see if you threw the ball in the basket, etc. In some sports, such as diving, KR is delayed a minute or so while the judges make decisions. Psychologists have found that a *KR delay interval* degrades learning, although how much is not firmly established.

With a speech biofeedback system, the stutterer receives immediate KR. A speech pathologist is usually polite and lets you finish your sentence before telling you what you did wrong on the first word. Immediate KR is one reason that biofeedback therapy is more effective than stuttering therapy with a speech pathologist.

PRACTICE SCHEDULING

The last area of motor learning concerns how to design *practice scheduling* and *practice composition* during *acquisition* to maximize *retention* and *transfer*.

Practice scheduling concerns the context of practice tasks, such as the order of tasks, or the schedule of practice/rest intervals. Practice composition varies the task or manner of practice. For example, executing a task with or without KR is a variance of practice composition.

Learning a motor skill is called *acquisition*. Executing the motor skill is called *retention*, even if conditions are altered. For example, you may learn fluency skills in a speech clinic, but then use these skills the next day at work. This is retention.

Transfer refers to using a skill for a task not experienced during acquisition. An example would be a child learning in school that 2 apples + 2 apples = 4 apples, and the child goes home and figures out that 2 oranges + 2 oranges = 4 oranges. School would be useless if skills didn't transfer. Speech pathologists use the term "transfer" to refer to using fluency skills outside the speech clinic. Psychologists would call this "retention." A psychologist might use the term "transfer" if you learned relaxed breathing in a yoga class, and then applied this in stuttering therapy.

Practice scheduling has a variety of parameters. *Massed practice* refers to practicing more than you rest, and *distributed practice* refers to resting more than you practice. Generally, distributed practice produces better results.

A 1978 study taught postal workers to type on a mail-sorting machine. All subjects received 60 hours of training, but the scheduling varied between four groups. One group had two two-hour sessions per day (for 15 days), a second group had one two-hour session per day (for 30 days), a third group had two one-hour sessions per day (for 30 days), and the fourth group had one one-hour session per day (for 60 days). The one-hour/one-session attained the performance goal in the least training time. The two-hour/two-session group had the worst performance. Interestingly, the postal workers preferred the two-hour/two-session schedule the best, even though this had the worst performance.

Stuttering therapy programs are usually either 8-10 hours a day for 15 days, or are one hour per week for months or years. Neither is ideal. Stuttering therapy programs appear to be optimized for failure and relapse.

Stuttering therapy would be more effective in one-hour daily sessions. This is another reason why speech biofeedback devices produce better results than non-instrumented stuttering therapy. The Dr. Fluency stuttering biofeedback computer system enables home practice. Users of the Desktop Fluency System anti-stuttering telephone device report that their stuttering diminishes over time. By leaving the device plugged into their telephones, the users get many short therapy sessions randomly spaced throughout the day. (See the chapter “Computers and Electronic Devices for Stuttering Therapy”.)

PRACTICE COMPOSITION

When several tasks are taught, you can schedule trials *blocked* (A-A-A, B-B-B, C-C-C) or at *random* (C-A-B, B-C-A, B-A-C). One study found the “blocked” subjects learned faster, but then forgot their skills. The “random” subjects learned more slowly, but their retention and transfer was dramatically better. The random scheduling forced subjects to store their new skills in long-term memory rather than short-term memory.

Brutten and Dancer (1980) found that stuttering frequency was reduced more during blocked practice (saying each word five times) then in random practice (saying the list of words five times). The researchers did not test which practice composition resulted in long-term retention of fluency.

Another practice parameter breaks down complex motor skills into simple tasks. This can be done in three ways:

1) *Fractionation*, or doing each simple task separately. For example, one day a tennis player might only practice serving.

2) *Simplification*, or reducing the demands of the task. For example, kids start baseball with T-ball, then with a pitching machine,

then slow-pitch softball, and finally move to baseball.

3) *Segmentation*, or doing one simple task before moving on to another.

Generally, part-whole practice is more effective than whole practice, unless the simple tasks interact. An example of the latter is controlling pitch and roll in a flight simulator.

Lastly, practice can be done alone or with other people. In many tasks, practicing with a group improves learning. Physiological stimulation caused by competition is a main reason for increased performance in a group. On the other hand, some tasks are performed poorly in front of an audience.

VARYING COGNITION IN PRACTICE TRIALS

Imagine practicing tennis returns with a tennis machine. The machine shoots the ball out perfectly time after time. You practice the same return again and again. An hour later, you have the return down perfectly.

Now imagine a broken tennis machine. Every serve is different. The timing varies, the speed varies, the balls go all over the court. Again you practice your returns, but after an hour of running around chasing balls, your return is far from perfect.

The next day you play in a tournament. Which practice leads to better performance?

Sir Frederick Bartlett once said about his tennis game, "When I make the stroke I do not, as a matter of fact, produce something absolutely new, and I never repeat something old." (Lee, 1991) The well-adjusted tennis machine produces better performance during the practice, but the broken tennis machine produces better retention and transfer, and better performance during real games.

Increased cognitive or mental effort during practice results in better motor learning. By varying the practice, you learn the invariable elements of the motor plans.

When observing the performance of a motor skill, you learn best by watching an unskilled person making mistakes. Watching a skilled person perform the task flawlessly doesn't do you much good. Watching an unskilled person involves higher cognitive effort.

In some stuttering therapies, your speech pathologist flawlessly demonstrates the therapy techniques to you. If your speech pathologist never stuttered, her effortless performance shows you none of the response selections a stutterer must make.

SINGLE VS. MULTICHANNEL PROCESSING

Stutterers sometimes complain that they can either pay attention to their therapy techniques, or they can pay attention to the conversation — but not both.

In the speech clinic, while reading word lists or talking about unimportant subjects, you can pay attention to the therapy techniques and talk fluently. But outside the speech clinic, when conversations are *pragmatic* or have a purpose, you pay attention to the purpose of the conversation, forget about your therapy techniques, and revert to stuttering.

Psychologists call this the *single channel theory*. In contrast, the *multichannel theory* suggests that the brain has several subsystems. You can use each channel for only one purpose, but you can use several subsystems simultaneously. For example, several studies have found that pianists can sight-read and play music, while repeating ("shadowing") a message heard on headphones. Typists can perform similarly.

There is evidence that multiple channels are learned. When you first learn to drive, you must devote all your attention to keeping the car on the road. But after some practice, you can drive and carry on a conversation at the same time. Of course, some drivers with cellular phones don't seem fully capable of multichannel processing! According to this model, if you practice your therapy techniques enough, eventually you should be able to pay attention to your speech and your conversation at the same time.

Research suggests that when two tasks are similar, it's harder to do the tasks simultaneously. When the tasks are different, you can do the tasks in parallel. But when two tasks are very similar, you can integrate the tasks (Kinsbourne, 1981). For example, a musician can dance while playing a saxophone. You must *integrate* or *differentiate:*

- Integrate your therapy techniques into your message. Relaxing your breathing and vocal folds lowers your vocal pitch and communicates that you are relaxed, confident, and authoritative. This also dramatically improves your fluency.
- Differentiate your therapy techniques from conversations by practicing them alone at home every day until they are as automatic as driving a car. In conversations, you would not have to think about your therapy techniques.

MALADAPTIVE MOTOR SKILLS ARE NOT "BAD HABITS"

When we think of "motor skills," and especially of learning new motor skills, we think of golf swings, hitting a tennis ball, or learning how to do a gentle onset. In other words, we think of positive goals, or things we want to do.

But motor skills can also be negative, undesirable, or suboptimal. Any coach can tell you about the “bad habits” his or her players use, e.g., an improper grip on the tennis racket. The coaches are mistaken in calling these "bad habits." A *bad habit* is something you don’t want to do — cracking your knuckles, picking your nose, etc.

A *maladaptive motor skill* enables you to do something, although not well as you could another way. Your improper grip on the racket enables you to play tennis, and you may even play fairly well, but not optimally. I type 45 word per minute with two fingers. I have a friend who took touch-typing in high school — and types 10 words per minute. He types the right way, I type the wrong way, but I type over 4 times faster. My typing is not a bad habit. My typing is a suboptimal or maladaptive motor skill.

Stuttering is similarly not a “bad habit.” Stutterers can talk, but not as well as they could if they had learned to speak fluently when they were children.

One way to distinguish bad habits from maladaptive motor skills is to ask whether you wished you’d learned something different as a child. I wish I’d learned to touch-type in high school. I wish that a speech pathologist taught me to talk fluently in early childhood. But you wouldn’t say about a bad habit, “I wish I’d learned a better way to pick my nose when I was a kid.”

EXTINGUISHING MALADAPTIVE MOTOR SKILLS

The problem with maladaptive motor skills is they enable you to do something desirable (e.g., talk or play tennis), so it’s hard to unlearn them and replace them with optimal motor skills. This problem could be called “one step forward, one step back.”

I learned to touch-type several times. The result was incredibly slow typing, about 10 wpm. After a week I gave up and go back to two fingers. If I continued to touch-type, my speed would increase to 45 wpm within a few weeks, and then surpass my two-fingered typing speed. After a few months I’d probably type 70 wpm.

In order to increase my typing speed (the step forward) I would have to type slower (the step back) for a few weeks or months. There are many analogies in tennis, golf, or other motor skills.

Retraining speech motor skills involves this same “one step

forward..." problem. In fluency shaping stuttering therapy, you use very slow speech for several weeks or months. Stutterers will do this in the speech clinic, but they refuse to use slow speech outside the speech clinic. The result is that they never move from the associative stage (conscious control) to autonomous or automatic fluent speech. To overcome stuttering, you must be willing to take "one step backward" before going forward.

To overcome stuttering, you must not only learn new fluent speech motor skills, but also forget your old stuttering motor skills. Psychologists call this process *extinction.* The usual method is punishment and reward. Typically the reward is removed, e.g., after training a rat to press a bar for food, it's relatively easy to extinguish this skill by not providing food when the rat pushes the bar. But "behavior that has been learned thoroughly is most resistant to extinction...Faults in motor performance that have been learned and practiced over a long period of time are the most difficult to eliminate." (Oxendine, 1984, p.125) The difference between knowledge of results (KR) and knowledge of performance (KP) is important for extinguishing undesirable habitual motor skills. Stutterers generally have KR, or know when they stutter. But stutterers lack KP, or awareness of movements. Eliminating behaviors you are unaware is impossible, so the first step in extinguishing stuttering is to develop KP, or awareness of your stuttering behaviors.

The opposite of retention is forgetting. The two main theories of forgetting are *fading* and *interference*:

Fading is simply disuse. Many users of electronic anti-stuttering devices report that their stuttering diminishing over time, and they no longer need the device. Several factors could affect this, and memory fading could be one factor.

Interference suggests that skills are lost when new skills interfere with the old skills. Learning fluent speech motor skills may alter or obliterate your stuttering motor skills. For example, stutterers learn new speech motor programs in fluency shaping therapy, which interfere with old stuttering patterns. Or in psychological stuttering therapy, you learn new stimulus-response translations to psychological cues.

Another theory of forgetting is Freudian *repression*, or your unconscious not wishing to remember a threatening event or activity. Stuttering often feels threatening, but stutterers don't repress it!

Neurology of Stuttering

Recent brain scan research has found brain abnormalities during stuttering, and promises new treatments for stuttering using drugs and computerized devices.

Most studies have found no differences between stutterers' and non-stutterers' cerebral activity have been found during silent rest and during fluent speech (Ingham, 1996).

But during stuttering, cerebral activity changes dramatically. The most striking difference is that left-hemisphere areas active during normal speech become less active, and areas in the right hemisphere not normally active during speech become active (Braun, 1997; Ingham, 1997).

This abnormal right-hemisphere dominance has produced a variety of speculative hypotheses from researchers. One hypothesis is that there is something wrong with stutterers' left-brain speech areas, and so right-brain areas not developed for speech take over. This seems unlikely, given that most stutterers are capable of normal, fluent speech in certain conditions.

Another hypothesis is that the right-hemisphere activity is the fears and anxieties that stutterers experience, generated by the limbic and paralimbic structures. But these areas don't seem to be abnormally active during stuttering.

Another hypothesis is based on the decreased central auditory processing during stuttering seen in almost all studies (Wu, 1995; Fox, 1996; Ingham, 1997). One study also found decreased activity in the area that integrates auditory and somatic (body) sensation (Braun, 1997). Stuttering reduces this rear-brain sensory processing, and reduces the left-brain communication of this sensory information to frontal speech and language areas. The abnormal right-brain activity may be an alternative pathway for rear-brain sensory information to travel to the front of the brain.

Another team of researchers believes that the key to stuttering lies in the different functions of the *lateral* and *medial* systems (Goldberg, 1985; Maguire, 1997). The lateral system is part of the cortex, where our consciousness is, and we have conscious awareness and control of lateral functions. This area produces and understands language (Wernicke's area), forms words (Broca's area), and forms muscle movements (supplementary motor areas). These areas can produce speech under *closed-loop motor control*. Even severe stutterers can speak fluently under closed-loop motor control, but high attention demands and abnormally-slow speech (Shea, 1993) make this an undesirable way to talk.

The medial or striatal system produces open-loop or normal speech. This system includes the caudate and putamen. Preprogrammed motor plans are retrieved from long-term memory and executed, without sensory feedback. Open-loop control can produce rapid movements, with little or no attention. The disadvantage is that there's no error regulation — if your speech motor programs contain stuttering, you'll continue stuttering rather than correct your speech. Open-loop motor control responds to stimuli, without conscious thought. Stutterers can speak fluently in certain situations, such as speaking to a pet, but when they experience stimuli such as time pressure or speak to an authority figure, their medial systems retrieve stuttering speech motor programs from long-term memory.

One study found that stutterers have decreased medial system activity during both stuttering and fluent speech (chorus reading). Stutterers have decreased lateral system activity during stuttering, and increased lateral activity during fluent speech (Wu, 1997).

Glyndon Riley, Joseph Wu, and Gerald Maguire (1997) propose that the medial system is affected by the D_2 dopamine modulation system. This includes the substantia nigra and its circuit to the striatum. Dopamine is the neurotransmitter that produces alertness, motivation, and mental acuity. In stutterers, excess dopamine may reach the striatum and reduce activation, making these areas less effective.

The dopamine system may explain why stutterers have "good days," when they easily speak fluently, and "bad days," when they can't get a word out without a hard block. Dopamine levels vary with diet and other factors. Genetic research has correlated stuttering with three genes that control dopamine in persons with Tourette's Syndrome and their relatives (Comings, 1996).

Riley, Wu, and Maguire point out that stuttering therapy works with the lateral system, teaching stutterers to consciously control their speech, stuttering behaviors, and feeling and attitudes. The result too often is fluency in the speech clinic, when the stutterer pays close attention to his speech, but when he returns to his normal environmental, cues to stutter cause him to lose control of his speech.

Because stuttering occurs in the medial system, they suggest developing therapies that work on the medial system. They suggest drug treatments, but electronic anti-stuttering devices also effect the medial system. The drug treatments are discussed in the next chapter, "Drug Treatments for Stuttering."

Delayed auditory feedback (DAF) electronic devices have been used to treat stuttering for over 30 years. The stutterer hears his speech in the headphones with a long delay, which forces the stutterer into closed-loop speech motor control, producing slow but fluent speech. More recently, researchers have explored short delays, which reduce stuttering about 75-80% without training, mental effort, or abnormal-sounding or slow speech. These researchers also discovered that shifting the frequency of the stutterer's voice in his headphones (FAF) produces the same effect (Kalinowski, 1993, 1994, 1995; Ingham, 1997; Zimmerman, 1997). For more on these devices, see the chapter "Computers and Electronic Devices for Treating Stuttering."

Electroencephalograph (EEG) brain scans found that DAF and FAF reduce right-hemisphere cerebral activity (Kalinowski, 1997). Apparently — and this is another speculative model — the rear-brain sensory areas notice that the auditory and somatic sensations are not matching. Extra blood flow is devoted to these areas, correcting stutterers' deficient auditory processing and integration. This information is sent with a "red flag" to the frontal speech and language areas. But the frontal areas don't check frequencies, and are too slow to detect a short delay, so they "OK" the information and your speech is not disrupted. The result is extra information for improved motor control and fluent speech.

Future stuttering therapies may begin with drugs and electronic devices to get the stutterer fluent, and then retrain speech motor programs and recondition psychological cues to stutter, reducing and then eliminating the stutterer's reliance on the drugs and electronic devices.

MORE BRAIN SCAN RESULTS

Different studies found different results because a variety of technologies were used (EEG vs. SPECT vs. PET, H2150 vs. FDG). Most studies were small, usually a half-dozen stutterers. The subjects were usually right-handed men — women and left-handed men may have different cerebral activity.

• Salmelin, 1998: "Neuromagnetic responses to monaural tones [found that] the basic functional organization of the auditory cortices was found to be different in stutterers and controls...and more severely by self-paced [stuttered] than accompanied [fluency induced by the chorus effect] speech."

* Braun, 1997: Language processing shifted to the right hemisphere, including the dorsolateral prefrontal cortices, middle temporal gyrus, and anterior cingulate cortex. Motor function shifts to the right hemisphere, including the "anterior forebrain regions and associated archicortical paralimbic areas." Visual processing also appeared to shift to the right hemisphere. Decreased sensory perception, including post-rolandic sensory areas and related paleocortical paralimbic regions. Increased somatosensory processing (sensation of the body), including the "dorsal region of the angular gyrus, adjacent to the superior parietal lobule, as well as somatosensory association cortices in the medial SPL."

• De Nil, 1995: During silent reading, increased activation in the left angular cingulate cortex, a "reflection of covert anticipation of stuttering."

• Ingham, 1996: "Present findings do not support recent suggestions that developmental stuttering is associated with abnormalities of brain blood flow at rest. Rather, our findings indicate an essentially normal functional brain terrain..."

• Ingham, 1997: "Diffuse overactivity throughout the cerebral and cerebellar motor systems...Deactivation of a verbal production circuit between left frontal (BA47) and temporal (BA22) cortex that has been previously identified in normal speakers."

• Kalinowski, 1997: Some stutterers showed the greatest reduction in the temporal-parietal area, and others showing greatest reductions in the right hemisphere posterior sites.

• Kroll, 1997: After fluency shaping stuttering therapy there is increased left-hemisphere activity, although large areas of activation in the right hemisphere remain.

• Watson, 1994: Abnormal right-hemisphere activity only in stutterers who also had language deficits.

Drug Treatments for Stuttering

The chapter, "Neurology of Stuttering," described how Glyndon Riley, Joseph Wu, and Gerald Maguire (1997) propose that the medial system is affected by the D_2 dopamine modulation system. Dopamine is the neurotransmitter that produces alertness, motivation, and mental acuity. In stutterers, excess dopamine may reach the striatum and reduce activation of speech motor control areas.

RISPERDAL

The dopamine D_2-receptor antagonist *risperidone* (Risperdal) is the most widely-prescribed anti-stuttering drug. One small study found that the drug reduced stuttering on average 55-60% in four subjects, without serious side effects (Maguire, 1997). Another study found a 48% reduction in stuttering (Riley, 1998).

Risperdal is FDA-approved only for short-term (6-8 week) treatment of schizophrenia. Side effects include insomnia, agitation, anxiety, somnolence, extrapyramidal nervous system disorders, headaches, dizziness, constipation, rhinitis (a breathing disorder), rashes, tachycardia (a heart disorder), and breast growth in men and women (due to increased prolactin), and neuroleptic malignant syndrome (potentially fatal).

One stutterer tried Risperdal, and couldn't leave his house due to severe anxiety. Another male stutterer wrote on the Internet, "I used Risperdal for about 6 months. It had a marginal (if any) effect on the intensity of my stutter. I had to discontinue its use due to hormonal side-effects (my right breast started to grow)."

Other stutterers have also reported no speech improvement. Some stutterers say that Risperdal improves their speech in situations where they are normally fluent, and does not affect their speech in difficult situations.

Risperdal has never been studied longer than 8 weeks. The drug may be useful during the first 6-8 weeks of a stuttering therapy program, with the dosages reduced and then eliminated as the stutterer progresses in the therapy program. Longer use should be scrutinized, due to unknown long-term side effects.

OTHER DOPAMINE ANTAGONISTS

The dopamine antagonist *haliperodol* (Haldol) has been proven to reduce stuttering in two double-blind placebo-controlled studies

(Bloodstein, 1995), but the side effects are severe. One stutterer took it for several days, then one night found his head rotating slowly back and forth 180 degrees — and there was nothing he could do to stop it! The effect on his speech had been minimal, so he stopped taking the medication.

Pimozide is another dopamine antagonist. Four out six stutterers studied had improved speech, but they would not continue the medication due to severe side effects (Stager, 1997).

The anti-psychotic *olanzapine* (Zyprexa) helped two stutterers (Daily Mail, 1998). It is a thienobenzodiazepine class selective monoaminergic antagonist with high affinity binding to a variety of receptors, including $dopamine_{1-4}$. Side effects include headaches, somnolence, agitation, insomnia, nervousness, hostility, dizziness, and rhinitis.

Tiapride is a substituted benzamide derivative with selective dopamine D_2-receptor antagonist properties, and preferential affinity for extrastriatal dopamine receptors, and anxiolytic properties. In a study of 14 children and teenagers, stuttering was reduced about 25%. Side effects were not a problem for any subjects, and five subjects opted to continue taking the drug after completing the study (Rothenberger, 1994). Tiapride is a German drug, not approved for sale in the United States. It is usually used to treat agitation, aggressiveness, anxiety, and sleep disorders in the elderly.

Dopamine levels can be altered by diet (Wurtman, 1986; Somer, 1995). Unfortunately, it's easy to increase dopamine levels (which in my experience increases stuttering), but reducing dopamine levels via diet results in feeling depressed and sluggish.

Diet can reduce dopamine in all areas of the brain, perhaps reducing stuttering but causing other problems. Drugs can reduce dopamine in selected areas, but still not selectively enough to avoid side effects. In the future perhaps there will be a drug that reduces dopamine only in the left caudate nucleus, where stuttering appears to originate.

Psychiatrist Gerald Maguire believes that stutterers avoid the use of cocaine and amphetamines, because these drugs increase dopamine levels (cocaine) and sensitivity (amphetamines) and increase stuttering. Caffeine also affects dopamine sensitivity, but no one has studied the effect of caffeine on stuttering. Dopamine receptor stimulation with the drug apomorphine failed to increase stuttering (Bloodstein, 1995).

ANTI-DEPRESSANTS AND STUTTERING

Prozac and other anti-depressants have been reported to increase stuttering. In a few cases, these drugs caused non-stutterers to stutter.

One stutterer wrote (Butcher, 1998):

> I was sitting in the hallway, in the dark. I had been crying and hitting my head on the wall, screaming to God, why me? I hated my stuttering and I suppose hated myself as well. From that point on it was as if when I remembered that incident all the feelings came back to me and wouldn't leave. Those angry, hurt, frustrating feelings from so long ago wouldn't go away. I was hiding my feelings from everyone around me, pretending to be super mom and super wife. I decided to seek professional help.
>
> We decided that I would try Wellbutrin. As my doctor put it, kill two birds with one stone, since Wellbutrin is also prescribed to help you quit smoking. The first week I felt like I had so much anxiety that I could explode. The second week I noticed my stuttering getting worse. By the third week the controls that I had learned in speech therapy were virtually unusable. It was so frustrating to not be able to control my stuttering at all. Needless to say we all agreed to flush the Wellbutrin and never go back on anything like that.
>
> Prozac, Trazadone and Effexor did not effect my speech at all.

Another stutterer wrote:

> I have tried 3 antidepressants: Prozac, Wellbutrin, and Zoloft. All increased my stuttering noticeably. The antidepressants that I have tried make me more able to get out of bed in the morning and restore my "get up and go"; however, they have caused me to go from being a person with a barely noticeable stutter to a more pronounced stutter.
>
> I went into my psychiatrist yesterday and explained that the current antidepressant is making my stutter significantly worse. However, in the 10 minutes we talked I was practically perfectly fluent. He then concludes that obviously "it's not that unmanageable."
>
> He prescribed 10mg Propanolol to take before I have to be in a difficult speaking presentation. It is supposed to "reduce performance anxiety." I don't feel like I have a tremendous amount of performance anxiety; stuttering just isn't very fun. I think he doesn't believe me about the severity of the stuttering.

Bloodstein's *A Handbook on Stuttering* lists a 1977 study of propanolol finding "no statistically significant effect on stuttering." The similar drug *oxprenolol* had a similar lack of effectiveness.

A stutterer/speech pathologist wrote:

> Antidepressants tend to not only increase the amount of stuttering I experience, but unfortunately significantly interfere with my ability to use easy, smooth modification techniques.
>
> Recently I've combined another kind of medication with my antidepressant. This new medication is in the family of drugs called neuroleptics. I found that on Risperdal my stuttering decreased significantly and I could now easily smooth out remaining stuttering when using small amounts of this drug. But after several weeks the side effects (difficulty with breathing) made me stop it. Now I'm trying thothixene (trade name: Navane) with good results. I'm almost back to normal with my speech abilities.

One stutterer/psychiatrist advises that stutterers in need of an anti-depressant ask for the dopamine antagonist Serzone instead of Prozac (Maguire, 1996).

Stager (1995) studied two other SSRIs. *Clomipramine* reduced stuttering about 5-10%, but side effects were severe. *Desipramine* was not effective.

RITALIN, ADHD, AND STUTTERING

A speech pathologist asked on the Internet:

> I'm treating an 8 year-old diagnosed ADHD and who suddenly began stuttering (advanced core and secondary behaviors) without any prior history of dysfluency, as a side effect of the medication Ritalin. He's had a whole neuro work-up which revealed nothing.

Another speech pathologist responded that many of the children he treated for stuttering were on Ritalin for ADHD.

Pharmacist Richard Harkness advises against Ritalin for children who stutter:

> Ritalin increases dopaminergic neurotransmission and is contraindicated for use in those with Tourette's disorder. Ritalin has also, in rare cases, brought on symptoms of Tourette's disorder. Tourette's disorder has been likened to stuttering in that it involves a flaw in dopaminergic neurotransmission.

Stuttering, ADHD, and Tourette's are genetically linked (see the section "Genetics of Stuttering").

OTHER DRUGS

Botulinum toxin (botulism) has been injected into stutterers' vocal folds. The toxin paralyzes your vocal folds, at least partially, and you can't get into hard blocks. You also can't talk loudly or forcefully. The toxin reduces stuttering somewhat, in most people. It wears off in a few months, and you get a second shot. The second shot reduces stuttering less than the first. By the third shot, the toxin usually has no effect on stuttering.

Calcium-channel blockers such as *nimodipine* (Maguire, 1995) and *verapamil* (Brady, 1989; Brumfitt and Peake, 1988, referenced in Bloodstein, 1995) improve fluency in some stutterers, but on average were not effective.

No studies have been done on the effects of *alcohol* on stuttering. Anecdotally, alcohol reduces stutterers' fears and anxieties, e.g., about talking to persons of the opposite sex, and so reduces stuttering. But alcohol reduces one's ability to use therapy techniques, so increases stuttering.

Tranquilizers, according to Bloodstein's *A Handbook on Stuttering*, have "more effect on the complexity or severity of the [stuttered] blocks than on their frequency."

Bloodstein lists several other ineffective drugs: thiamin, glutamic acid, carbon dioxide inhalation, and bethanecol chloride.

Theories of Stuttering Development

CHILDHOOD TRAUMA & CONDITIONING

Ivan Pavlov studied classical conditioning. Pavlov noticed that dogs salivate when they see their food. He sounded a tuning fork whenever he brought food to the dogs. The dogs salivated when they heard the tuning fork and saw their food. Eventually Pavlov could sound the tuning fork without providing food, and the dogs salivated as if they were about to eat.

The response, of the dog salivating at the sight of food, is called the unconditioned response. Salivating before eating is reflexive or "hard-wired," not learned.

Analogously, a child may be disfluent in a stressful speaking situation, such as an encounter with an angry parent, or a traumatic event. One man described his first stuttering experience:

> When I was six years old or so, I said good-bye to my parents on Christmas Eve, I watched them (through our living room window) pull out of our driveway; then they were broadsided by a drunk driver. My mother stepped out of the car and fell over (she was OK — just shaken up). I still remember this (I'm 35 now). My father said that when he came in to phone the police, I was overcome with concern for my mother and stuttered severely, for the first time! And...I continued to stutter, all the time.

A neutral or unrelated event occurs in conjunction with the unconditioned stimulus. The tuning fork was the unrelated event, and food was the stimulus for the unconditioned response (salivating).

In stuttering, the child associates unrelated events to his disfluency. This could be the sound or word he was disfluent on, or the room he was in. For the child above, the automobile collision was the stimulus, stuttering was the unconditioned response, and looking out the living room window, or seeing his mother get into her car was the unrelated event.

Later, the neutral or unrelated event triggers the response. The child stutters again when he says the word or sound he stuttered on in the traumatic event. Or he may stutter when looking out the living room window, or when seeing his mother get into her car.

Instrumental conditioning involves behavior followed by a reward (positive reinforcement) or punishment. Another type of instrumental conditioning is negative reinforcement or escape, in which certain behavior causes an undesirable situation to end.

Peters and Guitar (1991) believe that negative reinforcement contributes to the development of secondary symptoms. The child may try squeezing his lips, or nodding his head, and if the words pop out, he'll try the secondary behavior again.

JOHNSON'S DIAGNOSTOGENIC THEORY

Wendell Johnson developed the "diagnostogenic theory" of stuttering at the University of Iowa in the 1950s. His famous line was, "Stuttering begins, not in the child's mouth, but in the parent's ear."

In Johnson's early research (with Charles Van Riper in the 1930s), he was puzzled that beginning stuttering is often so hard to distinguish from normal childhood disfluencies. He hypothesized that certain parents are perfectionistic or overanxious, and make high demands for politeness, orderliness, etc., and also for fluency. Or parents came from stuttering families, believed stuttering to be hereditary, and listened to their child's speech too carefully for signs of stuttering.

These parents heard normal disfluencies in their child's speech, and told the child to stop it, or corrected the child's speech, or expressed displeasure in some way. The child began to think that something was wrong with his speech. He then became fearful of talking incorrectly, panicked when he couldn't say a word, and soon become a stutterer.

Johnson's theory could not be tested scientifically. We can't observe every reaction of a parent to everything a child says. We can't know what's going on the parent's mind or in the child's mind.

Johnson's theory is now not widely endorsed. Some studies found support for Johnson's model, but more studies did not find evidence to support to model (Onslow, 1992; Nippold, 1995).

However, speech pathologists now emphasize that parents make the child feel good about his speech, and reduce speech-related stress and fear.

Distortions of Johnson's theory produced a less positive result. Some speech pathologists told parents that ignoring their child's stuttering was the best course, and that stuttering treatment for a preschool child will make the child more concerned about his speech and make stuttering worse. This was never Johnson's view. Authorities in the field of stuttering agree that this is the worst possible advice, and that early intervention with a qualified speech pathologist is the best treatment for stuttering.

STARKWEATHER'S DEMANDS AND CAPACITIES MODEL

Woodruff Starkweather proposed the "Demands and Capacities Model" to explain why children begin stuttering. As a child develops, he or she improves four skill areas necessary for speech:

- Oral and speech motor coordination.
- Linguistic ability.
- Cognitive ability.
- Social and emotional maturity.

At the same time, expectations for the child's speech also increase. These demands include faster thought processing, complex language formulation, rapid speech and turn-taking behavior, and independent social behavior.

Starkweather believes that disfluencies occur when external demands exceed the child's speech capacity. "If the demands continue to exceed the child's capacities, stuttering occurs. If the demands are modified or the child's capacities improve sufficiently, stuttering disappears." (Gottwald, 1995)

Because a child may develop well in some of the four skill areas, but lag in one area, different children stutter in different ways. For example, some parents may speak too rapidly, and the child's speech motor coordination can't keep up. Another family may be more emotionally demanding, but the child's emotional maturity may be lacking.

Considerable evidence weighs against the Demands and Capacities Model. The section "Research On Parental Behavior" in the chapter "More Childhood Stuttering Therapy" summarizes more than a dozen studies finding that parental speech behaviors does not cause children's stuttering, and that changing parents' speech does not affect the child's stuttering. Children's speaking rates do not correlate with stuttering, suggesting that their stuttering is not due to exceeding a neurolinguistic speed limit (Yaruss, 1997). A series of studies by Kalinowski et al. found that stutterers have the ability to produce rapid fluent speech, showing that they have excellent oral and speech motor coordination. The section "Does Stress Increase Stuttering" in the chapter "Belief — Anticipation, Distraction, Stress, and Placebos" shows that social and emotional stress can reduce stuttering. There is no reason to believe that stuttering children lack linguistic or cognitive abilities.

NEUROPSYCHOLINGUISTIC THEORY

The "neuropsycholinguistic" theory of stuttering (Perkins, Kent, & Curlee, 1991) distinguishes between linguistic and "paralinguistic" systems. The paralinguistic system conveys emotion and intent via altering pitch, loudness, and duration (speaking rate). Normal or non-stuttered disfluencies occur when the linguistic and paralinguistic systems are dyssynchronous. "Dyssynchronous" means that either the linguistic system is delayed, or the paralinguistic system is delayed. Delays are caused by "competition for neural resources" resulting in parts of the brain becoming inefficient or slowing down. Different people have different "neural resources" due to genetics, brain injuries, or "competition for processing capacity" resulting from activities that use the same areas of the brain.

When the linguistic system is delayed, such as by uncertainty of word choice, the problem is "relatively available to awareness" and can be handled by the speaker. But when the paralinguistic system is delayed because of "self-expressive uncertainties" or limited neural resources, the result is disfluency. When the speaker is not experiencing time pressure, the result is a normal, non-stuttered disfluency. When the speaker experiences time pressure, the result is stuttering.

I agree with the distinction between linguistic and paralinguistic systems. I prefer to use the established terms "invariable characteristics" of a motor skill and "parameterization schema." Speech parameterization schema include volume, pitch, accent, intonation, and speaking rate — identical to the "paralinguistic" system.

In my view, stuttering is another parameterization schema, similar to an accent. Stuttering parameterization schema are chosen according to environmental stimuli. Perkins, Kent & Curlee would disagree with me, and instead say that environmental stimuli can make the process of combining invariable characteristics with parameterization schema break down.

Motor learning psychologists would not agree with Perkins, Kent & Curlee that the brain areas that produce the "invariable characteristics" and the "parameterization schema" can get out of step. If this were possible, we would see golfer and tennis players stuttering with their arms and legs. While any athlete can tell you that their arms and legs don't always hit the ball the way they'd hoped, the simpler explanation is that their brains selected the wrong parameterization schema.

Time pressure is a widely recognized environmental stimulus. Athletes blame failure on "time pressure" as often as stutterers blame "time pressure." In a panic situation, the brain may select older, deeply learned behaviors, rather than choosing recently- and poorly-learned behaviors.

COVERT REPAIR HYPOTHESIS

The *covert repair hypothesis* (Postma & Kolk, 1993) attempts to explain why stutterers are generally more fluent when speaking slower. They believe that

> individuals who stutter may attempt to use speaking rates that are too fast for their (assumedly) impaired phonological encoding mechanisms. (Yaruss, 1997)

Hypothetically, there is a monitoring function in the speech production system. This monitor detects errors in the grammatical, phonological, articulatory, and other stages of speech production. These errors could result from a variety of sources, such as conflicting rules for generating sentences or sounds. After an error is detected, the person interrupts his speech. The person then corrects the error by repeating the phrase, word, or syllable; by blocking; prolonging the sound; pausing; or breaking the word.

This hypothesis explains both normal disfluencies and stuttering — stuttering is quantitatively but not qualitatively different. Stutterers have something wrong with their speech generating functions that create more errors. If many errors are created, then many blocks, repetitions and prolongations are produced.

There are several problems with the covert repair hypothesis. The first is that the brain is too slow to produce speech under "closed-loop control," that is, listening to your speech and correcting your speech as you go. Postma and Kolk get around this problem by hypothesizing that you monitor pre-articulated speech. In other words, you check the grammar, order of sounds, etc., before you start talking. This is possible, but there's no evidence that your brain does this.

A second problem is, what does your brain check your speech against? Recalling a second copy of your stored motor program to compare to the first is pointless — the second recall would have whatever errors were in the first. Perhaps in recalling rules to create motor plans, some rules conflicted and produced errors, and you have some super-rules that can correct such conflicts. Again, why weren't the super-rules recalled in the first place, when the motor program was constructed? According to open-loop control theory, all you can do is recall stored motor programs and send them off to your speech-production muscles. Anything you could use to check the accuracy of a recalled information is also recalled, and there's no way to know which is right and or wrong.

A third problem is that the covert repair hypothesis doesn't explain why children develop from normal, fluent speakers into stutterers. Children's speaking rate does not affect stuttering (Yaruss, 1997).

A fourth problem is that the covert repair hypothesis is difficult to test scientifically. The existence of the monitor agent can't be proven, nor exactly what it monitors. As noted above in the subsection on stutterers' language skills, researchers have tested whether stutterers have problems assembling motor programs (using reaction time tests), and found that stutterers "do not...have problems in assembling motor plans for speech production or in building and retrieving memory representations of symbol-word combinations." (van Lieshout, 1996b)

Another study evaluated repeating three words ten times while adding numbers. No difference was found between stutterers and non-stutterers and this result "did not support the expectations derived from the covert repair hypothesis." (Bosshardt, 1997)

The "suprasegmental Sentence Plan Alignment model" is similar to the covert repair hypothesis in some ways. It

> suggests that speech disfluencies result when the suprasegmental or prosodic plan for an utterance needs to be adjusted and realigned with the remainder of the utterance. In the framework of this theory, reduced speaking rate allows time for this realignment and thereby reduces the likelihood of disfluency. (Yaruss, 1997)

LANGUAGE-LEARNING IMPAIRMENT

A recent article in *Science* suggests a new theory of the development of language-based learning impairment (LLI) in children (Merzenich, 1996). The research was not about stuttering, but there are some interesting parallels between stuttering and LLI.

A mother of a child with LLI described her son, on an Internet stuttering support group:

> I have a seven-year-old son whose speech is very delayed. He didn't start talking until he was almost four. He doesn't seem to 'pick-up' language like most kids do. His speech is very poor, maybe on the level of a typical three-year-old. His grammar is atrocious and doesn't seem to 'hear' the difference in certain words.
>
> He is officially (for school purposes) considered handicapped because of his speech. His hearing has been tested, seems fine. When his IQ was tested (at age 4 1/2), at first he ranked as retarded. But the tester said she didn't think that was right because when she asked him questions, he answered (often at great length) but she couldn't understand what he was saying and had to mark it incorrect. He was tested 6 months later, came out as average.
>
> In many things, he is very good. At age four he would put together incredible things with Legos. (Actually, I thought they were normal. His special ed teachers were the ones that couldn't believe it.) Physically, he's very well-coordinated. He's a wonderful loving child and has no inhibitions about his speech (the teachers considered this unusual also). If you don't understand something he says, he usually looks at you like you're an idiot, and repeats the same thing slowly. But it doesn't always sound like English.
>
> Now he can usually make himself understood, even to strangers (usually). But there are some odd things. He knows boy vs. girl, but the concept of referring to boys as 'he' and girls as 'she' seems to have escaped him. He uses them interchangeably. He'll say "I do's (pronounced dues) don't that" as opposed to "I didn't do that". The concept of tense (past, present, etc.) seems to have no meaning to him.

Children with LLI have difficulty learning language because they can't distinguish short-duration speech sounds. For example, the difference between /b/ and /d/ occurs in a few milliseconds. They can distinguish the sounds if the speech is slowed down, but at normal speaking rates the children can't understand certain sounds or words.

Such impairments can result when a middle ear disease muffles sounds. Other LLI children have normal hearing, but have neurological abnormalities. These brain abnormalities have been detected with evoked potential and imaging systems (such as positron emission tomography).

These facts have led to a theory that LLI is a learning deficit, and that it is a genetically-caused neurological disorder.

In this study, the subjects were seven children between six and nine years old. The researchers developed video games in which the children chose between phonetic elements (/b/ vs. /d/, for example). They also listened to tapes that had certain speech elements slowed down.

In 5-10 hours, all the children quickly learned what they supposedly have a neurological deficit preventing them from learning.

The researchers concluded:

> These studies…indicate…that there may be no fundamental defect in the learning machinery in most of these children, because they so rapidly learn the same skills at which they have been defined to be deficient. That finding suggests in turn that the physical differences and distributed functional response differences revealed in evoked potential and imaging studies of LLI individuals may substantially be effects of the learning histories of these special children.

In other words, these "learning impaired" children are perfectly capable of learning what they supposedly couldn't learn. Not learning language may have caused the neurological abnormalities, rather than the neurological abnormalities causing the children to not learn language.

What a child learns or doesn't learn can cause changes in his or her brain. The neurological abnormalities in adult stutterers may result from the person having not learned fluent speech motor skills as a child, as opposed to the conventional view that neurological abnormalities cause stuttering.

The article concludes:

> inherited factors contributing to LLI origin may relate to the initiation of a scenario that embeds, through learning, a defective representation of speech phonetics — and does not necessarily mean that these children have irreversible defects in the molecular and cellular elements of the learning machinery of their brains.

In other words, there may be a genetic component to language-learning impairments, but the genes only cause the child to learn to hear speech sounds incorrectly. This then causes the child to have difficulty learning language. If the problem is caught early and the child is trained to hear speech sounds correctly, the child then learns language normally and is cured of the disorder.

Learning speech and language is a long and complex series of steps for a child. If one of the early steps gets off on the wrong track, the child later develops all sorts of other problems. These later problems may not appear to be related to the original problem. In this case, children who appear to have an inability to learn language actually have no such deficit.

The genetic component in LLI appears to be irrelevant, if the disorder is treated early and the child set back on the right path. For more information about this treatment for LLI, contact the Scientific Learning Corporation at http://www.scilearn.com, 417 Montgomery Street Suite 500, San Francisco, CA 94104; (415) 296-1470.

Adult stutterers also have a speech/language learning deficit, although it is different from LLI. Ludlow, Siren and Zikria (1997) found that stutterers had difficulty learning nonsense words such as "abisthwoychleet." The researchers suggest that this may be because children who stutter fail to develop "an efficient speech and language production system." See the subsection "Language Studies" in the chapter "Physical Constitution and Personality of Stutterers." No research has investigated whether children who stutter have this speech/language learning deficit.

Even if there is no speech/language learning deficit in stuttering children, stuttering could develop from an apparently innocuous problem. A 3-year-old tries too hard to talk, overtenses his speech-production muscles, and gets stuck on a word. He pushes harder to get the word, tenses more, and gets more stuck.

This simple behavior, if repeated, grows and adds symptoms over time. The child gets onto a speech development track parallel to, but inferior to, normal speech development. If the child gets a nudge — or later a good shove — back onto the correct track by a well-trained speech pathologist and well-trained parents, he will develop normal fluent speech.

Even if there is a genetic component that causes that original stuttering behavior, early intervention can correct the problem, making the genetic component irrelevant.

But if the child stays on the stuttering track, he develops severe behaviors — including neurological abnormalities — that appear to have little commonalty with the original cause of his stuttering.

Measurement of Stuttering

Measuring stuttering is notoriously difficult. There are several aspects of stuttering you can measure:

• Frequency of disfluencies. I.e., disfluencies per hundred words. The "average" stutterer stutters on 10 percent of words. People who don't stutter have disfluencies on about 2% of words.

• Duration of disfluencies. The "average" disfluency lasts about 1 second.

• Speaking rate, or word per minute. The average speaking rate for people who don't stutter is 167 words per minute, with a range of 129 to 222 words per minute (Darley, 1940).

The average speaking rate for stutterers is 123 words per minute, with a range of 42 to 191 words per minute. The average stutterer speaks about 25% slower than the average non-stutterer.

• There are "stuttering severity scales" in which listeners subjectively rate a person's speech. These are used to categorize stutterers as "mild," "moderate," "severe," etc.

• Types of disfluencies. Wendell Johnson developed eight categories of disfluencies in 1959. The first three are common to both stutterers and non-stutterers. The last five are stuttering disfluencies.

1) Interjections ("uh," "er").
2) Revisions ("I was — I am going").
3) Incomplete phrases.
4) Part-word repetitions ("ba-ba-ba-baseball").
5) Word repetitions.
6) Phrase repetitions ("I was I was going").
7) Broken words ("I was g — (pause) — oing home").
8) Prolonged sounds.

• Psychological effects. Asking the stutterer about fears and anxieties related to speech.

The preferred test questionnaire for measuring stuttering is the "Stuttering Severity Instrument for Children and Adults," 3rd edition, by Glyndon Riley. This covers the above speech parameters. It is available for $79 from Pro-Ed, 8700 Shoal Creek Blvd., Austin, TX 78757-6897, (512) 451-3246.

A study by Young in 1961 found that ordinary listeners judged stuttering to be "severe" when there were part-word repetitions, prolongations, broken words, and a new category, "undue stress or tension." But many speech samples were judged "severe" with relatively few of these disfluencies, suggesting that there are yet more, unidentified types of stuttering disfluencies.

There are many electronic instruments that can measure aspects of stuttering. See "Instrumentation For The Assessment And Treatment Of Stuttering", by Klaas Bakker (1996) and "Automatic Recognition of Dysfluencies" (Howell, 1997).

PROBLEMS WITH MEASURING STUTTERING

1) Differences between judges. Different people listening to the same tape will hear different numbers of disfluencies, even if they are trained speech pathologists.

2) Counting normal disfluencies. Everyone has normal disfluencies. Does having lots of normal disfluencies make a person a stutterer? Or is stuttering something different? Should normal disfluencies be counted as stuttering?

3) Children vs. adults. Children stutter in different ways than adults: some disfluencies are normal for children but are abnormal in adults.

4) Hidden stuttering. Some stutterers can substitute words and appear to never stutter.

5) Speaking conditions. Some stutterers can read out loud perfectly fluently. Others stutter most severely when reading. Some stutterers are most fluent in conversation. Others are most disfluent. Some are most fluent in stressful situations, on telephones, etc., while others are the opposite. You can't judge how severely a person stutters from a single speaking situation.

6) Internal or psychological stuttering is difficult to quantify. For many stutterers the internal effects of stuttering are greater than their physical symptoms. Several stuttering therapies focus on improving the self-esteem and overall communication skills of stutterers, with little or no attention to improving physical fluency.

Additionally, the cost of paying trained speech pathologists to measure the stuttering of a large number of individuals over six months or more can run into several hundred thousand dollars.

Different people stutter in different ways, and each person has multiple ways of stuttering. There is no single behavior common to all stuttering. Be skeptical when anyone claims that a therapy reduced stuttering 85%, etc. Ask how stuttering was measured, under what conditions, etc.

Other Fluency Disorders

The following speech disorders are sometimes confused with developmental stuttering (stuttering that begins in childhood and develops as the child's speech and language develops).

CLUTTERING

A clutterer wrote on an Internet support group:

> Sometimes my mouth just doesn't want to do what it is told, words spurt out, mangled, interchanged syllables. I have tried to get help but it comes and goes and I, remarkably, have much better control when I am in front of strangers and uncomfortable. It's when I am with family that I become completely unintelligible.

Another clutterer wrote on an Internet support group:

> I just seem to rush through the words, and often slur words together and/or mumble — and as a result I often have to slow down, concentrate, and repeat myself.

Cluttering, also called tachyphemia, is defined as (APA, 1987)

> ...a disturbance of fluency involving an abnormally rapid rate and erratic rhythm of speech that impedes intelligibility. Faulty phrasing patterns are usually present so that there are bursts of speech consisting of groups of words that are not related to the grammatical structure of the sentence. The affected person is usually unaware of any communication impairment.

Cluttering usually includes repetitions, usually 6-10 units. Unlike stuttering, these are effortless, usually single syllables, short words, and phrases (stutterers only repeat initial sounds).

Cluttering may also be characterized by poor concentration and short attention span; perceptual weakness; and poorly-organized thinking, or speaking before clarifying thoughts.

Other symptoms include:

• Phonemes (speech sounds) dropped, condensed, or distorted, especially the /r/ and /l/ sounds;

• Grammar problems; and

• Monotone speech, that starts loud and trails off into a murmur.

Some clutterers have jerky respiration; delayed speech or late talking as a child; reading disorders; writing disorders, especially sprawling, disorderly handwriting, which poorly integrate ideas and space; musical inability, e.g., inability to imitate a simple rhythmic pattern; hyperactive, impulsive, careless, fidgety behavior; certain brain wave patterns detectable with an electroencephalograph (EEG); late maturation, clumsiness, uncoordination; and relatives with cluttering.

Stutterers feel as if they think faster than they speak. Clutterers speak fast, before their thoughts are organized.

Clutterers make slips of the tongue, substituting words without realizing their mistakes. David A. Daly writes of observing an adult clutterer make a short business presentation (Daly, 1993):

> …he said "At this plant in time" thinking he had said, "At this point in time." He also substituted…other words…He left the audience confused, and his proposal was [turned down]…More important, he did not receive the promotion he expected. Yet, this executive seemed oblivious to the mistakes he had made.

Kenneth St. Louis and Florence Myers provide the following example of a cluttering child vs. a stuttering child: (St. Louis, 1995)

Clutterer: "I want to go to the st…uh…place where you buy…market st-st-store and I don't have muh-muh ti-ti-time money."

Stutterer: "I want to go to the sssssssssstore and I don't have muh-muh-muh-muh-money."

Clutterers tend to do well in scientific careers. They appear to be of average or above-average intelligence, but not of low intelligence.

Cluttering is a rare disorder. However, many stutterers also clutter. "Pure" cluttering seems to be about 5% of fluency disorders, the majority being stutterers. The rest have symptoms of both stuttering and cluttering. The prevalence has not been established.

The cause of cluttering is unclear. There may a genetic component, but it could be a learning disability. The disorder is believed to be neurological.

Treatment for children who clutter is usually oral-motor coordination. Memory and attention span exercises may also be necessary. Story-telling is often a problem for clutterers, and commercially-available story-telling picture books may be used for practice. Therapy may also involve working on narrative structure in story-telling, emphasizing components such as *who*, *what*, *when*, *where*, and *why*.

Delayed auditory feedback (DAF) is sometimes used to slow down cluttered speech. The device makes cluttered speech more intelligible. DAF produces a more deliberate, exaggerated oral-motor response pattern.

If a DAF device is not available, a speech pathologist can play a "robot speech" game with children, talking in a drawn-out monotone with continuous phonation.

Turn-taking practice between speaker and listener is sometimes useful.

Another technique is pausing. Clutterers have a tendency to talk faster and faster (called "festinating"). Pausing effectively stops this before the clutterer's speech becomes unintelligible.

Getting clutterers to slow down and pause is notoriously difficult. The usual method is to begin with simple lists (e.g., steps to perform a routine task), then increase length and complexity into conversational speech.

Poor awareness of speech problems requires regular use of videotape in therapy. Recently, pocket-sized digital "tape" recorders have become available. A two-memory recorder enables recording the target slow speaking rate (from therapy) in one channel. The clutterer then records 20-seconds of speech into the second channel, and plays the recordings back to compare.

The speech pathologist may also treat the language component of cluttering. One exercise is "telegram," in which the person paraphrases or says only an outline of the message essentials.

Role-playing may be done, such as giving directions, or a job interview.

"Maze" speech, e.g., false starts and revisions, may be treated by making written transcriptions of the person's speech. The clutterer then "cleans up" the writing. Then the clutterer says the "cleaned up" message.

Childhood cluttering treatment should involve family members, because the clutterer may be unaware of symptoms.

Adult clutterers can be indifferent, belligerent, hostile, or even verbally abusive to speech pathologists.

Treatment for cluttering usually takes longer than stuttering treatment.

The September-December 1996 issue of the *Journal of Fluency Disorders* (*21*:3/4) has 21 articles about cluttering.

NEUROGENIC STUTTERING

Strokes and head injuries can cause stuttering-like symptoms in adults. Neurogenic stuttering has repetitions, prolongations, and blocks. However, these sound different from developmental stuttering (Helm-Estabrooks, 1993).

Neurogenic stutterers lack the facial grimaces, eye blinking, and fears and anxieties of developmental stuttering.

In some cases a person stuttered as a child or young adult, overcame stuttering, then had a stroke or head injury, and stuttering came back. For example, a successful high-tech executive stuttered as a young man but overcame stuttering. He then had a stroke in his early 40s, recovered from the stroke and soon was back to his full life, but his speech continued to be almost incomprehensible for years. He has now become a private pilot, even though his speech is poor.

In other cases, Alzheimer's and dementia bring back childhood stuttering.

On the other hand, there are a few cases of development stuttering disappearing after neurosurgery for brain tumors, and even after the development of multiple sclerosis. These appear to relate to changes in brain lateralism.

Neurogenic stuttering appears to result from damage to the pyramidal, extrapyramidal, corticobulbar, and cerebellar motor systems.

Assessment of neurogenic stuttering has six steps:

1) A complete case history, noting not only brain injuries but also all traumatic events, both physical and emotional, drug use, and other diseases, especially neurological diseases.

2) Testing whether the person also has aphasia (inability to find words).

3) Determining if the person only stutters on certain word classes, such as functional words (the, and, but) vs. substantive, informational words. Developmental stuttering occurs only on informational words. Neurogenic stutterers will stutter on all classes of words.

4) Test the "adaptation effect." In developmental stuttering, if the stutterer reads something over and over again, he will stutter less and less each time. Neurogenic stutterers are less likely to do this.

5) Check for disfluencies in "automated" speech tasks, such as saying the "Pledge of Allegiance," or counting to thirty. Developmental stutterers can do this relatively fluently. Neurogenic stutterers can't.

6) Distinguishing neurogenic stuttering from "palilalia," which is the repetition of whole words or phrases.

Neurogenic stuttering has been treated in a variety of ways:

- Brain surgery. Blood flow to a restricted hemisphere is improved.

• Drugs, such as anti-seizure medications. A variety of other drugs have also been used.

• In one case, a battery-powered electrode stimulator was implanted into a man's left centromedial thalamic nucleus, which improved fluency and reduced pain.

• In another case, a transcutaneous nerve stimulator in a woman's left arm reduced disfluencies.

• Delayed auditory feedback (DAF) and masking auditory feedback (MAF) help some patients.

• Electromyographic biofeedback helped one patient relax his speech-production muscles to talk more fluently.

• A "pacing board" is a low-tech way to help some patients. This is a board with six multi-colored squares. The patient taps her finger in each square as she says each syllable.

The wide variety of treatments shows that neurogenic stuttering is not one disorder, but is a symptom of a variety of neurological disorders. Because neurogenic stuttering varies from case to case, outcomes can't be predicted.

Parkinson's disease is not usually associated with stuttering. However, in some cases it can result in severe blocks, repetitions and prolongations. The preferred treatment for Parkinson's speech maximizes respiration and increases vocal fold adduction. The idea is to use a loud, good quality voice with sustained phonation. One exercise is to verbalize 10 to 12 "ah" sounds as long and as loud as possible. The exercise is done daily (Ramig, 1996).

PSYCHOGENIC STUTTERING

Adult psychogenic stuttering begins suddenly after an event causing extreme psychological stress. It's characterized by sudden onset; repetition of initial or stressed syllables, lack of conditions inducing fluency (including choral reading, delayed auditory feedback, and singing); no fluent speech, even for automatic responses; an indifferent attitude toward stuttering; and no secondary symptoms, e.g., avoidances, breaking eye contact.

Psychogenic stuttering is rare — less than two dozen cases have been reported. Cases include (Mahr, 1992):

•A truck driver was slowly crushed against his truck when another truck backed up. He recovered normal speech in 9 months of stuttering therapy, and his speech has been normal since.

• A "morbidly obese" assembly line worker was treated surgically under local anesthesia, and during the operation started screaming that the anesthesia had worn off. After the surgery her speech was "mildly disfluent," but within five months worsened into severe stuttering. "...psychological testing indicated a severe degree of psychopathology." 2.5 years of stuttering therapy did not affect her speech.

• A "32-year-old employed female executive" was admitted to a psychiatric institution for "an acute manic episode with psychosis." Psychiatric treatment went well, but brought out repressed memories of sexual abuse. As these memories emerged she started stuttering, from mild to severe in three weeks. As therapy continued over several weeks, her speech returned to normal.

I personally know only one case of psychogenic stuttering, a 35-year-old African-American woman. Her only stuttering symptom was rapidly-repeated initial sounds, 30 or 40 times. But she had no excessive muscle tension (I even connected her to an electromyograph, which showed relaxed muscles). She had no prolongations or hard blocks. She had no secondary symptoms, and never broke eye contact.

She said that she never stuttered until her last semester of college (although she refused to ask her parents if she stuttered as a child). She tried several treatment programs, with only temporary success. She tried one of my delayed auditory feedback (DAF) devices for twenty minutes, and was fluent for a week (this success is unheard of). She bought the device, but a year later it had no effect on her speech.

She complained about her job, was unmarried, and complained about dating problems. She was angry, and argued about racism on any pretext. I suspect that she had a psychological conflict. On the one hand, she was intelligent, attractive, hard-working, well-educated, and a devout Christian. She should have been successful in anything she wanted. On the other hand, she believed she would never be successful. For example, she often used "the n-word" and "slave girl" in reference to herself. When she was on the brink of success — graduating from college and starting a career — she developed a disability that helped her to fail.

SPASTIC DYSPHONIA

Spastic dysphonia is similar to stuttering, except that it is a repeated blockage of the larynx only, the onset is in middle age, and the disorder affects an equal number of men and women.

Speech pathologists are undecided over whether the vocal

"spasms" of spastic dysphonia are caused by a neurological disorder. Botulinum toxin is the only treatment that seems to help.

There are five types of spastic dysphonia. The most common are adductive (treatable with botulinum toxin), or abductor (less treatable with botulinum toxin, but responds to voice therapy better). People often have incipient spastic dysphonia for years without it really becoming noticeable. For more information, contact: Dystonia Medical Research Foundation, One East Wacker Drive, Chicago, IL 60601-2098, (312) 321-5710 FAX; National Spasmodic Dysphonia Association (NSDA), PO Box 1574, Birmingham, MI 48009-1574, (313) 645-9352 FAX; or *Our Voice*, 156 Fifth Ave., Suite 1033, NY, NY 10010-7002.

TOURETTE'S SYNDROME

Tourette's Syndrome is not a fluency disorder, but is similar to stuttering in many ways.

Tourette's is an obsessive-compulsive disorder. Abnormal breathing patterns are a common symptom. Touretters impulsively touch objects (e.g., the floor or walls) or people. About 20% of Touretters have verbal symptoms, such as impulsively barking animal noises, and saying obscenities. They can obsessively practice something over and over until they do it perfectly. They can have high levels of physical energy or hyperactivity.

Like stuttering, Tourettec "tics" or behaviors are embarrassing, but the more a Touretter tries not to do the behavior, the more he or she is compelled to do it. Touretters usually can substitute more acceptable tics and control the disorder. They enjoy support groups, where they can "let go" and do tics without worrying about social acceptability.

Like stuttering, Tourette's can be "switched off" for tic-free periods. For example, a New York actress never has tics on stage. Neurologist Oliver Sacks wrote about a surgeon with Tourette's in *An Anthropologist on Mars.* The surgeon's behaviors were wild everywhere but the operating room. During an operation he concentrates so completely that he has no tics. Similarly, stutterers experience fluent periods when acting or concentrating on something other than their speech.

Tourette's is related to abnormally high dopamine levels in some part of the brain. Some researchers believe that stuttering is caused by abnormally high dopamine levels in another part of the brain (see the chapter "Neurology and Drug Treatment for Stuttering"). Three genes have been associated with Tourette's.

The most effective drug for treating Tourette's — haloperidol, or Haldol — is also effective for reducing stuttering.

There appears to be a subgroup of Touretters who stutter, and stutterers with Tourette's (see the subsection on genetics in the chapter "Incidence and Prevalence of Stuttering"). If you think you have Tourette's, you should see a neurologist. The prevalence of Tourette's is about 0.05%.

Researchers at Johns Hopkins University suspect that Tourette's may be triggered by streptococcal or another childhood infection. The child's immune system may attack brain nerve cells in the putamen, an area of the brain that controls movement (ADVANCE For Speech-Language Pathologists, July 6, 1998, page 22).

The Tourette's Syndrome national support organization can be contacted at (800) 237-0717. They have a great videotape, called "Twitch & Shout," which my National Stuttering Project chapter enjoyed watching.

SOCIAL PHOBIA

People with social phobia experience anxiety and panic when going to parties, meeting strangers, performing public speaking, or even in minor social situations with a dentist or store clerk. The disorder has been distinguished from shyness, anxiety, and depression. The main symptoms include palpitations, trembling, and sweating. Less common symptoms include stuttering. Social phobia is sometimes treated with the anti-depressant drug moclobemide. In some cases Prozac-type drugs are used, or the older monoamine oxidase inhibitors.

One college student described his experiences with social phobia:

> My problem is that I have an extreme aversion to speaking. It's gotten to the point where I can barely even speak my name without having a horrible feeling completely overwhelm me. I'm seriously beginning to consider voluntary mutism because I just can't handle talking anymore. This aversion manifests itself both physically and mentally. I'm not sure how much of it is psychological and how much is biological. All I know is that it is ruining my life.
>
> The mere act of communicating orally with anyone (including close family members) has become a terrible chore for me. My voice tenses up and becomes all weak and unsteady. I run out of breath very easily when talking and by the end of a normal day, I'm completely exhausted

from the whole ordeal.

The worst part about this whole mess is that I naturally have a very talkative personality. I love to communicate with people and I feel as though this stupid problem I have with the physical process of speaking has turned me into someone I'm not. I end up getting so frustrated with it that I've actually turned into somewhat of a cranky, unpersonable person. I find myself getting angry at people who insist on talking to me even if their intentions are friendly, and I'm sure that the vibes I give off to the outside world say "stay away." I really don't want to be like this, but it's only a natural reaction to my situation.

A psychotherapy clinic can help you if you have social phobia.

There are other speech disorders, and support groups and therapy programs. For more information, call the American Speech-Language Hearing Association (ASHA) at (301) 897-5700, or write to 10801 Rockville Pike, Rockville, MD 20852. There are also many World Wide Web sites devoted to various speech disorders.

Conclusion — Nature And Origin Of Stuttering

The "Science" section began with the question "What causes stuttering?" The answer is, "A lot of things." Stuttering is a multifactorial disorder. At least five factors contribute to the development of stuttering:

Genetics. Comings, D., et al. (1996) found three genes that correlate with stuttering. These genes control levels of the neurotransmitter dopamine in the brain. Riley, Wu, and Maguire (1997) proposed that stuttering is caused by excessive dopamine in the left caudate nucleus speech motor control area.

But the three genes also correlated with ADHD, Tourette's Syndrome and obsessive-compulsive disorder. Why do some people with these genes develop Tourette's, but others develop stuttering? Why do some people with these genes not develop any of these disorders?

Triggers. Many children suddenly start stuttering severely, almost overnight. A *triggering event* may cause a child with these genes to develop one of these disorders.

Recent research has found such a trigger for Tourette's Syndrome (Singer, 1998). Children with sudden and severe onset of Tourette's were found to have recently had streptococcal infections. The children had antineuronal antibodies, which suggested that the child's immune system attacked his or her brain's putamen motor control area. The damage to the brain resulted in the sudden onset of Tourette's (see the chapter "Other Fluency Disorders").

It's possible that a similar autoimmune disorder could damage a child's caudate nucleus. But some healthy children start stuttering overnight.

Other stutterers report a psychological trauma as the triggering event. See the section "Childhood Trauma and Conditioning" in the chapter "Theories of Stuttering Development."

Vicious cycles and stimulus-response conditioning. Other children develop stuttering gradually, seemingly from normal disfluencies. If a child gets stuck on a word, and pushes harder to get the word out, the child will get more stuck. The child tenses his or her speech-production muscles. The child can get into a vicious cycle, making stuttering worse.

The child is most likely to get into this vicious cycle in situations where he or she most wants to speak well. This conditions the child to stutter when experiencing time pressure, when speaking to authority figures, etc.

In the past, the stimulus-response conditioning of the parents' reaction to the child's stuttering was believed to be the cause of stuttering. This theory is no longer popular, but the learned behaviors of *when* to stutter should be a focus of stuttering therapy, in addition to retraining *how* the individual stutters.

Neurological hardwiring. The way a child speaks becomes hardwired during the years that his or her brain is growing. The child's accent, grammar, and fluency become permanent neurological pathways. As the child's brain stops growing at puberty, these behaviors become increasingly resistant to change.

The development of speech and language is a long road, with many steps. A small misstep in early childhood can send a child onto the wrong track, and over time the problem compounds until it is a severe disability. See the section on language learning impairment (LLI) in the chapter "Theories of Stuttering Development."

Psychological factors. As stuttering develops, the child may develop fears, anxieties, and avoidances. These psychological factors were once seen as the cause of stuttering, but are now seen as an effect of stuttering. However, by adulthood these psychological effects can be more disabling than the physical stuttering.

Children learn many ways to speak — loud or quiet, fast or slow, questions or statements, etc. They learn *how* to speak in certain ways, and they learn *when* to use each type of speech. A child who stutters learns both fluent speech motor skills and stuttering motor skills — and learns in which situations to use each.

STUTTERING IS A DEVELOPMENTAL MALADAPTIVE MOTOR SKILL

Stuttering is a *developmental maladaptive motor skill.* The child learns how to speak, but it's not the right or best way to speak. Certain cues recall his stuttering motor skills — e.g., time pressure, or speaking to authority figures. Other cues recall his fluent speech motor skills — e.g., talking to pets or friends.

Whatever pattern of activity is practiced is the pattern that will be

> developed...volitional excitement [the stimulus of making choices or decisions] causes that pattern to occur in the manner in which it has been practiced. (Kottke *et al.* 1978, p.569)

Stuttering varies between individuals. For example, the *how to stutter* motor skill can tense any of one hundred speech muscles. The muscle movements may result in silent blocks, misarticulation, or prolongations and repetitions. Motor skills also involve emotional learning, and the stutterer experiences anxiety and panic during stuttering.

The *when to stutter* learning explains why stuttering occurs intermittently. Stuttering is a psychologically-conditioned choice of speech parameterization schema in response to environmental cues. In other words, different cues (e.g., time pressure, speaking to authority figures, or talking to friends or a pet) make you speak in different ways. Some cues make you stutter, and others make you fluent. These cues were learned, and this learning varies between individuals. For example, some stutterers stutter when reading out loud, when others are fluent when reading out loud.

This is analogous to typing with two fingers. I was never trained to touch-type, and I now type 45 words per minute with two fingers. I can type, and stutterers can speak. But I would type faster (and with fewer mistakes) if I had learned to touch-type at an early age. I have tried to learn touch-typing several times as an adult, but found it so slow that I gave up before becoming good at it.

Similarly, adult stutterers must start slowly when learning therapy techniques. Many give up and go back to using their old stuttering motor skills.

The chapter "Is Slow, Relaxed Speech a Means or an End?" presents research showing that the adaptation effect, which reduces stuttering about 70%, results from motor learning.

CHILDHOOD STUTTERING THERAPY

Childhood Stuttering Diagnosis and Treatment (2-6 years old)

Stuttering is a common childhood disorder, but poorly-understood by parents and physicians. Early diagnosis and treatment is likely to result in complete recovery. But leaving stuttering untreated can result in a lifelong disability.

Stuttering develops between the ages 2 and 6. The median age of stuttering onset is 30 months (Yairi, 1992).

Stuttering is the only communication disorder in which the child develops normal, fluent speech, and then loses it. Other speech and language disorders emerge when normal development fails to occur.

Speech and language are the most complex and difficult skills children learn. Most, if not all, children have problems with speech or language at some point. Parents should know how to differentiate normal childhood disfluencies from stuttering. Normal childhood disfluencies and stuttering are only slightly different at first, but as the child goes further on the wrong track, his stuttering develops in severity and becomes resistant to treatment.

65% of preschoolers who stutter spontaneously recover, in their first 2 years of stuttering (Yairi, 1993; Yairi and Ambrose, 1992). Finn (1997b) found that preschool and early-stage school-age children who recover from stuttering without therapy have speech indistinguishable from children who never stuttered.

However, children who stutter longer are less likely to recover without treatment. Only 18% for children who stutter 5 years recover spontaneously (Andrews, 1983).

The peak age of recovery is 3.5 years old. By age 6, the child is unlikely to recover without speech therapy. The earlier a child's stuttering is diagnosed and treated by a speech pathologist, the more likely the child is to outgrow stuttering.

If your child stutters, federal law requires that your school district provide speech therapy to your child. Your child can be as young as three years old — he or she doesn't have to be in school.

Stuttering develops in stages, but children do not always advance from one stage through the next — some children go from normal fluent speech one day into Stage 3 (beginning stuttering) or even Stage 4 the next day.

STAGE ONE: NORMAL DISFLUENCY (AGES 2-6)

Normal disfluencies tend to be single, such as "That my-my ball," or "I want some…uh…juice."

Normal disfluencies tend to be interjections (sounds or syllables), revisions (of words, phrases, sentences, or story), and whole-word repetitions (not part-word repetitions).

The child does not manifest struggle behaviors or visible tension, frustration or embarrassment. The child experiences disfluencies as if he stumbled while walking, and recovered his balance and continued walking.

Normal disfluencies occur when the child is planning a long or complex language structure. Brief silent pauses are considered normal. Normal disfluencies also occur under "pragmatic" conditions, such as when directing another person's activity, when concerned about the listener's reaction, and when interrupting or being interrupted.

Normal disfluencies may occur when the child's language skills exceed his speech motor skills. Or he may be so busy learning to walk or refine other motor skills that his speech skills don't develop rapidly enough.

Changes in the child's environment may also cause temporary normal disfluencies. This could involve parents' divorce, the birth of a sibling, or moving to a new home.

STAGE TWO: BORDERLINE STUTTERING (AGES 2-6)

The symptoms of borderline stuttering are:

1) Disfluency on more than 10% of words.

2) More than two disfluencies together ("That my-my-my ball").

3) More repetitions and prolongations, and fewer revisions or incomplete phrases.

4) No struggle behavior or fear of stuttering.

STAGE THREE: BEGINNING STUTTERING (AGES 2-6)

The symptoms of beginning stuttering are:

1) Part-word repetitions (not whole-word repetitions). Repetitions become rapid, tense, and irregular. A sound or word is repeated three or more times.

2) The child substitutes the neutral or schwa vowel ("uh") instead of the appropriate vowel (e.g., "luh-luh-luh-like").

3) Disfluency on more than 10% of words.

4) The child stutters for weeks or months, between periods of fluency. Stuttering for more than six months is a danger sign.

5) Stuttering when excited or upset, when having a great deal to say, or under high environmental demands.

6) Prolongations. Sounds are prolonged at least a half-second. Fixed articulatory postures occur (freezing of speech-production muscles).

7) Struggle and speech-production muscle tension, such as a rise in vocal pitch (caused by tensing the larynx), blocking airflow and stopping phonation, wide mouth opening or tongue protrusion, or irregular breathing patterns.

8) Stuttering only on the first word of a sentence or phrase.

9) Stuttering on both content and function words ("like," "but," "and," or "so").

10) Secondary or escape behaviors, such as eye blinking, nodding, facial grimacing, quivering lip, raising eye brows, flaring nostrils.

11) Frustration at being unable to get words out, but no fear or embarrassment about stuttering.

STAGE FOUR:
INTERMEDIATE STUTTERING (AGES 6-13)

1) Fear or avoidance of certain sounds or words. Word substitution begins.

2) Blocks become common, in addition to repetitions and prolongations.

3) Escape behaviors.

4) Stuttering becomes chronic, without periods of fluency.

5) Stuttering occurs on content words — major nouns, verbs, and adjectives.

6) Stuttering varies between situations, such as talking on the telephone, speaking to strangers, or when excited.

STAGE FIVE:
ADVANCED STUTTERING (AGES 14 - ADULT)

1) Vivid, fearful anticipation of stuttering.

2) Feared words, sounds, and situations.

3) Thinks of himself as a stutterer. Chooses his friends, social activities, and jobs to avoid talking.

4) Advanced stutterers may develop substitution and avoidance behaviors so well that you never know that they stutter.

ASSESSMENT OF BEGINNING STUTTERING

When a speech pathologist diagnoses a preschool child who is stuttering, she may:

1) Interview the parents. How do the parents talk about the child's stuttering? Is stuttering the main issue, or just one item in a list of behavioral, social, and emotional problems?

Were there problems in pregnancy or birth? Ask about development of the child's speech and language, and the child's motor development. Look for evidence of uneven development.

Does the child have problems sleeping, eating, or behavior problems such as temper tantrums? Ask about the child's personality, temperament, and interaction with other children.

Do other family members have speech or language disorders?

When were the child's first disfluencies noticed? Was anything unusual going on in the child's life at the time? Sometimes stuttering is tied to a traumatic event, often not.

Is the child is aware of or frustrated by his or her disfluencies? Ask about word substitutions or avoidance behaviors. What have the parents done about the child's speech?

2) Observe or make a videotape or audio tape of the parent playing with the child. She may ask the child questions about his or her siblings, likes and dislikes, etc. Sometimes a child won't talk to a speech pathologist. Other children are fluent with the speech pathologist.

3) Don't say anything about stuttering, but instead ask the child about "getting stuck on words." The speech pathologist evaluates how aware the child is of stuttering, how frustrated the child becomes, and whether the child is doing anything to get words out.

4) Note the child's stuttering symptoms, and measure the child's stuttering using the parameters described above in the chapter "Measurement of Stuttering."

5) Assess other speech or language disorders, and the child's overall speech and language development. If the child also has a language disorder, see the article, "Treating the Child Who Stutters With Concomitant Language or Phonological Impairment," by Nan Bernstein Ratner, *Language, Speech, and Hearing Services in*

Schools, Vol. 26, April 1995.

6) Assess any other factors, such as physical, cognitive, and social or emotional development.

The speech pathologist then assesses whether the child is normal, borderline, beginning stuttering, or more advanced.

Woodruff Starkweather suggests (Gottwald, 1995) evaluating the parents'

> ...fluency levels, rate of speech, and language characteristics...the number of open questions the adult asks, the verbal and nonverbal ways the adult responds to the child's stuttering, the number of topics the adult initiates, the frequency of negative comments the adult makes; the number of times the adult interrupts the child...

Starkweather suggests that the speech pathologist videotape interaction between the parent and child. He suggests that by watching the videotape, the parents may realize that the child has large numbers of fluent utterances, which will make the parent less anxious. Starkweather adds, "Parents have been amazed to realize that they physically froze, turned away, or closed their eyes each time their child stuttered." He also suggests that the speech pathologists help the parents talk to the child about stuttering in a way that reduces anxiety.

RECOMMENDED BOOKS AND VIDEOS

The Stuttering Foundation of America has published a variety of books and videos for parents, teachers, pediatricians, and speech pathologists that treat children. Prices are usually between one and five dollars. The SFA can be reached at (800) 992-9392, www.stutterSFA.org, or P.O. Box 11749, Memphis, TN 38111-0749.

See also the April 1995 issue of *Language, Speech and Hearing Service in Schools*. The issue is devoted to childhood fluency disorders, with eight articles on stuttering and one article on cluttering. Your school's speech pathologist may have a copy, or your university library.

Parents may want to join the e-mail discussion group about childhood stuttering. To subscribe, send the command "subscribe parents-w" (without the quotes) to majordomo@f-body.org. Post articles to parents-w@f-body.org. The list owner is Larry Burd, Larry_Burd@compuserve.com.

TREATMENT OF CHILDHOOD STUTTERING

There are two main approaches to treating childhood stuttering. The first — *indirect therapy* — focuses on changing the parents' speech or behavior. The second — *direct therapy* — focuses on improving the child's speech.

A study of 33 preschoolers who stutter found that 91% remained fluent after completing a therapy program with a speech pathologist. No control group was used (Fosnot, 1993).

Another study of preschoolers found that "near-zero stuttering levels were achieved post-treatment and were maintained in the long-term [2 to 7 years]" (Lincoln, 1997).

A study of fifteen 6-to-8-year-olds found that a 40-hour therapy program was successful for all the children. The children maintained their fluency over the next 18 months (Druce, 1997). The program was similar to "GILCU" (gradual increase in length and complexity of [fluent] utterances) programs.

INDIRECT THERAPY

Indirect therapy encourages parents to:

1) Refrain from criticizing the child's speech, or correcting, helping, or reacting negatively to the child's speech.

2) Be less demanding, restrictive, or perfectionistic.

3) Reduce situations in which the child is fatigued, excited, or expected to speak under pressure. Don't ask the child to confess guilt. Stick to a predictable daily routine.

4) Be a good listener. Put down what you're doing when the child wants to talk. Don't interrupt.

5) Parents should not talk too fast or use advanced vocabulary.

6) Wait two seconds after the child finishes speaking before answering the child.

7) Encourage fluent speech by speaking in chorus with the child (e.g., reading Dr. Seuss books out loud together), singing, rhythmic speech, or puppets.

8) Don't say "Slow down," "Take a deep breath" or "Think

about what you are going to say."

9) Praise your child, and let your child know how much you enjoy playing or talking with her/him, giving lots of positive nonverbal messages, like smiles and hugs.

While the above suggestions can't hurt, a literature review (Nippold & Rudzinski, 1995) found that indirect therapy (changing parents' behavior) doesn't do much. They found

> ...little convincing evidence...that parents of children who stutter differ from parents of children who do not stutter in the way they talk with their children. Similarly, there is little objective support...that parents' speech behaviors contribute to children's stuttering or that modifying parents' speech behaviors facilitates children's fluency.

Nippold and Rudzinski caution against only changing the parents' speech, and not directly working on the child's speech. They believe that "...direct intervention should begin with the onset of stuttering..."

More generally, psychologists now discount the role of parents in the development of children's character and personality. About 50% of the personality differences are attributable to our genes, and the rest due to the child's peers: "...what parents *do* seems to be nearly irrelevant" (Gladwell, 1998).

The evidence against altering parental behavior to change children's speech includes:

• Meyers and Freeman (1985a) compared boys who stuttered and their mothers to boys who don't stutter and their mothers. The researchers looked at positive statements (praise, encouragement, agreement), negative statements (criticism, reprimands), questions, topic initiations and terminations, etc. They found that "...it did not appear that children who stuttered and children who did not stutter were being treated in a way that was markedly different..."

• Meyers and Freeman (1985b) looked at interruptions, in the above data. "Results showed that there was no statistically significant differences between the two groups...It is also noteworthy that, when mothers interrupted, they did so *after* the child had begin to speak disfluently. a pattern which is *not* consistent with the view that parental interruptions cause a child to stutter."

• Meyers and Freeman (1985c) looked again at their data, comparing the mothers' speaking rate. "They found that mothers of children who stuttered talked faster to [both stuttering and non-stuttering] children than mothers of children who did not stutter…the children who stuttered spoke more slowly during fluent speech than the children who did not stutter…the faster the mother spoke, the slower the child spoke." This suggest that parents of children who stutter should talk faster to make their children talk slower — the opposite of what many speech pathologists tell parents! People get impatient and talk faster around stutterers. The child's slow speech may cause the parents to talk faster.

• Meyers (1986) looked at whether children who stutter and children who don't stutter spoke differently with an unfamiliar mother of a stutterer, an unfamiliar mother of a non-stutterer, and his or her own mother. No differences in stuttering were found. This suggests that parents of children who stutter do not make their children or anyone else's children stutter.

• Langlois et al. (1986) found that mothers of children who stutter use more questions and commands. Mothers of children who don't stutter use more statements. The researchers suggested that questions and commands might increase "communicative pressure" on children and cause stuttering.

• Stephenson-Opsal and Bernstein Ratner (1988) trained two sets of parents to slow their speaking rates. In both cases, their child stuttered less. However, the child's speaking rate increased.

• "Meyers (1990) reported that mothers and fathers both produced significantly more positive statements (e.g., praise, encouragement) and fewer negative statements (e.g. criticisms, disparaging remarks) than peers when talking with the child who stuttered." This could leads to the strange conclusion that parents' praise and encouragement causes children to stutter.

• Weiss and Zebrowski (1991) looked at conversational assertiveness and responsiveness. "…parents of children who stuttered did not differ significantly from parents of children who did not stutter…"

• Kelly and Conture (1992) looked at "response time latency" (RTL), which is the time between one person finishing speaking, and the other person beginning speaking. There were "…no significant differences between mothers of children who stuttered and mothers of children who did not stutter in number of interruptions, speech rate, or RTL."

• Kelly (1994) studied the same items, but with fathers instead of mothers, and "…no significant differences were found…"

• Winslow and Guitar (1994) studied one 5-year-old boy who stuttered, his 10-year-old brother, and their parents. "…at the dinner table, each boy was given a wooden block to hold, and was required to raise the block whenever he wished to speak. The boys were expected to wait until another speaker had finished...instances of appropriate turn-taking behavior were praised (e.g., 'Good job waiting)." After seven weeks, the boy's stuttering was reduced by about half.

• Yaruss and Conture (1995) found "No significant differences... between [stuttering and non-stuttering] groups in either mothers' or children's speaking rates or utterance lengths or in children's response time latencies, nor were any significant relationships found among these variables."

• Kloth, et al., (1995) conducted a multiyear study of 93 mothers of preschool children. At the start, none of the children stuttered. One year later, 26 of the children stuttered. The researchers compared the speech behaviors of the two groups of mothers, before their children started stuttering. No differences were found, except that mothers of children who would stutter had shorter, less complex utterances (the opposite of the capacities and demands model). "These findings suggest that the communicative behavior of mother of normally fluent children do not contribute to the development of stuttering."

• Howell, Kapoor and Rustin (1997) compared children's stuttering when interviewers spoke in a "formal" style vs. a "casual" style. The formal style had greater intensity, longer vowel durations, and differences between voiced and voiceless plosives were longer (i.e., the formal style was louder, slower, and clearer). No difference was seen in the children's stuttering.

• Rommel, *et al.* (1997) found that "illocution of the parents' utterances has no effect" on children's stuttering.

• Yaruss (1997) found that when children who stutter produce utterances faster, they are not more likely to stutter. He found that shorter response time latency did not correlate with increased stuttering.

Nippold and Rudzinski did not say that parents shouldn't be involved in the child's speech therapy. Research has shown the stuttering therapies administered by trained parents are more effective than therapy with a speech pathologist (Craig, 1996). Parents should administer the stuttering therapy, if they have been trained by a qualified speech pathologist. Nippold and Rudzinski's conclusion is that the focus of therapy should be changing the child's behavior, not on changing the parents' behavior.

DIRECT THERAPY

Speech pathologists increasingly advocate direct intervention to change the child's speech. Direct therapy is similar to adult stuttering therapy, in that it can teach *fluency shaping* techniques, or can integrate *stuttering modification* principles.

Fluency shaping skills teach the child to speak fluently. These skills include "easy speech" (also called "turtle talk") and stretching vowels. Fluency shaping therapy progresses from sounds to words and sentences, from a slow speaking rate to a normal speaking rate, and from the low-stress speech clinic to real-life conversations.

Stuttering modification is necessary when a child exhibits negative feelings or frustration in response to stuttering. In past decades, speech pathologists assumed that children never experience such frustration, but rather it was parents who expressed negative feelings about a child's speech. Parents were told to ignore their child's difficulties, instead of comforting the child.

Mary Wallace and Patty Walton give an example of a child's frustration and the clinician's response, in their book *Fun With Fluency: Direct Therapy With The Young Child* (Imaginart, 1998):

> Caitlyn, a four-year-old female who began to stutter in the midst of her parents divorce, was exhibiting significant struggle and tension behavior as well as secondary behaviors. Of most concern was her head-banging behavior during difficult moments of stuttering. After many sessions in which I attempted to eliminate this behavior through fluency-shaping principles, I saw no change. One day, shortly after Caitlyn banged her forehead on the table to interrupt a block, I modeled the same behavior. Caitlyn was shocked and ignored me. After I did this several times she asked me, "Why did you do that? Didn't that hurt?" I responded, "I don't know why I did it. But it sure didn't help me get my word out!" Caitlyn never again banged her head to help her talk. She has been out of therapy for six years and remains fluent.

Fun With Fluency is written for treating children ages 2.5 to 7 years old. Chapters include:

• "Is The Child Really Stuttering?" Normal disfluency vs. stuttering, the danger signs of stuttering, and stages of stuttering development.

• "The Movement From Indirect Toward Direct Therapy." When to use indirect and direct therapy methods.

• "The *Fun With Fluency* Direct Therapy Approach." Easy speech, easy bounces, self-corrections; contrasting to hard speech and pushing; following a hierarchy from simple words through sentences to storytelling; drawing the Speech Monster.

• "Issues Surrounding Progress, Transfer and Maintenance." Assessing progress, managing regression, counter-conditioning fluency disruptions, transfer outside the speech clinic.

• "Counseling Parents and Teachers." Involving parents and teachers in the therapy process.

• "Therapy Activities." Games from picture naming to Mr. Potato Head, sequence stories to "search and find" pictures.

Other speech pathologists use the following strategies and games for direct stuttering therapy:

• "Solo play." The speech pathologist has two boxes of toys, one for the child, the other for herself. At first, they silently play with their toys. Gradually, the speech pathologist starts, making car or animal noises as she plays. Then she adds single words. Then her toys start bumping into the child's toys, and they interact for short periods. Eventually she uses short phrases and sentences. This places no speaking demands on the child. The goal is to let the child verbalize little by little, as he or she feels like talking.

• "Turtle talk." The speech pathologist has a turtle hand puppet walk slowly when the child uses slow, relaxed speech. When the child uses fast, tense speech, the turtle stops and crawls into his shell. The child has to use slow, relaxed speech to ask the turtle to come out of his shell. If you don't have a turtle hand puppet, you can have a car slowly drive along a table, avoiding obstacles.

• "Say The Magic Word." The child tells the parents what he or she sees in a picture book or when looking out the window. When the child says the "magic word," the parent rings a bell or gives the child a peanut. No particular word is magic — the child is rewarded for fluent words.

• "Can't catch me." Each person gets a peanut when the other person asks a question. You then quietly eat your peanut before answering the question. If you answer the question before eating your peanut, you must put your peanut back. The parent should lose more peanuts than the child, by answering too quickly. This reduces the time pressure the child feels about quickly answering questions.

• "Response contingent stimulation" has the parent praise or reward the child for fluent speech, identify disfluencies and ask the child to correct the word. After a disfluency, the parent has the child "time out" or pause for 5 seconds (Onslow, 1992, 1994, 1997).

• "Restimulation." After the child has a frustrating disfluency, the parent casually reflects or paraphrases the child. This reduces the child's embarrassment of stuttering.

School-Age Stuttering (7-12 years old)

EFFECTIVENESS OF THERAPIES

An Australian study of 98 children, 9 to 14 years old, compared three types of stuttering therapy. (Craig, 1996) The three types of therapy were:

1) Intensive smooth speech. This trained relaxed, diaphragmatic breathing; a slow speaking rate with prolonged vowels; gentle onsets and offsets (loudness contour); soft articulation contacts; and pauses between phrases. The intensive program started with five hours of training in a speech clinic, followed by one week of six-hour therapy days (35 hours total).

2) Home-based smooth speech. This was similar to the first group, but parents were included, and encouraged to "take the role of clinician for their child." Therapy was done in a speech clinic, in a series of four weeks, once a week for six hours (24 hours total). Parents were required to "record details of the treatment regime carried out at home so that the clinician could appraise parental activities."

3) Electromyographic biofeedback. The children used an EMG biofeedback computer system about six hours a day for one week. The EMG system monitored the child's speech-production muscle activity. The children were instructed to tense and then relax their speech-production muscles, and so develop awareness and control of these muscles. The children then worked through a hierarchy from simple words to conversations, while keeping their speech-production muscles relaxed. After mastering this while watching the computer display, the children had to do the exercises with the computer monitoring but not displaying their muscle activity. The speech pathologists did relatively little with the children: "Constant clinician presence was not necessary as the computer provided feedback as to whether the child was performing the skills correctly."

A fourth (control) group did not receive any stuttering therapy.

At the end of each therapy program, all three therapies reduced stuttering below 1% on average.

One year after the therapy program, the percentage of children with disfluency rates under 2% were:

- 48% of the children from the "intensive" clinician-based program.
- 63% of the children from the "parent-based" program.
- 71% of the children from the EMG computer-based program.

In other words, the computers were most effective, the parents next-most effective, and the speech pathologists were least effective in producing long term fluency. The control group had no improvement in fluency.

The results for children with disfluency rates under 1% were even more striking:

- 10% of the children from the "intensive" clinician-based program.
- 37% of the children from the "parent-based" program.
- 44% of the children from the EMG computer-based program.

The follow-up was done in the speech clinic, on telephone calls, and at home. The average rate of stuttering increased from 1% to 3%, but speech naturalness improved. The children receiving stuttering therapy were also less anxious than the controls.

42 of these children were examined four years after completing their therapy programs. The 20 children in the control group were given speech therapy, so were not evaluated in the follow-up studies (Hancock, 1998).

The children treated with the EMG computers seemed to lose ground over four years, the home-treated children held steady, and the clinician-treated children gained ground. The result was that after four years, all three treatments were almost equally effective. The all three groups had average stuttering reductions between 76% and 79%.

For more about EMG biofeedback, see the chapter "Computers and Electronic Devices For Stuttering."

STUTTERING MODIFICATION THERAPIES

"The House That Jack Built" is a stuttering modification therapy for school-age children. (Ramig & Bennett, 1995) The therapy has four stages:

1) "Laying the Foundation of Knowledge." The speech pathologist helps the child learn what stuttering is, how fluent speech is produced, and the terminology she'll use.

2) "Installing the Plumbing." The speech mechanism is seen as "plumbing" and disfluencies as "clogs" in the system. This stages involves practicing "easy stuttering," or easy repetitions, prolongations, and blocks. One drill involves saying a word with hard stuttering, then saying it with easy stuttering. Or this drill can be three-part — fluent, hard stuttering, easy stuttering.

3) "Building Rooms and Walls." The child works on becoming an "architect" to "design his own house." The child may want to design the following "rooms": what to do when teased; being open about

stuttering; not avoiding speaking; voluntary stuttering; modifying stuttering with cancellations and pullouts; relaxation; positive self-talk; reducing time pressure. The child decides what goes into each "room."

The speech pathologist should discuss with the child why other children tease, how the child reacts, and other ways the child could react. Role-playing can be used here.

Negative thinking should also be addressed. Examples are "I can't," "Its never going to work," "I should talk better," etc. The speech pathologist helps the child recognize negative thought patterns, and shows how to replace these with positive thoughts.

This stage may also involve preparing for relapse by doing daily "inspections" (practice drills) or repairs with his "tool box" of therapy techniques.

4) "Building the Roof of Fluency." The "roof" is fluent speech, as a result of either using fluency-shaping techniques or easy stuttering. The walls, rooms, plumbing, and foundation must support the roof. The roof can't stand by itself.

FLUENCY SHAPING THERAPIES

Fluency shaping therapies are often used with elementary- and high-school stutterers. A recent study compared two types of fluency shaping therapies. Both types were effective, reducing stuttering to less than 1% of words, in only about eight hours of establishment therapy, plus about twelve hours of maintenance therapy over the next fourteen months (Ryan, 1995).

The first therapy used delayed auditory feedback (DAF) to train slow, prolonged speech. The child begins with extremely slow, fluent speech, and gradually increases speaking rate until he is fluent at a normal speaking rate.

The second therapy is "Gradual Increase in Length and Complexity of Utterance" (GILCU). The child starts with single words, first in reading out loud, then in monologue, and then in conversation. When he can say single words fluently, he gradually builds up to five minutes of fluent speech.

SPEECH-RELATED ATTITUDES

Several studies have shown that adult stutterers have poor speech-related attitudes. Few adult stutterers say "I like the way I talk," while many will say "It is hard for me to talk to people." But when children who stutter are asked to make wishes, they don't make speech-related wishes (see the subsection "Attitudes And Emotions Of Stuttering" in the chapter "Symptoms of Stuttering"). At what age do poor speech-related attitudes begin?

Luc De Nil and Gene Brutten studied 70 stuttering and 271 non-stuttering children, aged 7 to 11, using the Communication Attitude Test (De Nil, 1991). For the non-stuttering children, poor speech-related attitudes dropped steadily from a score of 10 at age 7, to a score of 6 at age 11 (positive attitudes had lower scores). For stuttering children, poor speech-related attitudes increased steadily from a score of 15 at age 7, to a score of 18, at age 11.

In other words, plenty of non-stuttering seven-year-olds think their speech is poor, and somewhat more stuttering seven-year-olds think their speech is poor, but the attitudes are fairly close between the two groups. But by age eleven, stutterers score three times worse than non-stutterers. This study suggests that stuttering therapy should include developing positive speech-related attitudes, even for children as young as 7.

CLASSROOM ACTIVITIES TO DEMYSTIFY STUTTERING

Speech pathologists are now considering classroom activities involving teachers and classmates, to "demystify" stuttering. See Cooper and Cooper's Collaborative Oral Language Fluency Program. (Cooper, 1991)

A teacher can call the National Stuttering Project for an adult stutterer to make a presentation to her class.

DIAGNOSIS AND COUNSELING

Diagnosing a school-age (7-14 years old) intermediate stutterer can be similar to evaluation of preschool stutterers and their parents, or similar to adult evaluations, depending on the child.

The major difference is that the speech pathologist interviews the child's teacher as well, and may observe the child in his classroom. The parent of a school-age stutterer could ask the child's teacher the same questions:

1) Does the child talk in class? Does he stutter?

2) Does stuttering interfere with the child's academic progress? Does he say, "I don't know" when he knows the answer to a question?

3) Do other children tease him about his speech?

4) How does the teacher react to the child's stuttering?

The speech pathologist also interviews the child. She asks about his family and friends, so that the child knows she is genuinely interested in him. She then asks about his speech.

1) Does he have trouble talking? She evaluates how aware the child is of his stuttering. If the child is unaware of his stuttering, the speech pathologist doesn't directly ask about stuttering, as this could give the child anxiety about his speech and make his stuttering worse.

2) She asks about "tricks" to get words out, about avoidances, and difficult speaking situations.

3) Does anyone tease him about his speech? How does he react?

4) How does he feel about his speech? Does he ever feel frustrated or mad?

5) What do his parents do when he stutters?

There are two questionnaires for school-age stutterers:

- The A-19 Scale of Children's Communication Attitudes, by Susan Andre and Barry Guitar (Peters & Guitar, 1991).
- The Children's Attitude Test, by Gene Brutten.

The speech pathologist also evaluates the child for other speech and language disorders, such as syntax, semantics, and pragmatics. She also evaluates the child's physical, cognitive, and social-emotional development.

Treatments for intermediate stutterers are combinations of treatments for beginning and adult stutterers, depending on the child's abilities and needs.

The speech pathologist also advises the teacher on ways to reduce speech-related stress for the child. This can mean not having children read out loud by their seating rows, and not requiring oral reports. But this can also mean not excusing the stutterer from all oral assignments — each individual case may be different.

The Stuttering Foundation of America (800/992-9392) has a brochure, "The Child Who Stutters at School: Notes to the Teacher."

STARBUCK FAMILY PROGRAM

The State University of New York at Geneseo offers a two-week intensive residential stuttering therapy program for children up to 12 years of age and their families. The program is usually the first two weeks of July, and costs about $1900. For more information, contact: Starbuck Fluency Clinic, Sturges Hall, SUNY Geneseo, 1 College Circle, Geneseo, NY 14454.

The clinic also offers a four-week program for teenagers and adults.

GAMES FOR SCHOOL-AGE STUTTERING

Here's a game I invented for my National Stuttering Project support group, which should also be fun for school-age children. You read passages from Winnie-the-Pooh, with each character using a different fluency technique:

- Winnie-the-Pooh hums a lot, so he uses continuous phonation;
- Piglet talks in a high, squeaky voice, which makes you fluent;
- Owl uses the Hot Airflow Method;
- Eeyore uses Dreary Auditory Feedback, which is tediously slow and depressing, but makes you fluent;
- T-T-T-Tigger b-b-b-bounces his words;
- Rabbit talks very fast, which makes him stutter, but he's too busy to notice; and
- the narrator articulates clearly and speaks slowly, in case children are listening, which makes him fluent too.

Another game we enjoyed was for two people to read Dr. Seuss books together.

A stuttering therapy group can also do role-playing. Watch a movie scene with a "high-status" character and a "low-status" character (e.g., *The Godfather*). What does each actor do to indicate rank? Role play the scene. One person pretends to be a low-status person, and talks fast, in a higher-pitched voice, repeating phrases, avoiding eye contact, and looking at the floor. Another person pretends to be a high-status person, and speaks slowly, calmly, with a lower-pitched voice, and maintains eye contact. Discuss how self-esteem affects fluency.

There are several board games for stuttering therapy. Check the mail order catalogs for speech pathologists.

BOOKS FOR YOUNG STUTTERERS

The *Mary Marony* series of books by Suzy Kline portrays a seven-year-old girl who stutters. Her parents, speech pathologist, and teacher support her. In *Mary Marony Hides Out*, Mary's favorite author comes to talk to her school. She is torn between her desire to talk to the author and her fear of speaking in the school assembly. When she gets up the courage to speak, a classmate makes fun of her, and Mary hides in the bathroom.

Fluency Services in the Schools

Speech therapy is provided under the federal Individuals with Disabilities Education Act (IDEA). Schools must accommodate any disabilities that interfere with the child's education.

The American Speech-Language Hearing Association's (ASHA) Special Interest Division on Fluency (Division 4) had a task force study fluency services in schools. The task force found that treatments varied from daily half-hour individual sessions to monthly group sessions of less than a half-hour. Most children received one or two group sessions per week, of about thirty minutes. Some districts had summer programs.

The task force found that group therapy sometimes means three children with articulation problems (far more common than stuttering) and one child who stutters being treated together. This can be a problem, as different speech disorders require different therapies. Techniques to improve articulation can make stuttering worse. You should check that your child is being treated specifically for stuttering.

Parents were concerned that their children were not receiving appropriate treatment. Some children continue in speech therapy year after year, without progress.

Parents felt that attention was not given to the impact of stuttering upon their child's social and emotional development. They disapproved of their child missing physical education and recess for speech therapy. Some speech pathologists find that working 12:00-6:00 is better, as some children prefer speech therapy after school.

The task force found that parents felt excluded from the speech treatment. They wanted books on stuttering available in the school library; stuttering treatment for preschool children; and summer treatment programs. They wanted to meet other parents of children who stutter, and to educate the public about stuttering, especially for how to identify stuttering in young children, and the importance of early intervention.

School speech pathologists complained about large caseloads, which force group therapy. They found that family participation was difficult in the school setting. They wanted to be trained better in counseling parents.

School administrators complained that speech pathologists are not trained in treating stuttering, and that health insurance doesn't pay for children to receive stuttering treatment from specialists outside of schools. Administrators also complained about the shortage of speech pathologists, especially in poor and rural school districts.

The task force also noted that some states allow schools to hire speech pathologists not certified by the American Speech-Language Hearing Association (ASHA). Most states require a masters degree in speech pathology, but some only require a bachelors degree. Sometimes the child is treated by an untrained "speech aid" who is more or less supervised by a speech pathologist.

Check that your child's speech pathologist has experience and training in treating stuttering. ASHA's certification requires no experience treating stuttering. If your child's speech pathologist knows little about stuttering, ask if your school district has a specialist in stuttering. Or look for a stuttering specialist at a speech clinic, university, hospital, or in private practice. (See the chapter "Choosing A Speech Pathologist.")

The ASHA SID4 task force can help you organize a meeting between your school district's speech pathologists, administrators, and parents of children who stutter. Or you may want to help the National Stuttering Project organize a "Youth Day" weekend workshop with specialists in childhood stuttering.

ADVICE FOR PARENTS

Magdalene Lima wrote the following advice for parents, on an Internet stuttering support group (reprinted with permission):

I am an SLP in private practice and formerly a public school therapist for 9 years. My suggestions to parents of children with speech problems are:

1) Do some research in these areas. Check out the communication disorders websites. You can find these by searching with any search engine such as Infoseek or Yahoo!. Look up stuttering or articulation disorders or language disorders. There are many resources for parents on these sites.

2) Go to your school speech pathologist with what you know and ask her what she thinks. The best approach is to treat her as the professional she is in a non-critical way with the attitude that you just want to understand all the treatments available for your son. Offer to help get information to her if she doesn't have it. Let her know you understand the position she is in and that you are on her team. This will get you much further in getting the appropriate services for your child than fighting your school.

3) If your insurance covers it or you have the funds, find a good private pediatric speech and language clinic in your area and AT

LEAST have an evaluation done. Just that information alone could really help the school SLP. If you can afford private therapy, get it. The main difference in service is that your child will receive individual therapy with a clinician that has the time and resources needed to provide the highest quality therapy.

As a former school speech pathologist, my skills and knowledge didn't suddenly changed when I switched over to private practice. The setting changed, and that makes a huge difference. I now serve 30 clients rather than 75, I see them all individually, and I am paid more than in the schools. In the hours I don't see clients, I am busy researching, giving parent support, writing regular and detailed reports, and planning innovative therapy rather than, going to bus duty, lunch duty, hall duty, faculty meetings that don't really apply to me and filling out massive amounts of government-required paperwork.

Is The Problem Ability Or Setting?

Now to those of you who think the worst of the public school speech pathologist: I'd like you to stand in her shoes for a minute. In the last 3 years of my public school experience my caseload became unmanageable, I had 75 students, including a severely and profoundly handicapped class, 4 autistic students and all other students in speech from grades K-5 at that school. I begged, cried and pleaded for help from my supervisors. I KNEW I could not provide the quality of service each and every one of these students and their families deserved. However, the answer was always: get creative, we don't have money in the budget. Please understand, in my situation, it was not a lack of caring, lack of skill or ability — there was absolutely nothing I could do. I became angry and frustrated at our administration. Why didn't they provide the training, time, personnel and support we needed to provide services to these students?

Speech Pathology: A Growing And Diverse Field

The disorders in our field and the therapies that have now been developed have become extremely specialized. In the schools I was expected by parents to be an expert in the following fields: stuttering, swallowing disorders, voice disorders, articulation disorders including tongue thrust, cleft palate, phonological process disorders as well as motor speech disorders, autism and PDD, traumatic brain injury, ADHD, language and learning disabilities, hearing impairments and social and pragmatic communication disorders. Excuse me, do you realize that just as physicians receive a basic foundation in medicine, so do speech pathologists receive a basic foundation in all of the above disorders. You graduate from college and through your experience and personal growth and research, you become an expert in a few areas. It would be virtually impossible for one person to have the time and energy it would take to become an expert in all those areas!

This is why our field is moving towards specialty certifications. What will public schools do then? I guess they will have to hire the specialists that their individual students require.

Many And Varied Problems In The Schools

More and more our district began hiring speech assistants (speech practitioners who are not required to meet the standards of education, clinical practicum and experience needed to be fully certified and licensed) to handle huge caseloads with minimal supervision from licensed speech pathologists. There is a shortage of qualified speech language pathologists willing to go into public school therapy when there are much more lucrative and attractive positions available in other settings. As I talked with administrators, I soon became aware of the pressure being applied to them from the state, parents and other agencies to meet all these educational requirements. For every parent who complains there is not enough money to provide quality special education services in the school, there is another parent complaining that their gifted and talented child is not being given the education THEY deserve because of all the money being poured into special education programs. Or what about the parents of children in sports programs, they have THEIR list of complaints. Everyone thinks that their cause is totally justified because they are arguing for their children, and nothing can convince anyone that their child doesn't deserve the best.

I left the public school system to go into private practice and now my problem is solved — I love my work and I'm giving quality services to clients with fantastic results! However, what's your solution? My final and personal resolution to this whole issue, is that in many cases — not all, but many — I truly feel that schools are doing the very best they can with the resources available to them to provide the services that our children need. However, sometimes, parents are right, it's not enough. So what are we going to do? Is every parent in America with a complaint going to file suit against the local school district? If this happens, our schools will begin focusing on preventing lawsuits rather than on how best to serve and educate our children.

Work With Your Administration/Educators

Sometimes all it takes is going to an administrator, such as the Director of Special Education, and pleading your case. Also give your specific suggestions at your child's IEP meeting. You'd better have some research and documentation to back up the necessity of your suggestions. The attitude and manner in which you present yourself is of utmost importance, if they perceive you are willing to make compromises and work with them they will be more willing to stick their neck out for you. Suggest specific things such as the district paying for an outside assessment, or hiring a consultant temporarily who can lend their expertise to your child's case. Get over any intimidation you feel in asserting yourself with these people, they are just people with children and jobs and stresses just like you. What they say to you is never written in stone.

Conclusion

I'm not saying you shouldn't fight extreme injustice or abuse. I'm saying it's a huge system with a lot of variables involved. The fight is societal and governmental — usually not your local educational facility. Become involved politically in your state with your speech and hearing association — they always have a branch that is lobbying for legislation to improve speech services in the schools. Meanwhile, you have a child that has needs for quality services in the area of speech pathology, do the best you can to get that service, whether it be private therapy through insurance or private pay, or school therapy, don't stop looking until you find what you need.

YOU take responsibility to research, learn things for yourself and communicate with those who affect your child's education.

Teenage Stuttering

I am a mother of a stuttering thirteen-year-old boy. Stuttering really had never bothered him until this year. It is very frustrating for him to talk on the phone. His friends call all the time but he has refrained from talking on the phone because his stuttering seems to get worse. My husband and I have noticed him withdrawing from his peers. We have always had an active role with his stuttering. He has been to a lot of speech pathologists and we have also tried the CAFET system. This was helping him. Unfortunately the closest center was more than two hours away. After one year it was too stressful on him missing too much school. Because of this we had to stop. Since then he wanted nothing to do with speech pathologists.

This common story usually has these elements:

- The teenager has been seeing his school's speech pathologists for five or even ten years.
- He is fluent in the speech pathologist's office, but stutters everywhere else.
- He has lost motivation to work on his speech.
- His social behavior has changed. He is withdrawing from social contacts.
- The parents have taken him to other speech clinics, without success.

The teenager is changing from childhood stuttering patterns to adult stuttering patterns.

Previously he saw himself as being like most other kids, doing the same things as other kids, although sometimes he had trouble talking. Now he thinks of himself as a stutterer, different from other teenagers. There are social activities that other teenagers do, such as dating or getting an after-school job, that he won't do because he stutters.

Previously he pretty much said what he wanted to say, even if stumbled on words. Now he fears and avoids certain words or speaking situations.

Previously he liked his speech therapist. Now he's making no progress in therapy and wants to discontinue therapy.

TEENAGERS ARE ADULT STUTTERERS

He's now an adult, in terms of stuttering, and you should look at adult stuttering therapies rather than relying solely on your school speech pathologist. The rest of this book is about adult stuttering. There are many aspects of adult stuttering, and many adult stuttering therapies. Your son should decide how he wants to approach stuttering:

• He may prefer cognitive therapy, to become conscious of the choices he has in every situation, rather than feeling that he can respond to social situations in only one way.

• He may prefer to continue with physical speech therapy, similar to what he's had in school, but to do it in an out-of-state, 3-week intensive therapy program. Getting out of the familiar family and school environment may be what he wants.

• He may want to join or even start a support group for teenagers who stutter.

• He may want to attend Indiana University's one-week "Speech Camp for Teens Who Stutter" (ages 13-17). The fee is $250 (the actual cost is much higher and Sertoma Clubs are picking up the balance). Contact Ann Densmore at (812) 855-6251; fax (812) 855-5531; adensmor@indiana.edu; Dept. of Speech and Hearing Sciences, Indiana University, 200 S. Jordan Ave, Bloomington, IN 47405; http://www.Indiana.edu:80:/~bradwood/sertoma.html

DEVELOP A PASSION

Read the chapter "Famous People Who Stutter" carefully. Note that many celebrities developed their talent during high school as a result of stuttering:

• Carly Simon developed her skills as a singer and a songwriter because she stuttered.

• James Earl Jones, Bruce Willis, and Peggy Lipton found they were fluent when acting.

• Bob Love and Greg Louganis focused on sports.

Teenagers can have incredible drive and focus in an activity that they feel passionate about. Help your teenager find an activity that he is passionate about. Ideally this should be something that improves his fluency. Such activities include:

• Singing.
• Acting.
• Debating.
• Foreign languages.
• Studying the science behind stuttering.
• Organizing a teenage stuttering support group.

Even if your family never does these activities, take your teenager to plays or concerts, or help him with science projects or organizing a support group.

Next best are non-verbal group activities, such as team sports or music, which will improve his self-esteem and enable develop of social skills in a peer group.

Third-best are non-verbal, individual activities such as computers, individual sports, writing or photography, which will maintain his self-esteem, but won't improve his fluency or social skills.

If your teenager was an introverted child, don't force him into extroverted activities, such as debating. The stress of extroversion may be too much. But conversely, if your teenager was an extroverted, outgoing, boisterous child, don't allow him to develop an introverted persona to avoid talking. The loneliness of introverted activities (such as computers or individual sports) will be stressful and could lead to depression.

STUTTERING IS NOT THE DRAGON

The mother of an 18-year-old stutterer called me. He'd come home in despair. He'd gone to the library for a video on homeless people for a school project. But he couldn't say "homeless," so he walked out without the video. He'd been accepted at an excellent university, but now he didn't know if he should leave home. Who would talk for him when he couldn't?

He'd had lots of stuttering therapy, so was fluent most of the time. But he'd get into situations where his hard blocks came back. We agreed that more therapy wasn't what he needed.

I told him that he was in the stage of ego development where young men have to fight dragons and rescue princesses. Even though our society now values feminine energy and pushes young men to be co-operative and empathetic, young men first have to prove their strength to the world, before they can move onwards. I'm 36, and I'm stuck in this stage too. I haven't killed many dragons. More often I've been wounded, or I backed away without a fight.

The dragon was the librarian, and the princess was the video. The psychic pain he was experiencing showed that his ego had been forced a step backwards, when it wanted to grow.

Stuttering was not the dragon. Dragons make you so aware of your weaknesses that you think they are the dragons. But your weaknesses, including stuttering, are never the dragon. If you fight stuttering, you won't win, because it's not the dragon.

Most dragons aren't good fighters, so they hide or disguise

themselves. The young man didn't see that a dragon had disguised itself as a librarian. If you can't see the dragon, you can't slay it.

Dragons' other defense is to make you terribly aware of your weaknesses. You scrunch down behind your shield, so that no part of you is vulnerable.

But with both hands clenching your shield, you've dropped your sword. You've spent long hours practicing stuttering therapy, getting that sword razor-sharp. But then you drop the sword. You can't use your therapy skills to fight the dragon.

Stand up straight, throw away your shield, and tell the dragon where your weaknesses are. Say to the librarian, "Excuse me, I stutter and I'm having trouble saying a word." By pointing out your weaknesses, you're really saying that you're so strong that you are daring the dragon to attack. Most dragons will back down.

But some dragons will attack you. Instead of meeting strength with strength, use aikido to make the dragon's own energy throw it off-balance. If the person laughs when you stutter, smile and tell a joke about stuttering.

If the dragon thinks you're mentally-retarded and handicapped, acknowledge your disability and begin with, "My speech therapist wants me to talk to people more..."

If someone questions you abrasively, turn on your charm and smile. If your strength is in using technology, several companies make electronic anti-stuttering devices.

When your verbal aikido has thrown the dragon off-balance, lift up your sword and slay the dragon. Use your humor, charm, or your other strengths. Then take a moment to listen to all the princesses in the world cheering, before you grab your princess and ride off into the sunset.

HIGH SCHOOL STUTTERING PROJECTS

I've put a variety of science and other projects for high school students on my website at

http://www.casafuturatech.com/Science/daf.html

The main project is building a delayed-auditory feedback (DAF) stuttering therapy device. Six experiments using the device are presented.

Eleven other projects are listed, including

• Building a frequency-shifted auditory feedback (FAF) and masking auditory feedback (MAF) stuttering therapy devices.

• Writing a report on the history of stuttering therapy, using *Stuttering: The Search for a Cause and Cure* by Oliver Bloodstein, Ph.D.

• Write a report about a famous person who stutters. If the person is alive, ask a librarian how to find the person's address, and write to him or her.

• Interview a speech pathologist about the cause of and treatments for stuttering. Describe the techniques and goals of two therapies. Observe the speech pathologist treating a preschool child. Learn to use any therapy devices, such as a computer-based biofeedback system, that the speech pathologist has.

• Help your school's speech pathologist organize a "Youth Day" weekend workshop for children and teenagers who stutter in your area. The National Stuttering Project has a book explaining how to organize a "Youth Day" workshop.

• Interview a successful adult who stutters. This could be an accountant, a lawyer, or a teacher. Ask how stuttering affected the person's youth, education, career, and relationships. Ask about therapy the person has had. The National Stuttering Project (800/364-1677) can help a student find an adult to interview.

• Draw a family tree showing relatives who stutter.

• Compare stuttering to another student's disability.

• Repeat Wendell Johnson's 1937 studies of adaptation and anticipation (see the chapter "Belief: Anticipation, Distraction, Stress, and Placebos").

Stuttering Therapy for Mentally-Retarded Individuals

Oliver Bloodstein writes in his *A Handbook On Stuttering* of "ample evidence" that stuttering is especially prevalent among persons with mental disabilities. Stuttering seems to be especially common among persons with Down Syndrome. There is some debate about this, as the stuttering symptoms among the developmentally-delayed can be different from stuttering in adults of normal intelligence.

Developmentally-delayed individuals tend to have other speech and language problems as well. A speech pathologist treating a mentally-retarded person will probably use more than just stuttering therapies. There are books devoted to this, such as *Communication Strategies for People with Developmental Disabilities: Issues for Theory and Practice*, edited by Ken Linfoot, Ph.D. (1995, Baltimore: Brookes Publishing Company, $33, 800/638-3775).

Eugene Cooper suggests that "reducing the number of abstract concepts the clinician uses" is paramount in treating mentally-retarded stutterers. He also emphasizes that therapy should focus on helping mentally-retarded stutterers "identify and express their feelings and attitudes about the problem." Too often, speech pathologists act as if mentally-retarded persons lack feelings and emotions, as well as intelligence. Cooper also writes that the stutterer should be "capable of verbalizing the goal of the procedure and their desire to achieve that goal" (Cooper, 1986)— good advice with any stutterer.

If the person likes to play video games, you may want to try some of the speech therapy computer games. See the list of companies in the chapter "Computers and Electronic Devices for Stuttering." MicroVideo's "Video Voice" has some games that require the player do relatively little to make a lot happen on the screen.

ADULT STUTTERING THERAPY

A stutterer returned from a two-week intensive stuttering therapy program in a distant city. His friends asked how the therapy had gone.

"Peter Piper picked a peck of pickled peppers," the stutterer said, completely fluent. His friends expressed amazement.

"Y-y-y-yes, b-b-b-but it's h-h-hard t-to w-w-work th-that into a c-c-c-conversation," he said.

Why Do Stutterers Avoid Therapy?

Perhaps 99% of adult stutterers never seek treatment for their stuttering (see the chapter "Incidence and Prevalence of Stuttering").

Many stutterers don't know that stuttering treatments are available. If a stutterer is unsuccessful with one therapy program, he probably won't try another therapy — again, due to ignorance that there are many types of stuttering therapies available.

Many therapy choices are available to stutterers. Never think that you have reached a "dead end"!

Stutterers seek speech therapy at life changes — when graduating from college, looking for a job, wanting to marry, etc. When life is unchanging, stutterers see no reason to change their speech.

Getting stutterers to practice 20 minutes a day is difficult. Getting stutterers to use therapy techniques in conversations can be impossible. There are several reasons for this:

1) Stuttering is a developmental disorder. You've stuttered as long as you can remember. People who start stuttering later in life (from a stroke or head injury) almost always seek treatment. To these people, the ability to talk is a major loss. But if you've never talked fluently, you don't know what you're missing. Stutterers may not realize that their stuttering is a problem. See the subsection "Poor Awareness of Stuttering" in the chapter "Symptoms of Stuttering," and also see the chapter "About the Author."

2) Some cultures assume that stuttering is "God's will" or punishment for misdeeds in an earlier incarnation. Other people assume that suffering is the human condition, and they live with difficulties rather than try to solve their problems. An economist once wrote: "Aristotle thought that slaves were the ordination of Nature — the devil of it was, the slaves thought so too."

3) Denial — stutterers are embarrassed about stuttering, and so don't want to think about it. Failure at stuttering therapy can support denial — a stutterer goes to a therapy program, the therapy "doesn't work," and now he has an excuse to never try again.

Sally Ballard wrote about her *fear of speech therapy* for the British Stammering Association newsletter. After describing several bad experiences with speech pathologists as a child (due more to her temper than the speech pathologists), Ms. Ballard describes taking her children to a speech clinic:

> I am terrified of [my children] stammering...Even though it did not look as if they would stammer, I took them to a speech therapist. I was petrified of her...She told me that my children were fine, and asked me if I would like help for myself. I said thanks but no thanks, and almost ran out of the room.
>
> Years later, I realized that I could not carry on as I was [having her husband make telephone calls, walking because she couldn't tell the bus driver where to stop]...Even though I was scared of speech therapists, I decided I had to get over my fear...I worked out that it was two main things: the fear of being unable to gain respect [fear that speech pathologists would treat her like a child or a mentally-retarded person], and the fear of being a failure [and continuing to stutter].
>
> I went to my local health clinic and asked (eventually) to see a speech therapist...I went into a flat panic. I could not decide what to do. What if they could not help me? What if I would always stammer or, worse still, what if she helped me overcome my speech problem? I would not have an excuse any more and, if I failed in life, I could no longer put it down to the fact that I stammered. I would have to accept the blame myself.
>
> When the fateful day of my appointment arrived, I was a nervous wreck. I wouldn't let my husband come with me in case I chickened out and didn't go at all, but in the end I went. My palms were sweating by the time I arrived...

The speech pathologist taught Ms. Ballard to "stammer more fluently." The speech pathologist then asked how stuttering affected Ms. Ballard's life. She said that stuttering

> had stopped me from doing the one career that I wanted. Teaching. With terrific support from my husband, children, friends, and my speech therapist, I applied to the local college...

Despite rejections from several universities because of her stuttering, Ms. Ballard eventually was accepted. She concludes,

Never give up. If things don't go the way you wanted them to, don't look on the down side of life. Try to look at all the things you have achieved in life. Everyone will be surprised at how much that really is.

Stuttering Modification Therapy

Stuttering modification therapy is primarily associated with Charles Van Riper. The therapy is also associated with Oliver Bloodstein, Edward Conture, and Joseph Sheehan. These men were stutterers, who became speech pathologists.

The goal of stuttering modification therapy is not to eliminate stuttering. Instead, the two goals are:

1) Modify your moments of stuttering, so that your stuttering is less severe.

2) Reduce your fear of stuttering, and eliminate avoidance behaviors associated with this fear.

The therapy has four phases: identification, desensitization, modification, and stabilization.

Stuttering is a vicious cycle. In situations where you want to speak well you try too hard, tense your speech-production muscles, stutter, try harder, tense more, and stutter more. Stuttering modification therapy takes you out of this vicious cycle. When you stutter, you stop, sense what muscles are tense, relax these muscles, sense your fears and anxieties, eliminate these fears, and go on. This isn't an instant cure for stuttering — making this reaction automatic takes years. But as time goes on you stutter less and less.

IDENTIFICATION

You begin by identifying the core behaviors, secondary behaviors, and feelings and attitudes that characterize your stuttering.

Your speech pathologist points out your "easy or effortless stuttering" first. You learn to identify when you do these behaviors. The goal is to improve your awareness of what you do when you stutter.

Next, your speech pathologist trains you to identify and become aware of your avoidance behaviors, postponement behaviors, starting behaviors, word and sound fears, situation fears, core stuttering behaviors, and escape behaviors.

Finally, you learn to identify feelings of frustration, shame, and hostility associated with your speech.

At first, identifying these behaviors is done in the speech clinic. Later, your speech pathologist takes you out of the clinic, to identify what you do in everyday conversations.

Edward Conture suggests beginning the "identification" process with recordings of other stutterers, then moving to recording of your speech, and finally moving to identification as you talk.

DESENSITIZATION

Van Riper called this "toughening the stutterer to his stuttering." You do this in three stages. The goal is for you to become comfortable with all three of these aspects of your stuttering.

1) Confrontation, or accepting that you stutter. If you've read this far, you've probably accepted that you stutter. But reading a book or enrolling in a therapy program is not enough. You are expected to tell people that you stutter, and talk about what you are doing in therapy to change your stuttering.

2) Freeze your core behaviors — repetitions, prolongations, and blocks. When you stutter, your speech pathologist raises a finger. You hold what you are doing, until she drops her finger. For example, if you were repeating a syllable, you have to continue to repeat that syllable. Your speech pathologist will make you freeze these core behaviors for longer and longer periods. The goal is for you to become less emotional or more tolerant of these behaviors.

3) Voluntary stuttering, or stuttering on purpose. This helps you remain calm when you stutter.

MODIFICATION

This is where you learn "easy stuttering" or "fluent stuttering," in 3 stages:

1) Cancellations. When you stutter, you stop, pause for a few seconds, and say the word again. You say the word slowly, with reduced articulatory pressure, and blending the sounds together.

2) Pull-outs. After you master freezing and cancellations, you use your "easy stuttering" while you are in a stutter, to pull yourself out of the stutter and say the word fluently.

3) Preparatory sets. After mastering pull-outs, you look ahead to words you're going to stutter on, and you use "easy stuttering" on those words.

These techniques are difficult if you have severe physical stuttering. Some stutterers lack the vocal control to do these techniques. Additionally, preparatory sets can reinforce your fears of certain words and sounds.

STABILIZATION

The last stage of stuttering modification therapy seeks to stabilize or solidify your speech gains. This is accomplished through sub-goals:

The first is for you to become your own speech therapist. You take responsibility for making your own assignments and prescribed therapy activities.

"Becoming your own speech pathologist" doesn't mean reading books about stuttering, taking a class, going to conventions, or learning about new research and therapies. "Becoming your own speech pathologist" means motivating yourself to do therapy activities indefinitely. There's a presumption that you wouldn't do these therapy activities on your own, because you don't perceive resulting benefits. You need a speech pathologist to get you to do the activities.

Another sub-goal is "the automatization of preparatory sets and pull-outs." Unfortunately, stuttering modification therapy was developed before motor learning theory. Stuttering modification therapies just tell you to practice, and don't include any techniques to maximize autonomous motor learning.

The last subgoal is for you to change your self-concept from being a person who stutters to being a person who speaks fluently most of the time but who occasionally stutters mildly.

STUTTERING MODIFICATION SELF-THERAPY

Stuttering modification can be done as self-therapy, as opposed to going to a speech clinic. There is an excellent book for this: *Self-Therapy For The Stutterer*, by Malcolm Fraser.

The book is short and extremely easy to read. You work on your feelings and emotions, on relaxation, speaking slowly, stuttering easily, eliminating secondary behaviors and avoidances, listening to your voice, and talking more. You also do voluntary stuttering, cancellations and pull-outs.

I met a stutterer who bought the book, did the exercises, and was cured. I bought the book, tried to do the exercises, and wasn't helped a bit. Hopefully you'll have better luck.

Your local library probably has the book. If not, it is available for $3 from the Stuttering Foundation of America, P.O. Box 11749, Memphis, TN 38111-0749, 800/992-9392.

PROBLEMS WITH STUTTERING MODIFICATION THERAPY

One reviewer criticized this book for being "unbalanced" with more pages about fluency shaping therapy than about stuttering modification therapy. This edition corrects that problem, if you count the recommendation to read Malcolm Fraser's *Self-Therapy for The Stutterer* as equivalent to the self-therapy chapter "Fluency Shaping Techniques." This leaves the chapter "Problems with Fluency Shaping Therapy" without an analogous chapter about problems with stuttering modification therapy (aside from the minor criticisms included in this chapter).

There have been few published critiques of stuttering therapy programs, by other speech pathologists. The exceptions are the two papers referenced in the chapter "Problems With Fluency Shaping" (Kuhr and Perkins). To my knowledge, there have been no published critiques of stuttering modification therapies, so this book remains "unbalanced" in that respect. Whether this book is unbalanced for or against stuttering modification therapy or fluency shaping therapy I will leave to the book reviewers!

Fluency Shaping Therapy

Fluency shaping therapists believe that stutterers can learn to speak fluently. In some fluency shaping therapy programs, fears, anxieties, and avoidances are not treated because these psychological issues should disappear after you develop normal, fluent speech. Other fluency shaping programs include some psychotherapeutic time.

The first stage of fluency shaping therapy is to establish fluent, but abnormal-sounding speech in the speech clinic. This fluent speech is then shaped into normal-sounding speech. Lastly, you transfer this fluent speech outside the speech clinic, to everyday conversations.

William Perkins and Richard Curlee developed the first fluency shaping programs. Einer Boberg (ISTAR), Bruce Ryan (Monterey Fluency Program), George Shames and Cheri Florence (Stutter-Free Speech), and Ronald Webster (Hollins Precision Fluency Shaping Program) have developed other programs.

Perkins believes that stuttering is a discoordination of phonation (vocal fold vibration) with articulation (lips, jaw, and tongue) and respiration (breathing). He believes that stuttering is a disorder of timing. He believes that stutterers are constitutionally limited in their ability to talk fluently, although he notes that no organic basis for stuttering has been found.

Perkins' therapy develops compensatory skills that enable stutterers to talk fluently (Peters & Guitar, 1991). You can't use all these fluency skills in every conversation. Using fluency skills demands considerable attention and mental effort. You have the fluency skills for difficult speaking situations. The rest of the time, you talk spontaneously. For some people the fluency skills become habitual and effortless. But for most people, only parts of the motor skills become habitual. Still, this produces improved, if not perfect speech.

Because Perkins believes that stuttering is a disorder of timing, his therapy emphasizes slow speech. The therapy uses delayed auditory feedback (DAF) to electronically force you to talk extremely slowly (see the chapter "Computers and Electronic Devices for Stuttering Therapy").

Perkins first set the DAF delay to 250 milliseconds, or 30 words per minute, or 5-10 times slower than normal speech.

You don't stutter when you talk this slowly. You start with reading out loud, then use slow speech in conversations in the speech clinic.

You don't use this slow speech outside the speech clinic.

After establishing extremely slow, fluent speech, you work on five "breath flow" motor skills. These are:

1) Phrasing. You limit your phrases to 3-8 syllables. This is prevents running out of air.

2) Phrase initiation. You start each phrase with an easy vocal onset. In other words, you relax your vocal folds on the first sound of the first syllable.

3) Soft contact. You articulate consonants softly, keeping your lips, tongue, and jaw relaxed.

4) Breathy voice. This is a soft or breathy speaking style.

5) Blending. You maintain a continuous airflow from the beginning of each phrase to the end. You blend each syllable into the next.

The last fluency skill improves your prosody, or rhythm. The slow-motion speech produces a monotonous, droning speaking style. Now you work on adding inflections, intonations, and emotions to make your slow speech sound normal.

When you master these seven fluency shaping speech motor skills at the extremely slow speaking rate, you then work on increasing your speaking rate, while continuing to use your fluent speech skills. The DAF delay is reduced to 200 ms, or 45-60 words per minute. Then the delay is reduced to 150 ms, or 90-120 words per minute. Then the DAF volume is reduced, then one earphone is removed, and finally DAF use is discontinued.

At this point, your speech in the speech clinic is fluent and sounds normal. You are now ready to transfer this fluent speech to conversations outside the clinic. Perkins does this in four steps:

1) Evaluate your speech. You make tape recordings of your speech, and rate your speech in terms of fluency, rate, breath flow, prosody, and self-confidence. If you miss any of these targets, you are expected to practice the appropriate fluency shaping motor skills.

2) Speaking hierarchies. This a rating of speaking situations from easy to difficult. This ranges from conversations in the speech clinic to conversations outside the speech clinic; one-to-one conversations to speaking to an audience; etc. When you can use your fluent speech in an easy situation, you move on to using it in more challenging situations.

3) Social and vocational changes. You are encouraged to take responsibilities at work that require talking, and to participate in social activities that require talking.

4) Prepare for relapse. There are times when your fluent speech will relapse, and your stuttering will return. To prepare for this, your

speech therapist has you speak without each of the fluency shaping motor skills, until you stutter. For example, your talk as fast as you can, until you stutter. Then you start again, using your fluency shaping speech motor skills to regain your fluency.

Fluency Shaping Techniques

There are three groups of fluency shaping techniques, centered on the three main speech-production muscle groups:

1) Respiration, or using relaxed, diaphragmatic breathing instead of speech breathing.

2) Phonation, or vocal fold relaxation and control. These techniques include gentle onset and stretched vowels.

3) Articulation, or relaxing your lips, jaw, and tongue.

You can see that fluency shaping assumes that stutterers tense their speech-production muscles too much, and so trains you to speak with these muscles relaxed.

RELAXED BREATHING

There are two kinds of breathing: relaxed breathing and speech breathing.

Relaxed breathing uses your diaphragm muscles. Put one hand on your stomach. You should feel your stomach move out as you inhale, and in as you exhale. You take more, smaller breaths, resulting in lower lung pressure and respiratory muscle tension. You should have equal time for inhaling and exhaling.

For speech breathing, you quickly take a big breath, then you hold it as long as you can, letting out just enough air to talk. You hold back the air so that you can keep talking without taking another breath.

Speech breathing uses upper chest (thoracic) muscles. You take fewer, larger breaths. The result is higher lung pressure and tense muscles. Worst of all for stutterers, you increase laryngeal tension to hold back the air.

Relaxed breathing shortens your phrase length to about five words. You have pauses between phrases while you slowly inhale. Your speech sounds relaxed, confident, and clear. The hard part is avoiding the impulse to say long sentences on a single breath.

When you exhale, let out all your air, then pause a moment to release tension in your diaphragm.

The common advice "take a deep breath before you talk" is bad for stutterers. Taking a large breath increases lung pressure and respiration muscle tension, and may increase your vocal fold tension. It's better to take a smaller breath, gently using your diaphragm muscles to inhale, keeping lung pressure low and your muscles relaxed, and then gently exhaling and beginning to talking.

To learn more about the mental and physical health benefits of relaxed breathing, see *Conscious Breathing*, by Gay Hendricks.

VOCAL FOLD AWARENESS AND CONTROL

To understand how your vocal folds work, put your fingers on your throat and say "ah." You should feel your vocal fold vibration. You produce vowels by vibrating your vocal folds.

Now try saying *voiceless* consonants, such as /p/ /t/, and /s/. Your vocal folds do not vibrate for voiceless consonants.

There are also voiced consonants, such as /b/ and /d/. Your vocal folds vibrate to produce these consonants. They come in pairs, each with a voiceless consonant. Say /b/, /p/. Your lips and tongue do the same motions, but you feel your vocal folds vibrating with the /b/, but not with the /p/.

Try other consonant pairs, such as /d/ and /t/.

For example, let's say "coffee." Put your fingers on your throat and say the initial /k/ sound. You should not feel your vocal folds vibrating, because /k/ is produced in your mouth, not in your throat.

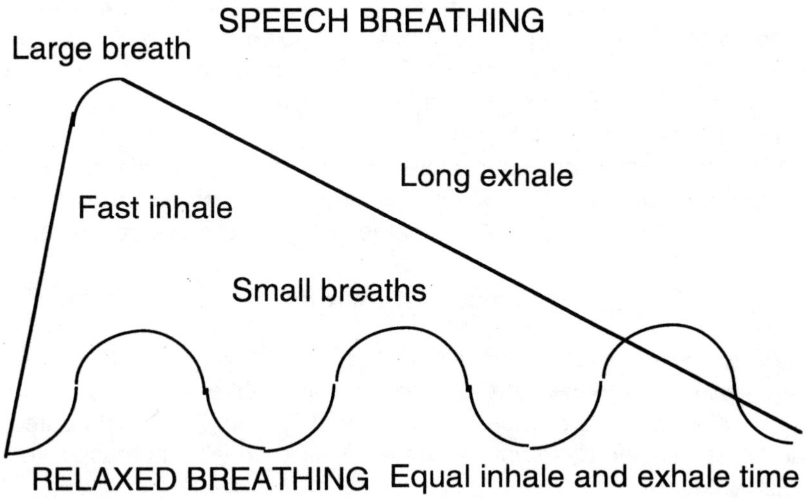

Now say the middle /aw/ sound. You should feel your vocal folds vibrate.

Then say the /f/ sound. Again, your vocal folds should switch off.

Lastly, say the final /ee/ sound. Your vocal folds should vibrate again.

Put it all together and you have /k/ /aw/ /f/ /ee/. Your vocal folds start off, switch on, switch off, and switch on.

Vocal fold vibration is the only muscle movement not directly controlled by your brain. Male vocal folds vibrate about 125 vibrations per second, and female vocal folds about 250 times per second. This muscle movement is too fast for your brain to control. Instead, your vocal folds vibrate through a combination of other muscle activities.

First, you have to let some air flow through your throat, from your lungs.

Then you have to tense your vocal folds slightly, so that they catch in the air flow. Then your vocal folds should vibrate.

If you tense your vocal folds too much, you block the air flow and can't say anything.

If you relax your vocal folds too much, you whisper.

If you have too much air flow, you'll run out of air before you can say anything.

Stuttering includes problems switching on your vocal fold vibration. You tense you vocal folds too much, or tense your vocal folds before you let some air out of your lungs. Then you hold this tension too long, while you struggle to speak. However, there's nothing physically wrong with stutterers' vocal folds (see the subsection "Laryngeal Disorders" in the chapter "Symptoms of Stuttering").

Put one hand on your throat and feel your vocal fold vibration. Put your other hand on your stomach and feel your diaphragmatic breathing. You should be able to talk fluently as long as you continue to vibrate your vocal folds and breathe with your diaphragm.

GENTLE ONSET

After you understand how your vocal folds work, practice *gentle onsets.* Take a relaxed breath, let out a little air, and stretch the first vowel sound of the phrase. Begin vibrating your vocal folds quietly, and gradually increase your volume. This gradually increases vocal fold tension.

When a word starts with a consonant, lightly touch your lips or tongue to make the sound, for a moment, quietly, and then stretch the vowel and increase your volume on the vowel.

For example, say "dog." The right way is to lightly say the /d/, stretch the /aw/ while gently increasing the volume, and lightly end with the /g/.

The wrong way is to make a hard /d/, with lots of tension in your tongue. Don't try to say the /d/ loudly. You'll tense your speech production muscles, and you may be able to repeat d-d-d-d-d, but your vocal folds will be too tense to move onto the vowel /aw/ sound.

Note that you're not having a problem say /d/ — you're having a problem moving onto the vowel after the /d/.

Some fluency shaping programs use biofeedback computers to display your *loudness contour.* These programs include Hollins, CAFET, and Dr. Fluency. The computers also give you error messages when you make a mistake. A visual representation of "dog" is presented below.

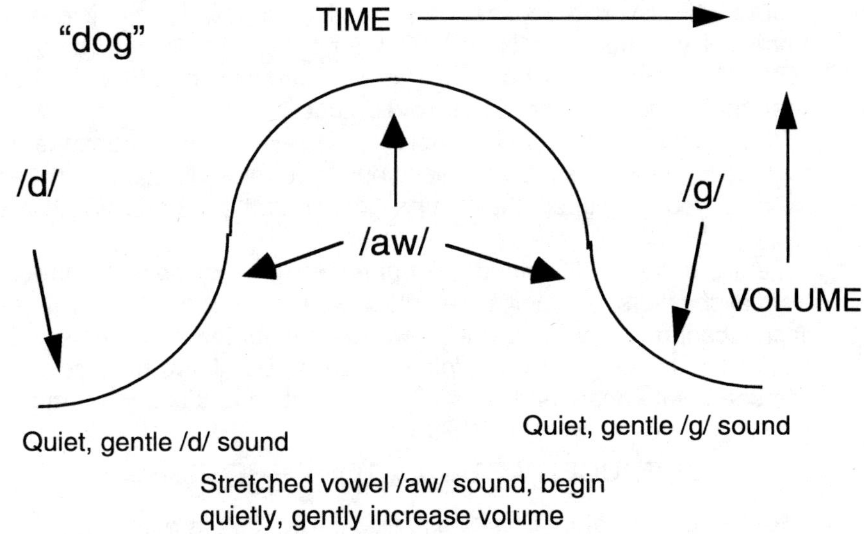

STRETCHED VOWELS & CONTINUOUS PHONATION

Note that the /d/ and /g/ consonants are short, but the /aw/ vowel is stretched. *Stretched vowels* are usually the most effective fluency technique.

With gentle onset, you stretched the first vowel of a phrase. With the stretched vowel target, you stretch all your vowels. Because your vocal folds vibrate to produce vowels, stretching your vowels keeps your vocal folds vibrating, and you don't stutter.

If you listen to a tape your stuttering, you may notice that you shorten the syllable before a stuttered block. You speed up to get a running start into a feared word. The result is a shortened vowel before you lock your vocal folds. Stretching vowels prevents shortening syllables, and prevents stuttering.

You can stretch your vowels a lot, so that you talk abnormally slowly. Or you can stretch your vowels a little, and talk at a "slow-normal" rate. The choice depends on how severely you stutter, and what therapy program you choose. Delayed auditory feedback (DAF) devices are highly effective in training the stretched vowel target.

Continuous phonation is like gentle onset and stretched vowels, but now you join your words together. This is also called "blending."

Start a phrase with gentle onset, stretch your vowels, and join your words. If you put your fingers on your throat, you'll feel that your vocal folds never stop vibrating. This is continuous phonation. If you keep this vibration going, you'll never stutter.

You have to stop vocal fold vibration to say voiceless consonants such as /t/, /p/, and /s/. If you keep your vocal folds vibrating for these sounds, you'll produce their voiced consonant partners, which are /d/, /b/, and /z/.

Gentle onset and continuous phonation are not normal speech. Normal speakers turn their vocal fold vibration on and off many times each second. You recall that we demonstrated this by saying "coffee" and feeling our vocal fold vibrations. But if you practice, you can use gentle onset and continuous phonation and sound normal.

REDUCED ARTICULATORY PRESSURE

Reduced articulatory pressure is also called "soft targets."

Lightly touch your tongue for the /t/. Lightly close your lips for the /b/. Keep your speech production muscles relaxed for all sounds.

The wrong way is to tense your lips and tongue and jaw too much, and hold this tension too long. This forceful speech leads to stuttering.

After you stretch and emphasize vowels, you must next de-emphasize consonants. If you stretch and emphasize vowels, and de-emphasize consonants, you should be able to speak fluently.

Is Slow, Relaxed Speech a Means or an End?

Non-speech motor learning is associated with increased performance speed. A tennis pro executes responses faster than a novice tennis player. But improvements in fluency result from decreased speaking rate. Why does a tennis pro move faster as she improves her game, but a stutterer speak slower as he improves his fluency? Ludo Max and Anthony Caruso (1998) investigated these contradictory hypotheses.

The researchers had eight adult stutterers read two 300-word passages. The first passage was read out loud solo six times. The second passage was read out loud in unison with a fluent speaker five times, and then solo five times.

The researchers then measured the speed of different aspects of speech production. These aspects included articulation rate, word duration, vowel duration, and consonant-vowel transition extent.

The sixth readings had on average 70% less stuttering than the first solo readings. The subjects also executed speech movements faster on the sixth reading:

> participants in the present study showed a statistically significant increase in articulation rate and a statistically significant decrease in word and vowel duration in their perceptually fluent speech during the sixth reading of a 300-word passage as compared to the first reading of the same passage. Additionally, for most participants, adaptation was also associated with reductions in the duration of word-initial consonant-vowel transitions.

This research shows that as fluency improves, stutterers talk faster, not slower. Why then do many stuttering therapy programs train stutterers to talk slower? And why do stutterers report that this slow, relaxed fluent speech is easy to do in the speech clinic, but they have difficulty using slow, relaxed speech outside the speech clinic?

Slow speech switches speech production from *open-loop* motor control to *closed-loop* motor control (see the chapter "Motor Learning Theory").

Open-loop motor control – used for normal speech — retrieves pre-programmed speech motor programs from long-term memory and executes them without sensory feedback. Open-loop motor control is fast and requires no attention or conscious mental effort — to paraphrase the Nike ads, you "just do it." The problem is that there's no error-correction — if you retrieve a defective speech motor program from memory, you'll execute the mistakes, and may not even be aware that you made mistakes.

Closed-loop motor control — what is taught in speech clinics — uses sensory feedback (what you hear, feel, or see) to control your muscle movements. The result is improved accuracy and the ability to produce unpracticed movements. You consciously control your muscles, and even severe stutterers can be 100% fluent under closed-loop motor control. The problem is that closed-loop motor control is slow, and requires mental effort and attention.

Stutterers report that slow, fluent speech feels abnormally slow, even when their speaking rate sounds normal. They report that they are easily distracted by the conversation and forget to maintain the slow speaking rate. This self-consciousness and unmaintainable mental effort is characteristic of closed-loop speech motor control — no matter how much you practice, closed-loop fluency will never become automatic and effortless.

The problem here is that speech pathologists and stutterers confuse the *associative* and *autonomous* stages of motor learning. The exercises and goals of these two stages are different, even opposite.

In the *associative* stage, you learn to perform a new motor skill. The goal of this stage is slow, mentally-concentrated performance. Whether you're learning a golf swing, to touch-type, or to speak fluently, you begin practicing slowly.

In the *autonomous* stage, you learn to perform the motor skills quickly and effortlessly. The goal of this stage is fast movement, without mental concentration.

Slow speech is the goal of the associative stage, but not the goal of the autonomous stage. You should work to master slow, fluent speech, but then you should increase the speed and decrease the mental effort until your speech is close to normal.

Slow speech enables you to learn fluent speech motor skills, such as integrated breathing and vocal fold movements. Using slow speech without practicing a motor skill is like hunt-and-peck typing — the result is a finished letter that may look acceptable, but you'll never develop into a smooth, fast, effortless typist unless you also practice the correct finger placements and other skills of touch-typing.

IS RELAXATION A GOAL OF STUTTERING THERAPY?

Relaxed breathing and speech-production muscles are another goal of the associative stage that is not a goal of the autonomous stage. Motor learning begins with relaxed, slow muscle movements, but as you improve your skill, you must increase both the speed and the intensity of execution:

> Performance should be at the maximal level at which the patient can be continually successful, and practiced at a level just below the peak of performance. Performance is improved only by successful near-maximal performance...the effort, speed or complexity [should] be increased to the point where failure occurs [and then diminished slightly for consistent success]. (Kottke, 1978; see also Doman, 1974)

This confuses stutterers because stuttering is characterized by overtense speech-production muscles (Starkweather, 1995). Relaxed speech feels good and sounds good. Listeners prefer slow, clear, relaxed speech (especially if English is not your or their first language). You should learn slow, relaxed speech. You may be so happy with this speech – at least at first – that you feel you have reached your goal of fluency.

But after you master slow, relaxed speech, you should work on increasing the speed and intensity of practice so that your fluency becomes automatic and effortless.

If you don't increase speed and intensity of practice, you won't develop motor programs that can be executed in automatic, effortless open-loop motor control. Your speech will be fluent when you remember to relax your breathing and vocal folds, but soon your attention will be distracted and you'll switch to open-loop speech motor control. Without the fluent speech motor programs in your memory, you'll retrieve your old stuttering speech motor programs.

Fluency-shaping stuttering therapy is not finished until you master the autonomous stage of motor learning — fast, automatic, effortless fluent speech. If you've mastered fluent speech at a slow speaking rate in the speech clinic, you're only halfway.

Pharmacist Richard Harkness stuttered severely until he was about 40. He overcame stuttering by practicing speech sounds and words, with prolonged sounds, loudly and forcefully, and abrupt phonation onset. After 2-3 weeks, he no longer stuttered. In the five years since, Harkness has remained fluent, although he does "refreshers" of his therapy every few months. (I'm not surprised at the effectiveness of Harkness' self-therapy, but other stutterers should not expect to develop fluency as rapidly as Harkness. Several months or a years is more realistic for most stutterers.)

Harkness emphasizes that his self-therapy produced automatic, effortless fluency, unlike some stuttering therapies (Harkness, 1996):

> Fluency shaping courses attempt to make you responsible for consciously controlling all the small details of synchronizing movements of the speech articulator muscles. That's not really feasible. That's the brain's job. The brain is designed by nature to take care of these details automatically. Plus, if you are constantly concentrating on the muscle movements, it's difficult to think about what you want to say.

For more information, see Harkness' website at http://members.aol.com/rharkn.

Problems With Fluency Shaping Therapy

Fluency shaping stuttering therapy is a form of "operant conditioning" (Kuhr, 1994). "Operant conditioning" is also called "behavior modification" or "Skinnerian conditioning" (after psychologist B.F. Skinner). The idea is to reward desirable behaviors, and punish negative behaviors.

There were a few experiments in the early 1960s with punishing stuttering behaviors, but these were soon abandoned*.

Fluency shaping programs teach you new behaviors, and then reward you for doing these behaviors. For children, the reward may be getting to pick a toy from the speech pathologist's treasure box. For adults, the reward is your speech pathologist saying that you did the behavior right. If you use a biofeedback device, the reward is a green light, and the punishment is a red light.

So far, operant conditioning makes sense, and is widely-practiced and respected.

But operant conditioning therapists also believed that a scientific approach should focus only on observable behaviors (such as breathing or vocal fold control), and must ignore internal, invisible psychological factors. This aspect of fluency shaping is now no longer endorsed.

Fluency shaping has a number of problems:

1) Fluency shaping is effective at producing fluency in the speech clinic, but too often the graduates relapse a few weeks or months after the program ends. Most of these therapy programs ignore motor learning theory, which could improve the retention of fluency techniques.

Some clinicians overstated the effectiveness of their programs. As other speech pathologists saw large numbers of graduates of certain programs relapsing to stuttering, these claims became questionable.

2) Fluency shaping therapies can produce abnormal-sounding speech, or fluency that is so mentally-demanding that you can't pay attention to both the conversation and your speech. The goal is use

---

* The delayed auditory feedback (DAF) effect on stuttering was discovered in one such experiment, by Israel Goldiamond. Hearing your voice delayed in headphones is annoying for people who don't stutter. Dr. Goldiamond set up an experiment in which he punished the subjects whenever they stuttered by switching on DAF in their headphones. To his surprise, the DAF caused his subjects to talk fluently. His subjects liked the punishment, and asked him to keep the DAF on! Dr. Goldiamond abandoned his punishment experiment, and instead explored why DAF eliminated stuttering.

this abnormal-sounding speech only in the clinic, and use normal-sounding spontaneous speech outside the clinic, but many stutterers never achieve this goal.

Fluency shaping therapy does not train normal speech. Non-stutterers use speech breathing, a fast speaking rate, switch their vocal fold vibration on and off many times a second, etc.

3) Fluency shaping therapies are boring, repetitive. You sit in a little room at the speech clinic, saying word lists over and over for hours. You do this for weeks or months before you see any results. A typical program costs about $2500, plus taking several weeks off from work and flying across the country may cost you several thousand dollars more.

4) Fluency shaping therapies are "one size fits all," but stutterers are heterogeneous (we're all different). Fluency shaping therapies teach everyone the same skills, going through the same exercises, regardless of age, severity, or individual needs.

Newly-graduated speech pathologists like using therapy programs that are highly-structured, with a manual showing what they should be doing each minute of the therapy session. But after a few years of experience, speech pathologists realize that different people have different needs, and prefer to tailor therapies for each individual.

Current thinking is that there are many subgroups of stutterers. For example, some stutterers also have language disorders. Some stutterers fear speaking, but others don't. Different stutterers have different therapy needs.

5) Stuttering therapies (both operant and otherwise) are based on little research. The bulk of research articles study controlled laboratory experiments, which can be done in an hour or two per subject. Therapy studies have too many variables to control. Long-term studies can cost one hundred thousand dollars or more. See the chapter "Effectiveness of Stuttering Therapies."

PERKINS' "FLUENCY CONTROLS AND AUTOMATIC FLUENCY"

William Perkins described how he and Richard Curlee developed their fluency shaping program (Perkins, 1992). Their clients could talk fluently in their speech clinic, but encountered problems with their speech outside the speech clinic.

Their clients tried to use the fluency-shaping speech outside the clinic, but soon found that practicing all the fluency skills demanded too much mental concentration and attention. They also found that to talk completely fluently, their speech sounded monotonous and droning. They said, "I'd rather stutter than talk like this."

> So subjects stopped controlling their rate and went back to speaking spontaneously. Then came the miracle. They felt and spoke like normal speakers — at least for a few hours, usually for a few days, sometimes for a few weeks, rarely for a few months, and only once for a few years. They had no control over this spontaneously fluent speech. They could not make it happen, and they could not prevent its disappearance. They called it "lucky fluency."

Perkins expected that this spontaneous, fluent speech resulted from the fluency shaping speech motor skills becoming habitual. His clients' spontaneous fluency didn't last. Perkins concluded that fluency shaping speech motor skills can never become automatic or permanently habitual.

Perkins then changed his therapy goals:

> …those who were most satisfied with therapy were those who found that they could use their fluency skills to warm up each day, and also have them available for emergencies. The remainder of the time they forgot about controls and spoke naturally. This made them vulnerable to some stuttering, but by facing up to their avoidances, stuttering progressively lost its sting. These clients gained confidence in their ability to speak out freely, even though that included stuttering occasionally.

Perkins differentiates two types of speech:

1) "Warm up" or speech exercises.

2) Spontaneous speech.

The "warm up" speech can sound abnormal, or require mental concentration, or involve an electronic device. None of these "downsides" matter if the "warm up" speech produces carryover fluency or improved spontaneous speech.

Perkins believes that no stutterer is ever cured. He concludes that you will have to practice "warm up" techniques every day, to continually improve your spontaneous speech.

Perkins points out that the key issue in fluency shaping stuttering therapy is why this fluent speech too often doesn't become habitual and automatic.

Stuttering Therapy Programs

This chapter describes a variety of currently-practiced stuttering therapy programs . There is no attempt to categorize them as "stuttering modification," "fluency shaping," "behavioral," "cognitive," etc. Most speech therapy programs incorporate a variety of elements.

Therapy programs are included in this chapter for a variety of reasons. The biggest programs — Hollins and Martin Schwartz — are included. Some small but innovative programs are included. Other programs are included because the clinician wrote a good description of what he or she does.

I'm not recommending these therapy programs, but rather presenting these therapy programs to show the variety of stuttering therapies available. The reader is encouraged to consider his or her needs and goals, and to investigate therapy programs further, before choosing a stuttering therapy program.

WEBSTER'S HOLLINS FLUENCY SYSTEM

The Hollins Fluency System™ is a "pure" fluency shaping program. It uses computer biofeedback devices. No desensitization of fears or anxieties is included.

The program was developed by psychologist Ronald Webster. Webster believes that the cause of stuttering is interference between bone- and air-transmitted perception of your speech (Hollins, 1993).

Hollins is an intensive residential treatment program. You work eight hours a day for 19 consecutive days. With over 3,900 graduates since 1972, it's one of the largest stuttering therapy program.

The Hollins program uses speech biofeedback computers to train fluency skills. The biofeedback computer monitors vocal onset. The computer also assesses your skill level as you move through the program. This computer analysis helps the speech pathologists determine how well you are progressing. The computer-based training leads to "reduced muscle tension levels."

The program also uses a biofeedback device to train diaphragmatic breathing.

In the first two weeks you learn fluency skills. Webster lists these as:

- Initial articulatory positions.
- Completion of articulation gestures.
- Diaphragmatic breathing.
- Control over laryngeal muscles.

In this stage, as "the stutterer is first taught to use an exceedingly slow rate of speech [using]...stretched syllable, smooth transition, slow-change, and full-breath targets...the stutterer learns to hold each syllable for two seconds." (Bloodstein, 1995) This is ten times slower than normal speech.

After mastering slow speech, you work on gentle onset. You read long lists of one- or two-syllable words, with the computer telling you if your vocal onsets were correct.

In the third week, you reduce the two-second stretch to faster, normal-sounding fluent speech. Then you work on transfer, first with telephone calls and then in shopping malls.

Hollins states that 90% of clients have "3% or fewer disfluencies" at the end of the 19-day program.

In a follow-up study of 200 graduates, an average of ten months after therapy, 72-75% of the graduates were fluent, in both reading and conversation. An additional 15% had improved fluency, compared to before therapy.

The cost of the therapy program is $3,195, plus your hotel and meal costs, travel to Virginia, etc. The Hollins program can be reached at (540) 362-6528.

The therapy is also practiced at other speech clinics, under the name Precision Fluency Shaping Program (PFSP). Be aware that the program could produce different long-term results depending on whether it is practiced intensively (eight hours per day for 19 days) or is done less intensively over a longer period (e.g., two weekly one-hour clinical sessions and an hour of homework each night, for a year). See the chapter "Motor Learning Theory."

SCHWARTZ'S INTENT THERAPY

The National Center for Stuttering in New York City is operated by speech pathologist Martin Schwartz.

Schwartz believes that "the physical source of all stuttering is a locking of the vocal cords." He believes that if you can reduce vocal fold tension before you start speaking, your speech will be fluent.

"Intent therapy" involves two intentions: the intent to rest, instead of speak; and the intent to start speaking slowly.

In this therapy he trains two physical techniques, three stress-reduction techniques, and three nutritional approaches (herbs to take and foods to avoid) .

Physical Techniques

The first physical technique is to relax your vocal folds, by using relaxed breathing instead of speech breathing. Schwartz trains you to "exhale just before speaking as if one were not going to speak at all but were simply quietly breathing. The passive airflow keeps the vocal folds apart and relaxed prior to speech."

This technique "subtracts" tension from your vocal folds prior to speaking. Schwartz believes that stutterers' have a critical threshold level for vocal fold tension. Once you go over the threshold, you go into the vicious cycle of stuttering.

You say the first word slowly. You use normal emotional inflection and intonation.

Then you pause. During the pause, whether you continue to exhale doesn't matter. Then you say the rest of the phrase as fast as you want. If the rest of the sentence is at a normal speaking rate, listeners don't notice that the first word is slow.

Schwartz likes to say that your fluency techniques are done before the sentence begins. The techniques subtract tension from your vocal folds before the start of a sentence. As you speak you can tense for a feared word in mid-sentence, and not enough tension is developed to reach the critical vocal fold locking threshold, and no stutter ensues. If you've done the techniques before you start talking, you don't need to use fluency techniques during talking.

If the first word has two or more syllables, say each syllable slowly, with equal time for each syllable. You can then go on to the rest of the sentence. You don't have to pause at the end of the first word.

The second technique is "low energy speech." This also reduces the tension on the vocal folds by lowering the air pressure beneath them. You use a "confidential" tone of voice, and you reduce your articulation muscle movement (you move your jaw, lips, and tongue less). This low-energy speech is only used in high-stress situations. Pretend you're Marlon Brando in *The Godfather*, confidently making "an offer you can't refuse."

Stress-Reduction Techniques

The three stress reduction techniques are:

• "Education and Demonstration," which shifts the stutterer's locus of control from external to internal during the speaking act.

• "Recalibration," which reduces the speed demands from

listeners.

• The "Bathtub Technique," which is a form of meditation using *affirmations* or positive statements. Examples include, "As I practice I become more and more relaxed," and, "My confidence is growing higher and higher each day."

Therapy Program

Schwartz prefers working with groups of up to fifteen stutterers. Group therapy increases stress and adds an element of competition. He prefers to work with a group all day, rather than one-hour sessions. The workshops are usually two days, followed by several months of follow-ups. The initial two-day workshop is $900. However, after the first day, if you are not satisfied you don't have to pay anything and any deposit is refunded.

The follow-up sessions cost four $300 monthly installments. You can choose to discontinue the therapy at any point and stop paying. The total cost is $2,100.

The first few hours involve learning relaxed breathing and the airflow technique. Then Schwartz introduces the "contract" exercise. You talk for one minute, and every time you block you have to pay $1. This may seem harsh, but Schwartz says that this motivates people and almost no mistakes are made. A rich young Texan once insisted that he pay Schwartz $50 for each disfluency!

"Contract" starts with one minute per day, then is gradually increased. For home practice, Schwartz suggests you throw your dollars out the window! He adds that the thought of this defenestration motivates people to devote complete attention to their speech.

Another exercise is called "toughening." This trains you to ignore the speed that other people talk, and maintain your own relaxed, comfortable speaking pace. In this exercise, your partner asks you a question, and in the middle of your answer, asks you a second question. You have to stop speaking in mid-answer, listen to the second question, and answer again, using your calm, relaxed speech. In the middle of your second answer, your partner interrupts with a third question, and so on.

Schwartz emphasizes daily practice for the first four weeks.

For the next four or five weeks, you do "nickel-and-dime practice." This refers to the many times in the day when you have five or ten minutes to spare. Examples are while driving or doing household chores. Here you practice saying strings of unrelated sentences, either out loud or silently. (Makes you wish you were schizophrenic, so you'd have someone to talk to.)

Schwartz uses a device called the "MotivAider" in this phase of the therapy. The device is something like a beeper, in that it vibrates at random intervals. Whenever it vibrates, you are supposed to pay attention to your speech and use your physical techniques.

For the last four or five weeks, Schwartz has his clients move up through a hierarchy of more-difficult speaking tasks. You begin with conversations on a simple or unemotional topic with people. For example, you could discuss baseball.

Next, you work on telling jokes. Lastly, you move on to debates, arguing with people about emotional subjects.

Schwartz writes:

> Many patients report that following the twelve-to-fifteen week period of basic training, the habit is both automatic and strong. But it is not always that simple. Patients' use of the technique is frequently compromised by the extreme stress associated with certain sounds, words, and situations…it is the elimination of these speaking fears and scanning behaviors, rather than the initial fluency produced by mastering the airflow technique, that signals the permanent result.

Schwartz employs a psychological technique called "systematic desensitization" to overcome these situation fears. You again work up through a hierarchy of more difficult speaking tasks. These tasks are tailored to the individual. A successful, but unmarried, automobile dealer stuttered most severely when meeting women socially. Schwartz took the man to a series of bars, and had the client buy drinks for and engage in short conversations with women. He began with a "bag lady" in a disreputable bar, whom he had no interest in and was completely fluent with, and then worked up to better locales and more attractive women.

If you fear saying your name, then Schwartz prepares a hierarchy of people to say your name to, from friends to strangers. He adds that you must say your name at least one thousand times.

12-36 months after completing Schwartz's program, about 95% of the clients that his staff contacted by telephone said that the program had been successful.

For more information, read *Stutter No More* (Simon & Schuster, 1991), by Martin F. Schwartz, or call the National Center for Stuttering at (800) 221-2483, or visit http://www.stuttering.com/, or write to 200 East 33rd St., New York, NY 10016.

SHEEHAN'S "APPROACH-AVOIDANCE" THERAPY

In the 1940s, behavioral psychologist Neal Miller tied strings to rats, and sent them scampering down a runway towards food. He measured how hard the rats pulled on the strings to get to the food. He called this force the "gradient of force."

He then put an electric shock at the end of the runway, instead of food. The rats scampered away from the electric shock, and Miller called this the "gradient of avoidance."

He put the food and the electric shock together at the end of the runway. The rats wanted to scamper to the food, but away from the electric shock. They ended up running back and forth in a narrow space somewhere in the middle of the runway. This was called the "approach-avoidance conflict."

This reminded psychologist Joseph Sheehan of stutterers' repetitions and prolongations. In 1953, Sheehan developed the theory that stutterers want to say a word, but also want to avoid the word.

Why would stutterers wish to avoid saying words? Sheehan suggested that stutterers dislike the listener, or fear certain words, or fear certain situations, or feel guilt or anxiety about the emotional content of our message.

Sheehan believed that "stuttering is not a speech disorder, but a conflict revolving around self and role, an identity problem." He based this view on the fact that most stutterers have difficulty saying their names, and that many stutterers are fluent when acting (Sheehan, 1970).

Sheehan developed a stuttering modification therapy program based the reduction of avoidance. First, in the "self-acceptance" phase, you are trained to accept yourself as a stutterer. You are encouraged to maintain eye contact with listeners, and discuss your stuttering with friends and acquaintances.

In the "monitoring" phase, you improve your awareness of what you do when you stutter.

In the "initiation" phase, you seek out feared situations, and feared words, and stutter openly.

In the "modification" phase, you stutter openly and easily. You let the listener know that you are having trouble with a word. You do a prolongation on the first sound of the word. You do a "smooth release" onto the next sound.

Lastly, in the "safety margin" phase, you develop a tolerance for disfluency.

Sheehan did not believe that stutterers could or should speak fluently. In his therapy, "No practicing of special techniques for achieving fluency are involved — only openness and honesty and a changing role of self-acceptance as a stutterer will lead to overcoming the tyranny of stuttering" (Culatta and Goldberg, 1995).

Sheehan's stuttering therapy is practiced at the University of California — Los Angeles (UCLA).

BREITENFELDT'S SUCCESSFUL STUTTERING MANAGEMENT PROGRAM

The "Successful Stuttering Management Program" (SSMP) is practiced by Dorvan Breitenfeldt and Dolores Rustad Lorenz at Eastern Washington University in Spokane, Washington. It's a three-week, intensive, residential group therapy program. The program is mainly stuttering modification therapy, emphasizing avoidance reduction.

The program begins with "confrontation of stuttering." The aim is to develop awareness of your stuttering, reduce use of avoidance techniques, and eliminate word and situation fears. The techniques are voluntary stuttering and stuttering surveys.

In a "stuttering survey," you go to a shopping mall, stop strangers, and ask them questions about their reactions to your stuttering. You stutter on purpose. You do 200-300 stuttering surveys in the program.

In the second phase, you learn the stuttering modification techniques: preparatory sets, cancellations, and pull-outs. This differs from other stuttering modification therapies, in which preparatory sets are learned after cancellations and pull-outs.

The second phase also includes changing your self-concept and lifestyle.

You also substitute continuents for plosives. You substitute /w/ for /b/, /s/ for /t/, and /z/ for /d/. For example, you say "wank" instead of "bank," and "zollar" instead of "dollar." You also add sounds with prolongations. For example, "water" becomes "oowater."

Other speech pathologists are skeptical of this technique (Dé Nil, 1996):

> this type of substitution behavior seems to go against the original philosophy of nonavoidance...the idea of teaching stutterers to substitute...strikes us as [an avoidance "trick"]...it may even strengthen clients' tendencies to scan ahead in anticipation of sounds that are feared

and should be avoided.

In the third phase, you transfer your new skills to face-to-face and telephone conversations. You are also encouraged to do voluntary stuttering.

One graduate of the SSMP writes (Carpenter, 1996):

> The "magic" of the program for me...was its emphasis on self-exploration and insight. It really challenges you to learn about yourself, your stuttering, and the "emotional side" of the disorder. Dr. B's most central technique [is] "advertising" that you are a stutterer.

MONTGOMERY'S TOTAL IMMERSION FLUENCY TRAINING

Catherine Otto Montgomery practices an "in-depth body/mind" fluency shaping stuttering therapy in New York City. She began her fluency specialization at the Hollins Communications Research Institute. She then developed her holistic treatment process.

Montgomery uses intensive treatment. 4 to 6 clients work for 8 hours per day, five days per week, for three weeks. The intensive therapy is followed up with telephone contact, evening group practice sessions, individual one-hour sessions, full-day "tune-up" sessions, or one-week refresher courses.

Montgomery believes that stuttering results from "miscoordinated speech-muscle movements." The program begins with retraining respiration, phonation, and articulation. She educates her clients about the physical speech mechanism. She states that her fluency techniques are "normal and natural," and do not result in "artificial" sounding speech.

Her training focuses on the internal, kinesthetic feeling of muscle movements. She does not believe in trying "to sound a certain way" or listening to your speech. She does not believe that biofeedback devices can improve muscle control.

The training begins with diaphragmatic breathing. This leads to vocal fold control. The stutterer "learns to coordinate his muscles and the result is fluent speech. Confidence comes from this base of knowledge and physical skill."

Montgomery believes that "people who stutter walk through life with far greater degrees of tension and tightness throughout the body than the rest of us." To reduce this tension, she trains "a form of body movement that looks similar to yoga. The client learns to release tension, open the chest and shoulders, lift the torso, align the head and neck, open and align the body to allow the speech mechanism full freedom of movement." The result is that the stutterer "has more energy, feels more powerful and more confident."

After the physical training, Montgomery works on changing "years of conditioned learning...[including] expectancy, fear, and avoidance...Unless this mental/attitudinal aspect is dealt with and somehow strengthened and changed, our client won't hold onto the newly-learned, fragile speech muscle coordination."

Montgomery believes that childhood stuttering begins when "excitement and anticipation," for example, of the first day of school, puts the child's "body and neurology...in high gear." The child stutters, and then goes into a fight-or-flight response. The child learns that saying his name, for example, produces the fight-or-flight response. By adulthood, this response is "strongly-conditioned."

Montgomery trains her clients to be aware "that we are in constant dialogue with ourselves...At the same time, we unconsciously create mental pictures or images that coincide with the thought process." She uses Neurolinguistic Programming (NLP) to consciously create new mental imagery or visualization. The stutterer "learns to visualize himself speaking with ease and confidence."

She also teaches her clients "a very simple form of meditation." The meditation produces an "alpha" state, "a deeper level of consciousness that allows our minds to be more open and receptive to the changes we are wanting to make."

In the third week of therapy, Montgomery takes her clients "to stores and restaurants and puts them on the telephone, literally to do hundreds of phone calls."

Montgomery also asks her clients "to take a look at the downside of fluency. How has he benefited from stuttering? What will he be giving up? What might his fears be about becoming a fluent speaker?"

In a 1989 study, "91% of 200 past participants surveyed reported that the program was highly worthwhile for them. About 81% reported a substantial increase in self-confidence. To me, these measures are much more meaningful than simple measures of fluency."

Total Immersion Fluency Training may be reached at 27 W. 20th St., Suite 1203, New York, NY 10011; (212) 355-7111.

DAHM'S GENERATING FLUENT SPEECH

Barbara Dahm's "Generating Fluent Speech" therapy trains stutterers to not

> monitor words and speech sounds…[in this program] their language development process is simplified and becomes subconscious. In addition, they learn to give up control of their speech muscles. Articulation becomes an automatic process that works efficiently at a rapid rate.
>
> Instead of trying to be fluent, Generating Fluent Speech students learn to detach themselves from the result of the activity of speaking…Without conscious effort, artificial monitoring of speech, and using intentional or subconscious controls, speaking becomes natural and effortless.

The therapy program also includes exercises training stutterers to "vibrate their vocal folds in an easy effortless manner." For those who need it, the program includes "extensive work on changing attitudes and beliefs."

In the chapter "Becoming a Speech Clinician," Ms. Dahm describes her 20 years treating stuttering, using Gestalt psychology and fluency shaping therapies.

The program is offered at the Stuttering Center of New Jersey, and Israel's Communication Therapy Institute (5 HaMa'apilim Street, Kfar Shmaryahu, Israel 46190; voice 972-9-506218; fax 972-9-561837; dahm@netvision.net.il).

PERSONAL CONSTRUCT THERAPY

One study found that even when therapies reduced stuttering to normal levels of fluency, stutterers maintained poor speech attitudes (Andrews, 1974). For example, stutterers continued to believe that there speech was worse than non-stutterers, or that they couldn't do things such as make presentations. A later study found that stutterers who improved their speech attitudes had better speech a year after completing therapy, as compared to stutterers who maintained poor attitudes (Guitar).

Personal construct theory (PCT) is used in a wide variety of psychological treatments, including some areas that have proven resistant to other forms of psychological therapy.

PCT assumes that your universe is the product of countless *bipolar personal constructs.* E.g., foods are fattening or not fattening, temperatures are hot or cold, etc. People can be tall or short, young or old, honest or deceptive; hard-working or lazy, etc.

You react to your environment according to your personal constructs. If you believe that you like people who wear glasses more than people who don't wear glasses, you'll react to a person wearing glasses differently from a person not wearing glasses.

George Kelly, the developer of PCT, believed that all personal constructs can be altered, and by doing so you alter your universe. PCT uses the repertory grid test and other tools to help you become aware of your personal constructs. You then work on role playing and other techniques to change your personal constructs.

PCT is used to treat stuttering in the United Kingdom. One method for eliciting personal constructs is to create a description of yourself, and then create a description of who you expect to be in five years. Or you describe yourself as a stutterer, and then describe what you'd be like if you didn't stutter. The differences in your self-descriptions point out personal constructs crucial to your stuttering. For example, assertive vs. shy, or popular vs. lonely.

You then consider how these personal constructs affect situations in your life. You work on imagining other ways you could handle these situations. PCT emphasizes the stutterer "releasing his imagination and discovering novel ways of helping himself to deal with the issues that confront him." (Botterill, 1987) For example, you could use role playing to imagine buying a bus ticket. You imagine different ways you could handle each step in the situation, and test out new strategies. You are trained to see "alternatives in situations" and "arrive at a choice" of actions from amongst the alternatives.

Instead of stuttering forcing you to react to situations in only one way, PCT shows that you always have alternatives. Kelly wrote that "no one needs to be completely hemmed in by circumstances; no one needs to be the victim of his biography" (Kelly, 1955).

Trudy Stewart compared two adults, after completing a stuttering therapy program. One man maintained his fluency, the other man did not. Using repertory grid analysis, she found that the "good maintainer" changed his personal constructs more than the "poor maintainer." The constructs included confidence, relationships, and worrying about speaking situations (Stewart, 1996).

The question "who would you be if you didn't stutter" is a good conversation topic at stuttering support groups. People initially say, "I'd be more successful at work," "I'd be more assertive with my husband and family," and other *negative* aspects of stuttering.

After 10 or 15 minutes, people start saying, "If I didn't stutter, I'd be less compassionate," "I would never have developed my writing talent," or "I'd be a less-interesting person." People realize that they chose a career in a "helping profession" (e.g., nursing or teaching), or they developed non-verbal skills, such as athletics or music, because they stutter. They then realize all the *positive* aspects of stuttering.

RICHARDSON'S INTERACTIVE FLUENCY TREATMENT PROGRAM

Marcelle Richardson's "Interactive Fluency Treatment Program" (San Diego State University) emphasizes cognitive psychology. Richardson states that, "Stuttering is viewed as a behavior that is responsive to an individual's beliefs and perceptions. As beliefs and perceptions change, so do the stuttering behaviors."

The "Interactive Fluency Treatment" program explores five cognitive areas:

1) Beliefs, or how you view yourself. Examples include, "I feel helpless when I talk," "I must be perfect in all performance areas," "If I just tried harder, I could control the stuttering," "I should hurry when I speak and not waste the listener's time."

2) Predictions, or beliefs in action. Examples include, "I've stuttered with this person, in this situation, or on this word before, I will stutter again."

3) Strategies, to cope with threatening communication situations. These strategies include avoidances, rehearsals, starters, circumlocutions, averting your eyes, or secondary symptoms such as head jerks.

4) Evaluation, or beliefs that reinforce your self-concept as a stutterer. Examples include, "I knew I would have difficulty and I did," "I stuttered and it was my fault," "If I would have done something better or differently, things would have turned out better."

5) Emotions, such as embarrassment, humiliation, anger, fear, anxiety, panic, and shame.

The program's procedures and activities include counseling, desensitization, peer guidance, contracting, role playing, visualization, charting, writing, and reading.

Psychological Self-Therapy

BE OPEN ABOUT YOUR STUTTERING

If you fear listeners finding out that you stutter, this anxiety partly causes your stuttering. If you tell people that you stutter, you'll be less anxious and stutter less.

Ironically, when you stutter severely you don't want to think or do anything about stuttering. But after you've made progress on your fluency, stuttering becomes easier to talk about.

Some people have a "fear of success" holding them back. You want to be successful, but you fear being visible and people seeing your faults. This fear is sometimes called "fear of success/fear of failure," because you are afraid that success will show people that you are also a failure. E.g., a better job would require talking to more people, and listeners would think you are a failure because you stutter.

Here are some suggestions for being open about your stuttering:

1) The National Stuttering Project used to have buttons that said, "If you stutter, you're not alone." The buttons were the final issue that forced John Ahlbach to resign after fourteen years as Executive Director. The board of directors said that few people wore the buttons, and were expensive to give away. John said that people *should* wear the buttons, and save themselves thousands of dollars of therapy.

2) Have your speech pathologist give you a few of her business cards. Ask her to write down one therapy technique on the back of each card. Give one of the cards to the listener, explain what the technique is (e.g., slow, relaxed speech), and ask the listener to hold up the card whenever you forget to use the technique. If you're making a speech, give the card to a friend in the front row.

3) Buy a roll of quarters. Tell people that you will give them a quarter every time they catch you stuttering. When I do this, I don't stutter.

4) Put stuttering on your business card. Geoffrey Mangers, of the San Jose NSP chapter, lists his specialties as "PC Instr & ATE • Software • Stepmotors • Stuttering." If you are an officer of your National Stuttering Project chapter, put this on your business card.

LISTENING SKILLS, REDUCING TIME PRESSURE

Listening is as important as speaking. Your listening affects your speech.

Don't interrupt people until they finish speaking. Let them finish what they're saying. This helps you eliminate the time pressure that makes stuttering worse. Also, people will like you more if you don't interrupt them.

TALK MORE

Jerry Vimont wrote on an Internet stuttering support group:

> I've been a stutterer for almost 30 years (I'm 36). There have been 2 times in my life when my stuttering literally went away — once when I was an Assistant Manager for a bowling center in the early 80s and now I'm an Assistant Manager for a Walgreens. Both have something in common. I'm required to speak so much that the vocalization starts to become a sub-conscious act. During periods of time when I wasn't required to speak so much, my stuttering increased. For some reason I would start to become more aware of my vocalization instead of it letting it be a subconscious act. The more I talk the less I'm aware of the vocalization and the less I stutter. It's that simple.

Many stutterers have developed careers and relationships which minimize talking. They may hardly talk at all outside the speech clinic. Developing fluent speech requires talking a lot — but how much is enough?

A variety of studies have been done on the learning of manual (hand) skills (Kottke, 1978). In one study, beginner cigar-makers worked three times slower than experienced cigar-makers. Becoming fully skilled required making 3 million cigars!

3 million repetitions were also needed for Japanese pearl handlers to become proficient. The Suzuki method of teaching violin-playing to children requires the production of about 2.5 million notes. Basketball, football, and baseball throws (and punts in football) require about a million practices. Gymnasts practice every day for 8 years to become proficient.

Normal speech produces over 10,000 syllables per hour. If you talk one hour per day for a year, you will produce over 3 million syllables. In other words, developing fluent speech probably requires about one hour per day talking with your therapy techniques, for one year.

My biggest breakthrough in fluency was at the 1994 American Speech-Language Hearing Association convention in New Orleans.

From 10 a.m. until 5 p.m., for three days, I showed my company's biofeedback devices to speech pathologists. I talked seven hours straight each day, staying on target to show how the biofeedback worked.

Each evening I put away the devices and went out with friends*. Every night I was fluent, without thinking about my speech. After the convention, I flew home and was so busy I didn't have time to unpack the electronic devices. I continued to talk fluently, without thinking about my speech, for several more days. Eventually my stuttering returned, but not as severely as before the convention.

You must use your therapy techniques correctly during practice time. "Failures do not result in learning" (Kottke, 1978). For practice away from the speech clinic, the stutterer should use an electronic speech biofeedback device to monitor his speech and alert him when his speech is "off-target" (as I did in New Orleans).

Many stutterers have jobs that require minimal talking, and hobbies and social lives that don't have much talking. Ask your supervisor for tasks that require talking. You could do volunteer work that requires talking. One of my customers volunteers at a hospital information desk every Saturday, directing people where to go.

BE MEAN TO TELEMARKETERS

A person on an Internet stuttering discussion group wrote:

> I have about a 100% success rate when I use prolongation during my therapy sessions, but I don't use it outside of therapy because I think people may think it's as weird as stuttering. I know that these thoughts are illogical. I mean, when I prolong on a word, it's so much easier to say...and much quicker. I just can't get over the "not quite normal" mindset.

To get over these feelings, exaggerate your stuttering therapy techniques with people you dislike, such as telemarketers.

If your speech therapist taught you slow-motion speech, talk really slowly. If your speech therapist wants you to "bounce" or do "voluntary stuttering," bounce or stutter on every word. Try to keep the telemarketer on the phone as long as possible by asking stupid questions.

Most stutterers are afraid of wasting listeners' time. They talk as fast

---

* Hint: when visiting New Orleans, call the local National Stuttering Project chapter and get a native to take you out!

as possible, which increases their stuttering. Stop thinking that you are wasting listeners' time by intentionally wasting a telemarketer's time.

Stuttering increases when you think you are inferior to the listener. Find people who are inferior to you — the people who interrupt your dinner trying to sell you something you don't want. Think of all the pain and suffering people have caused you because you stutter. Inflict that pain back onto telemarketers, switchboard operators, or anyone who annoys you.

OK, I doubt this idea will make it into an SFA brochure. But I'll bet that Joseph Sheehan would have liked it. Fred Dietrich also liked it:

> I used to have feelings of tension, anticipation and panic as I was flooded with thousands of mini-decisions to make before talking on the phone, just to reach some elusive "comfort" level. Then, in spite of all my preparations, the stutter would come, triggered by some new, uncharted factor I had not prepared for. Panic and fear would deepen.
>
> I discovered that the primary factor was the overpowering fear of what unseen horror was taking place on the other end of the call. I would project all manner of hideous reaction, ridicule, boredom, confusion and embarrassment that was undoubtedly affecting the listener, and I had no power to respond or even mitigate the impact on the unsuspecting caller.
>
> The breakthrough for me came when I accepted myself, recognized my own self-worth, and realized that *I* could control what was happening on BOTH ends of the conversation. Of course, it took a wide variety of techniques, materials and dialog, as well as a lot of assertive communication.
>
> The suggestion to "work-over" the telemarketing rep is an excellent one. Those creeps think nothing of disturbing your life, so they deserve anything you dish out. Think of it as a learning experience for them too, only this time *you're* the teacher. As you gain more experience, you'll be able to handle more phone calls with confidence.
>
> One of my software clients is a very nice doctor who stutters. When he would call for technical support, my staff was uneasy talking to him because it took so long and they were not sure he understood what they were telling him. Once, when they passed the call to me, I started by telling him that I was also a PWS. He immediately became calm and fluent, and we had a wonderfully smooth and warm conversation. He still stutters a lot if anyone on my staff answers, but is totally fluent talking to me.
>
> Now, I have a new problem. Yep, you guessed it, he is enjoying himself so much that he doesn't want to hang up. Oh sigh!

WRITE YOUR STUTTERING AUTOBIOGRAPHY

Write an autobiography of your stuttering, answering the following questions:

1) When did you begin to stutter? What is your first memory of stuttering? What stuttering behaviors did you have as a child?

2) Describe your parents and how they affected your stuttering.

3) Does anyone else in your family stutter?

4) What do you believe caused your childhood stuttering?

5) Describe stuttering therapy you've done.

6) Are there times or situations in which you stutter more, or less?

7) Describe feared words and speaking situations.

8) Do you use any "tricks" to get words out?

9) Has your speech affected your school or career choices or success?

10) Has your speech affected your relationships with people? Do you find social interactions difficult?

11) Describe any feelings of frustration, shame, or hostility associated with your speech.

12) Has your stuttering caused you more problems recently? Why do you now want to change your speech?

13) Lastly, describe your speech goals. How do you want to talk in ten years? Do you have a role model, someone you want to talk like?

This "autobiography" will be longer than you expect. You'll be surprised how big stuttering is in your life.

If you want to share your stuttering autobiography with others, the Stuttering Homepage has a section for such stories (http://www.mankato.msus.edu/dept/comdis/kuster/stutter.html).

IMPROVING AWARENESS OF STUTTERING

Videotape of yourself talking. Pick a 5-minute segment of the tape. Measure your stuttering (see the chapter "Measurement of Stuttering"):

1) Frequency of disfluencies, i.e., disfluencies per hundred words.

2) Duration of disfluencies. Time your three longest disfluencies with a stopwatch.

3) Speaking rate, or words per minute.

4) Types of primary disfluencies, e.g., repetitions, prolongations, and blocks.

5) Secondary behaviors, such head jerks, eye blinks.

Watching your videotape, transcribe every word and every sound you make.

• For repetitions, count the number of repetitions, and write all these down. If you have four repetitions on the word "car," write down "c-c-c-car."

• Time each prolongations with a stopwatch, and write down the time.

• For silent blocks, write "<block>".

• Write down every head jerk, facial grimace, eye blink, etc.

When you are finished, read back your transcription, repeating your stuttering exactly. Try to perform your stuttering exactly as you did on the tape.

Consider filling out the "Stuttering Severity Instrument for Children and Adults," by Glyndon Riley. ($79, Pro-Ed, 8700 Shoal Creek Blvd., Austin, TX 78757, 512/451-3246.)

Buy a pocket tape recorder (less than $30 at Radio Shack) and tape conversations. After a conversation, note how fluent you thought you were. Then listen to the tape and see if your perception matches reality.

Record conversations with and without therapy techniques. You should develop an ability to hear and feel when your voice is right or "balanced," versus when your voice is tense and fast.

POSITIVE COMMUNICATION SKILLS

Speech is only one aspect of communication. Non-stutterers can communicate poorly. By improving your non-verbal communication skills, you can become a better communicator than many non-stutterers.

A speech pathologist once told me to never say anything negative about myself. Don't tell people about stupid mistakes you made, or bad luck that happened to you. When you feel like saying something negative about yourself, think of something positive to say instead. An event may feel like a disaster, but later becomes minor and forgettable. Or it becomes laughable. Or the dark cloud has a silver lining.

Mention your stuttering. Making a *minor* revelation about yourself creates intimacy. If the person respects you, he or she will like you more for showing that you're not perfect.

Dale Carnegie's *How To Win Friends And Influence People* (1936, New York: Pocket Books) has given millions of people practical advice to improve their communication skills. His suggestions include giving praise and appreciation, and avoiding criticizing, complaining, or condemning; developing awareness of other people's needs; being a good listener; and respecting other people's opinions, even when you disagree. Stutterers can do the communication skills that Carnegie presents.

Effectiveness of Stuttering Therapies

THE REALITY OF RELAPSE

Two studies of "smooth speech" fluency shaping found that about 95% of stutterers were "very satisfied" or "satisfied" with their speech at the end treatment.

A year later, their satisfaction dropped to 43%.

- 41% said their fluency was good.
- 47% said their fluency was adequate.
- 12% said they were disfluent.
- 73% said they had experienced relapse of stuttering.

Of the 73% who'd experienced relapse, 93% said they'd overcome this relapse, 22% said the relapse was due to embarrassment of smooth speech, and 61% said the relapse was due to pressure to speak faster (Craig, 1991).

Howie (1981) found that all stutterers who had completed a 3-week intensive "prolongation technique" therapy program had "near normal" fluency, but one year later 40% reported relapse.

COMPREHENSIVE STUTTERING PROGRAM

Einer Boberg and Deborah Kully followed 42 stutterers (17 adults and 25 adolescents) for two years after therapy. All subjects completed the three-week intensive Comprehensive Stuttering Program at the Institute For Stuttering Therapy And Treatment (ISTAR) in Edmonton, Alberta, Canada.

The program is fluency shaping, based on slow, prolonged speech, starting with 1.5 seconds per syllable stretch, and ending with slow-normal speech. The program also works on reducing fears and avoidances, discussing stuttering openly, and changing your social habits to increase speaking. The program includes a maintenance program for practicing at home.

Boberg and Kully made considerable efforts to accurately measure fluency. For example, they included surprise telephone calls to the subjects at home or at work.

The therapy program reduced stuttering from about 15-20% stuttered syllables to 1-2% stuttered syllables.

12-24 months after therapy, about 70% of the stutterers had satisfactory fluency. About 5% were marginally successful. About 25% had unsatisfactory fluency.

Most speech pathologists and stutterers agree that these numbers seem right — the best stuttering therapy programs help 70-75% of stutterers.

In a self-reported questionnaire, 93% of the stutterers expressed satisfaction with their speech immediately after treatment. 12-24 months later, 80% of the subjects reported satisfaction. 85-90% said they could use fluency techniques control their stuttering or sound fluent. 96% said they were sometimes able to talk fluently without thinking about their fluency techniques.

Boberg and Kully offer five reasons for relapse after their therapy program:

1) Adult stutterers have difficulty adopting new attitudes and behaviors after years of embarrassment and frustration, and poor feelings of self-worth.

2) Stuttering is cyclical — the "good days and bad days" syndrome. (See the chapter "Conditions That Increase or Decrease Stuttering.")

3) Life can be stressful at times, negatively impacting upon stuttering.

4) Monitoring fluency techniques can require constant attention, at least for the first few weeks and months. People give up if the fluency skills don't become automatic and habitual.

5) There may be an undiscovered neurological cause of stuttering in some individuals, which is not corrected by therapy.

PROLONGED SPEECH

Onslow (1996) reported that in a "prolonged speech" fluency shaping program, all 12 subjects who stayed in the 2-3 year program achieved and maintained zero or near-zero stuttering. The program began with 2-3 weeks of intensive residential treatment (7 days a week in a speech clinic). The stutterers then moved to weekly visits until they'd achieved near-zero stuttering levels. The stutterers continued weekly therapy sessions for two years.

The study began with 18 subjects, but 6 dropped out. The dropouts were doing well in the program, but had other time commitments.

This study suggests that near-zero stuttering can be achieved by combining an intensive program with weekly maintenance.

The Australian government paid for the program. In the United States, the program would cost around $15,000 ($3,000 for 2-3 weeks of residential treatment; $12,000 for 150 weeks of one-hour sessions at $75-100 per hour). If you add your time lost from work, etc., the program might cost $30,000. It's not surprising that one-third of the stutterers didn't have time for this therapy.

THREE THERAPY AREAS AND SIX TREATMENT MODELS

Andrews and Craig (1988) reported that when stutterers in "intensive group therapy" mastered three areas:

- Fluent speech motor skills.
- Internal locus of control ("the extent to which a person perceives events as being a consequence of his or her own behavior").
- "Normal attitudes towards communication."

97% maintained fluency ten months later. However, no subject who failed on one of these was able to maintain fluency.

However, another study found that locus of control could not predict success in stuttering therapy or fluency two years after therapy. (De Nil, 1995)

Andrews, Guitar and Howie (1980) reviewed 42 studies and found "six common principal treatment models." These were, in order of effectiveness:

1) Prolonged speech.
2) Gentle onsets.
3) Rhythm.
4) Airflow.
5) Attitude therapies.
6) Systematic desensitization

OTHER STUDIES

Oliver Bloodstein's *A Handbook On Stuttering* reports dozens of studies of fluency shaping stuttering therapies, or therapies using fluency shaping techniques (slow speech, gentle onsets). Most showed good results, similar to Boberg and Kully's results (although some studies had questionable methodologies).

Bloodstein does not report any long-term studies of stuttering modification therapies, except for four studies of "systematic desensitization." These studies found that 50-75% of subjects were helped. One study found that stuttering was reduced on average 35-40%.

The general agreement among speech pathologists is that fluency shaping therapies produce better fluency, but stuttering modification therapies produce "better-adjusted" stutterers.

Some therapy programs claim 85%, 90%, even 95% success rates.

You should be skeptical of these claims. Too often this means that the stutterers are fluent in the speech clinic immediately after treatment, but no long-term study was done.

Sometimes such claims are implied but not stated. For example, one therapy program sends out videotapes showing people stuttering severely before treatment, and then shows them talking fluently two weeks later. This does not mean that the program has any long-term effectiveness, or that it will help you.

There are several reasons for the lack of stuttering therapy effectiveness studies:

1) Measuring stuttering is difficult (see the chapter "Measurement of Stuttering").

2) Some therapy programs help you reduce fears and avoidances. These are important parts of stuttering, but can't be measured scientifically.

3) Stutterers can be difficult to reach after treatment. Many stutterers are still embarrassed to talk about their stuttering even with the speech pathologist who treated them.

4) A careful therapy study costs about $100,000. There are no grants available for studying stuttering therapies, according to ASHA's list of grant-providing agencies. There are only a few grant sources for studying etiology (the nature and origin of stuttering).

THERAPY OUTCOME PREDICTIONS?

If most stuttering therapy programs only help 70-75% of stutterers, can speech clinics predict which stutterers will be helped and which will fail? No one has studied this. If this were possible, it would save stutterers a lot of time and money!

It would be interesting to see if the 25-30% of stutterers who are unsuccessful in one therapy program are also unsuccessful in other therapy programs. Eugene Cooper raised this hypothesis in his idea of "chronic perseverative stuttering."

My cynical view is that no speech clinic will ever turn away a stutterer willing to pay them several thousand dollars.

My other views are that:

• Severe physical stutterers fail therapy because they lack speech motor control to do the therapy techniques outside of the speech clinic. If they can develop improved motor control, they will be successful.

• Stutterers who fear listeners discovering that they stutter, and are unwilling to alter their speech or acknowledge that they stutter, will not benefit from stuttering therapy that does not change these attitudes.

• Stutterers who relapse after completing one stuttering therapy program should not repeat that program or do a "refresher," but rather should look at other stuttering therapy programs that will better suit their needs.

UNASSISTED RECOVERY FROM STUTTERING

Woodruff Starkweather (1996b) wrote,

> In my experience, the people who have succeeded in recovering from stuttering on their own have a more complete recovery than those who have recovered through therapy of any kind. This may be because they have taken responsibility for their recovery

or because different therapies work for different people.

Patrick Finn studied 14 adults who recovered from stutterers without therapy (Finn, 1996). Their average age was 47, with a range from 24 to 74 years old.

8 of the ex-stutterers were men, and 6 were women. Finn also studied 14 men of similar ages, who have persistent stuttering. He did not comment on the sex ratio, but it's interesting that so many women had recovered from stuttering.

Finn found the following factors contributing to recovery from stuttering:

• 79% of the ex-stutterers reported using a modified speech pattern. This broke down into 55% speaking more slowly; 55% altered "speech formulation," including thinking before speaking, substituting words, or rearranging the word order of a sentence; 46% altered their breathing, including diaphragmatic breathing or exhaling slightly on the first sound; 27% paused before speaking, or paused and then repeated a stuttered word; 18% spoke in a rhythmic manner; 9% affected a different accent; and 9% worked on public speaking.

• 43% reported motivation to improve their speech. Some described an event that was a turning point.

• 28% reported an environmental change. This included moving away from home or family, or a change in occupation.

• 28% reported a change in attitude towards self. This included changing self-image and self-esteem.

•14% reported a change in attitude towards speech. This also included being open about stuttering, or judging stuttering as less formidable or uncontrollable.

• Other factors mentioned included two people learned to play a wind instrument (a trumpet and a trombone), being prepared in speaking situations, and practicing speaking.

The subjects expressed opinions on the effectiveness of stuttering therapies. Four subjects had received "nonsystematic" stuttering therapy, such as a doctor giving advice. Three of the four said this was ineffective, and the fourth said that any improvement was indirect. Eight subjects had completed a systematic stuttering therapy program. Half of these subjects said the therapy had no effect. One subject said he experienced temporary improvement in his fluency. The other three subjects said that any improvement was indirect.

In another study, Finn (1997) found that listeners were generally (but not always) able to judge whether an adult had recovered from stuttering without therapy, or had never stuttered.

Computers and Electronic Devices for Treating Stuttering

This chapter is available on a 60-minute video.

MASKING AUDITORY FEEDBACK

White noise masking reduces stuttering 35% at 85 dB to 55% at 90 dB (Kalinowski, 1993; Stager, 1997). Increased volume appears to improve fluency. 85-90 dB noise should not cause hearing damage (Dewar, 1979). An old hypothesis was that stutterers don't stutter when they can't hear themselves speak. This doesn't make sense, because many stutterers experience silent blocks. Also, stutterers anticipate stuttered words before they hear themselves speaking.

Sine wave masking appears to be more effective than white noise masking, at lower volumes. A 125-Hz sine wave mimics vocal fold vibrations, and so may fool your brain into thinking that your vocal folds are vibrating. This technology was used in the Edinburgh Masker device in the early 1980s. The device reduced stuttering without training, mental effort, or abnormal-sounding speech. Unlike DAF and FAF, MAF can pull stutterers out of silent blocks.

A large study followed 67 Edinburgh Masker users for six months. 82% of the subjects said the device continued to be highly effective. 67% said that, "as the result of using the device, their unaided speech fluency had improved" (Dewar, 1979). The average volume was 78 dB.

Other users reported that their stuttering diminished or disappeared over time:

> I am in contact with over 500 people who use or have used the Masker [out of 2500 devices sold]. In most cases the end result is the person uses the device less and less as time passes due to less need for it…[a person who does not experience carryover fluency] is exceptional. (Goldberg, 1994)

The Edinburgh Masker did not train therapy techniques. Instead, the carryover fluency may have been due to reduced fears and anxieties. E.g., a stutterer may have feared using telephones, but when using an Edinburgh Masker, he was not afraid of telephone calls. When he discontinued using the device, he no longer experienced fear and anxiety on telephone calls. The Edinburgh Masker can't teach you how to talk fluently or make you forget *how* to stutter, but it could help you forget *when* to stutter.

DELAYED AUDITORY FEEDBACK

Delayed auditory feedback (DAF) delays your voice to your headphones a fraction of a second. Six studies found the following % reductions in stuttering:

				Delay (milliseconds)				
Study	Task	*n*	Time	4	25	50	75	195
Webster 91	Reading	6	20	28%				
Kalinowski93	Reading	9	1			55%		
	Reading, fast	9	1			83%		
Sark 1996	Reading	14	3		50%	71%	75%	
	Reading, fast	14	3		50%	76%	76%	
Brenaut1995	Telephone	7	4				34%	
Zimmerman	Telephone	9	2				59%	
Stager 1997	Reading, slow	10	2					85%
Average	All studies	55	4	28%	50%	71%	62%	85%
Average	Reading	39	4	28%	50%	71%	76%	85%
Average	Telephone	16	3				47%	

n is the number of subjects.

"Time" is average speaking time per subject with DAF, in minutes.

Webster (1991) tested ten delays between 3.31 and 5.56 milliseconds, for two minutes each.

Brenaut's (1995) subjects made ten telephone calls to businesses using DAF. Total speaking time was not noted, but was probably double the speaking time of Zimmerman et al. (1997). The authors miscomputed the stuttering reduction. They averaged the seven subjects' stuttering frequencies with and without DAF, then computed the stuttering reduction. It is more accurate to compute the stuttering reduction for each subject, and then average these.

Zimmerman et al's (1997) subjects made five telephone calls to businesses using FAF. Each call required asking three questions, or about two minutes total speaking time with FAF. Zimmerman has a typographical error for mean stuttering frequency under FAF. The correct mean in 12.8.

49 is the total number of individuals in the nine studies, not the average number of individuals per study.

These studies suggest that stuttering is reduced as delay length increases. Delays in the 50- to 75-ms range reduce stuttering on average 60-80%, at normal and fast speaking rates. A 195 ms delay appears to be only slightly more effective than a 75 ms delay, with an undesirable 60% slowing of speaking rate.

DAF appears to be slightly more effective when subjects are instructed to talk fast, which is a more stressful speaking situation. But DAF appears to be less effective on telephone calls to strangers than in reading. This suggests that DAF is more or less effective under different types of stress.

The above studies were done without training or speech therapy. DAF is also widely-used in stuttering therapy programs. Longer delays (90-220 milliseconds) are used, and the stutterer is trained to stretch his vowels and slow his speaking rate. This can almost 100% eliminate even severe stuttering, but can sound robotic or emotionless. After mastering fluency at very slow delays, the device is adjusted to faster delays, which increases speaking rate, until fluency at normal speaking rates is mastered. DAF therapy is effective for school-age children (Ryan, 1995) and adults (Ryan and van Kirk, 1974).

DAF is also a preferred treatment for cluttering.

FREQUENCY-SHIFTED AUDITORY FEEDBACK

Frequency-shifted auditory feedback (FAF) shifts the pitch of your voice in your headphones, typically one-half octave up or down. Like DAF, this immediately reduces stuttering about 60-80%, at normal and fast speaking rates, without training or mental effort.

The effect of FAF on a stutterer, and what FAF sounds like to the user, can be heard at http://www.ecu.edu/csd/audio.html.

FAF is usually combined with DAF for increased effectiveness, especially with severe stutterers. For example, if a stutterer only gets a 60% reduction on stuttering from DAF alone, he may get an 80% reduction in stuttering using DAF and FAF.

One advantage of FAF over MAF and DAF prosthetic devices is that FAF interferes less with one's hearing. A wearable anti-stuttering device should switch on when you talk, and switch off when you stop talking. No device will do this perfectly in every condition (e.g., when you whisper or talk loudly; if you're in a quiet office or a noisy concert). Also, some people talk while you are talking. When a masking device switches on, you can't hear anything but the masking tone. DAF is better because, with a well-designed microphone, it picks up background noise at a lower volume than your voice, but hearing speech and sounds twice makes hearing difficult. FAF has the advantage that even if the microphone picks up background noise,

you hear in real-time, so there is less interference with your hearing.
The effectiveness of FAF is supported by a review of eight studies.

				Octaves					
	Task	*n*	Time	+1	+0.5	+.25	-.25	-0.5	-1
K	Reading, normal	9	1		62%				
	Reading, fast	9	1		81%				
H	Reading, normal	14	4	70%	68%			69%	71%
	Reading, fast	14	4	71%	72%			69%	72%
B	Telephone calls	7	4					79%	
S	Reading, normal	12	4		59%	53%	53%	65%	
	Reading, fast	12	4		58%	38%	38%	54%	
Z	Telephone calls	9	2					60%	
I	Reading	3	25	80%					73%
	Monologue	3	73	60%					55%
A1	Public speaking	9	3					74%	
A2	Reading	12	10			47%	35%		
	Monologue	12	10			10%	11%		
H	Reading, adults	8	3		66%				
	Reading children	8	3		39%				
Av	All studies	93	11	70%	63%	37%	34%	67%	68%
Av	Reading	66	60%						
Av	Monologue	15	34%						
Av	Public Speaking	9	74%						
Av	Telephone calls	16	70%						

Notes: K = Kalinowski (1993); H = Hargrave (1994); B = Brenaut (1995); S = Stuart (1996); Z = Zimmerman (1997); I = Ingham (1997); A1 = Armson (1997); A2 = Armson (1998); Howell (1999); Av - Average

n is the number of subjects.

"Time" is average speaking time per subject with FAF, in minutes.

Hargrave et al.'s (1994) and Stuart et al.'s (1996) subjects read about one minute for each of four FAF settings at a normal speaking rate. The procedure was repeated at a fast speaking rate, for a total of eight minutes speaking with FAF.

Brenaut et al. (1995) used FAF combined with 13-millisecond delayed auditory feedback (DAF). Subjects made ten telephone calls to businesses using FAF. Total speaking time was not noted, but was probably double the speaking time of Zimmerman et al. (1997).

Zimmerman et al's (1997) subjects made five telephone calls to businesses using FAF. Each call required asking three questions, or about two minutes total speaking time with FAF.

Ingham et al. (1997) data is for subjects F.G., A.G., and E.O.

This review suggests that stuttering decreases as FAF pitch-shift increases, although most of the effectiveness is reached by one-half octave. Upshifts and downshifts seem to be equally effective (the one-octave downshift may be slightly less effective because of poor bass response in headphones).

FAF is effective for reading, public speaking, and telephone calls. Armson et al. (1997) found that FAF was equally effective in public speaking to audiences of two, four, and fifteen persons. This suggests that FAF effectiveness is not related to the difficulty of a speaking situation.

FAF appears to be less effective in monologue speaking tasks. With only three subjects, Ingham et al. (1997) could be anomalous. Armson and Stuart (1998) used a quarter-octave frequency shift, instead of Ingham et al.'s full-octave frequency shift. The result was an average stuttering reduction of 26%, with the standard deviation at 38%. The less-effective quarter-octave pitch shift produced effects within the variance of the data, so the greater effectiveness in reading could be anomalous.

THE FLUENCY MASTER

The Fluency Master is a hearing-aid size device. The device picks up your vocal fold vibrations via a microphone contacting your skin. It amplifies your vocal tone and provides the sound to your ear. Ronald Webster, the developer, believes that the device reduces stuttering by modifying how your hear your bone-transmitted voice. A study of 21 adult stutterers found that stuttering in conversations was reduced on average 14%. Webster then provided 10-12 hours of fluency shaping therapy, and the device reduced stuttering on average 38%. He did not have a control group do the therapy without the device. Although the average effectiveness was not great, some individuals found the device/therapy combination to be effective. He adds that, "several stutterers have been using the devices for three to four years with no decrease in the fluency effect." (Webster, 1991)

METRONOMES

Stager (1997) found that speaking with a metronome 100%

eliminated stuttering in all 10 subjects, at a very slow 92 syllables per minute (about three times slower than normal speech).

The Pacemaster is a hearing aid-size metronome. Franklin Silverman reported that the effectiveness "wore off" after he used the device several years. Other stutterers have reported using the PaceMaster effectively for many years. The clicking stays on all the time (it doesn't switch off when you stop talking).

Three hypotheses have been proposed why metronomes reduce stuttering:

• Slowing your speech. Two studies found that metronomes could make stutterers talk faster than normal speaking rates. Stuttering was decreased at the fast speaking rates, although not as much as at the slower rates.

• "Syllabification," or breaking up speech into separate syllables reduces stuttering. This "less complex motor plan" may reduce mental demands.

• "Rhythmicity." One study found that a rhythmic metronome beat reduced stuttering, but an arhythmic (irregular) beat did not reduce stuttering.

BRAIN SCAN RESEARCH ON AAF

Aerodynamic measurements (Stager, 1997) revealed that volume, air pressure and air flow increased with white noise masking; stayed relatively constant with DAF; and decreased with a metronome. Vowel duration increased with DAF and the metronome; but was constant with white noise masking. This suggests that fluency is increased when air pressure, air flow, and volume are reduced and vowel duration is increased.

The decreased speaking rate with 195 ms DAF and metronome suggests that these devices force the stutterer to use closed-loop speech motor control. Closed-loop motor control can eliminate stuttering, but produces abnormally-slow speech (see the chapter "Motor Learning Theory").

These physiological changes don't explain the effectiveness of altered auditory feedback at normal and fast speaking rates. Electroencephalograph (EEG) brain scans found that DAF and FAF immediately correct the abnormal cerebral activity associated with stuttering (Kalinowski, 1997). Because this research is new, the following model should be seen as tentative.

Brain scan studies have found decreased central auditory processing during stuttering (Wu, 1995; Fox, 1996; Ingham, 1997).

Any noise should increase blood flow to central auditory processing, explaining the (limited) effectiveness of white noise masking.

Braun et al. (1997) found decreased activity in the area that integrates auditory and somatic (body sensation) processing. The researchers concluded that stuttering involves reduced sensory processing, and reduced transmission from sensory areas to language areas.

Auditory processing is one of the fastest brain functions, capable of detecting events of only a few milliseconds duration. Areas of conscious control — including language processing — operate more slowly, taking over 100 milliseconds to execute an event (Shea et al. 1993). A 50-millisecond delay can be detected by the auditory processing and integration areas, but is not detected by the language processing areas. In other words, auditory processing and integration areas will notice speech that is heard 50 milliseconds out of sync with speech-production muscle proprioception. Blood flow should increase to these areas, correcting the abnormally-low blood flow found during stuttering.

But a short delay is undetectable by consciousness and language areas, so speech is not interrupted. The increased sensory information may be used for improved speech motor control.

Similarly, FAF is detected by auditory processing and integration, but not by language processing. E.g., if a person walks up to Bob and says, "Hi, Bob," and doesn't say, "Hi, Peter," the person's language areas won't find anything wrong.

When masking auditory feedback synthesizes a sine wave at the frequency at which the person's vocal folds vibrate, the person's brain hears phonation, but doesn't feel the sensation. This should also increase neurological resources to auditory processing and integration, and also explain why sine wave masking appears to be more effective than white noise masking (Dewar et al., 1978; Kalinowski et al. 1993).

Speculatively, altered auditory feedback introduces subtle errors detected by certain areas of the brain, increasing cerebral blood flow to those areas, but the errors are not detected by other areas of the brain, and so don't disrupt those functions.

CAFET AND DR. FLUENCY BIOFEEDBACK DEVICES

The Computer-Aided Fluency Establishment and Trainer (CAFET) and Dr. Fluency are computer-based stuttering biofeedback systems for clinical use. Both provide similar hardware:

• A chest strap to monitor breathing. Dr. Fluency uses two chest straps, to differentiate diaphragmatic (relaxed) breathing from thoracic (upper chest) breathing.

• A microphone to monitor vocal volume, as a surrogate for vocal fold activity.

You see your breathing and your vocal volume displayed on the computer screen, along with instructions or error messages.

The computer systems train similar speech motor skills:

1) Relaxed, diaphragmatic breathing.

2) Continuous breathing. The computer alerts you if you hold your breath more than 1/3 of a second.

3) Gradual exhalation, as opposed to the rapid, uncontrolled exhalation associated with stuttering.

4) Pre-voice exhalation, or letting a little air out before you begin tensing your vocal folds.

5) Gentle onset, or gradually increase vocal volume. The computer alerts you if your vocal volume changes too rapidly. The computer also alerts you if your voice is too quiet for your air flow (which sounds breathy).

6) Continuous phonation. Breaks in vocal volume are shown on the computer monitor.

7) Adequate breath support. The computer alerts you if you continue to talk after the point at which you should take another breath. Stutterers too often try to finish a phrase with insufficient air in their lungs.

8) Phrasing. Each of the above seven speech targets is taught first with vowels, then progressing to monosyllabic words, then to marked-length phrases. Stutterers too often pause to breathe at feared words or when they run out of air, rather than pausing to breathe at linguistically-appropriate points.

An unpublished study of the CAFET program with 197 adults and teenagers found that 82% met fluency criteria six months after completing the program; 89% were fluent after 12 months; and 92% were fluent 2 years post-therapy. Nearly every client reported satisfaction with the therapy. The criteria for fluency was three or less disfluencies per minute, a speaking rate of 175-200 syllables per minute, and normal intonation and volume.

The CAFET and Dr. Fluency provide the following advantage over non-instrument-based stuttering therapy:

• The computer provides instant, accurate information on what you are doing right or wrong. According to motor learning theory, fast, accurate *knowledge of results* is the most important factor in learning motor skills. A speech pathologist can't give you as precise or fast feedback.

• The computers are always paying attention, and never get tired of helping you practice.

• The computers provide step-by-step instructions. Dr. Fluency has animated graphics showing what your speech muscles should do for each exercise.

• With the computer training the physical speech motor skills, the speech pathologist can spend more time on the psychological aspects of stuttering.

• If you learn *visually* rather than *aurally*, you may learn faster with the computer displays than by listening to your speech on a tape recorder.

• Dr. Fluency is designed for home practice use as well as clinical use. According to motor learning theory, practicing one hour per day is optimal. Practicing more hours per day or fewer days per week produces poorer results in the long run.

ELECTROMYOGRAPHY (EMG)

Electromyography (EMG) measures muscle activity via electrodes taped to your skin. The device directly shows what your speech-production muscles are doing. Several studies have found EMG to be effective in treating stuttering (Craig, 1982; Manschreck, 1980).

A large study compared stuttering therapy with speech pathologists to stuttering therapy with EMG biofeedback computers. One year after the therapy ended, 48% of the children from the clinician-based program were still fluent. 71% of the children from the EMG computer-based program were still fluent (Craig, 1996). See the subsection “Effectiveness of Therapies” in the chapter “School-Age Stuttering Therapies.”

Electromyography is not widely-used because the devices are expensive ($600 to several thousand dollars); you have electrodes taped to your throat and face, so you can't use the device in public or for quick telephone calls; placing the electrodes requires training; and the electrodes don't work well on people who are fat or wear beards.

CASA FUTURA TECHNOLOGIES DEVICES

Casa Futura Technologies makes three devices:

• The Desktop Fluency System provides DAF, FAF, and MAF. It

has a "gentle onset" monitor. It also provides vocal tension biofeedback, training you speak with relaxed breathing and relaxed vocal folds. The device monitors vocal tension via the frequencies in your voice. An electromyographic biofeedback option is available to monitor specific muscle activity. The biofeedback display is five green, yellow, and red lights. The device plugs into telephones, or can be used in a speech clinic or for home practice. It is the size of a paperback book.

• The Pocket Fluency System provides FAF and MAF. A Lycra/Velcro neckband holds a throat microphone and the earphone wires. The neckband looks like part of your collar when worn with a t-shirt, or is hidden when wearing a dress shirt. FAF is used because it causes minimal hearing interference. A masking manual button is provided to pull stutterers out of silent blocks. Wireless hearing aid-style earphones are also available.

• The School DAF is a budget-priced portable DAF device for school speech pathologists.

Two university studies tested the Desktop Fluency System on telephone calls. In the first, 7 adults made 30 calls each, with and without the device. With combined DAF and FAF, the device reduced stuttering on average 79%, with a range from 53% to 100% (Brenaut, 1995).

In the second study, 50 ms DAF alone reduced stuttering 59%. FAF alone reduced stuttering 60% (Zimmerman, 1997). Combined DAF/FAF wasn't tested, but choosing DAF or FAF (whichever was more effective), the device reduced stuttering on average 73%.

ANTI-STUTTERING TELEPHONES

As noted above, the Desktop Fluency System plugs into telephones. Anti-stuttering telephones can be highly useful:

• Some stutterers only have problems on telephone calls. They are able to handle face-to-face conversations in one way or another. If a stutterer only wants to improve his speech on telephones, or if his employer only cares about his speech on telephone calls, there is little reason to spend $2500+ and weeks of effort on stuttering therapy, especially considering the 25-30% failure rate of most therapy programs. A $500 anti-stuttering telephone solves the problem more effectively.

• Most stutterers find it difficult to set aside time every day to practice therapy techniques. An anti-stuttering telephone can help the stutterer use therapy techniques on every call (such as slow speech or relaxed vocal folds). Most people spend an hour or more on the telephone each day, so no additional practice time is needed.

• Doing your therapy practice on telephone calls randomizes when you do therapy practice, and the length of time for each practice session. Regularly-scheduled therapy sessions may be best for developing new fluency skills in the associative stage of motor learning, but a randomized practice schedule should be more effective to make fluency skills automatic in the autonomous stage of motor learning.

• If a stutterer does therapy practice alone, he'll develop his ability to talk to himself fluently — hardly a useful skill! Therapy practice should be done in real conversations, such as telephone calls.

USING A DEVICE WITH THERAPY

In 1974, on the occasion of his retirement, Charles Van Riper speculated on the future of stuttering therapy. He predicted the development of a stuttering biofeedback computer that would make "adult stutterers completely fluent after just a few hours." The stuttering biofeedback computer would monitor "air pressure in the mouth and trachea, tension and gamma loop mistiming," and reward or punish the stutterer for performing correct or incorrect muscle movements.

After training with the clinical stuttering biofeedback computer, the stutterer would wear a portable version. After a month, stutterers would be cured! Van Riper predicted that some stutterers would refuse to wear the device, and that speech pathologists would oppose use of the device. He expected development of this stuttering biofeedback computer to take 75 years (Van Riper, 1974).

Van Riper wrote that to be cured of stuttering, you must do three things:

1) You must become "desensitized" to fears and anxieties about stuttering.

2) You must learn the motor skills of fluent speech.

3) You must spend a month using these fluent speech motor skills correctly, with your speech constantly and accurately monitored, with rewards and punishments for correct and incorrect speech.

I add a fourth point: you must talk a lot! Too many stutterers have jobs, hobbies, and relationships that require minimal talking. In my experience, you must talk at least 6 hours a day for fluent motor skills to become automatic. You should ask your employer for new job responsibilities, such as calling customers, or develop a new interest that requires talking.

Psychologists in the field of motor learning theory define three stages in learning a motor skill:

1) In the *cognitive stage*, you learn how the motor skill is performed and its objective, usually by watching someone else.

2) In the *associative stage*, you learn to perform and refine the motor skill.

3) In the *autonomous stage*, the motor skill becomes automatic and effortless.

The CAFET and Dr. Fluency effectively train the cognitive and associative stages of fluent speech motor skills. They are Van Riper's stuttering biofeedback computer, except that the training takes weeks, not hours (and you don't get electric shocks for punishment!).

Many stutterers learn to speak fluently in the speech clinic, but lose control of their speech in real-world conversations. DAF, FAF, and MAF devices enable these stutterers to use their fluency skills anywhere. They should turn off the device for short periods and continue to use their fluency skills, and then gradually increase the time with the sound off, until they no longer need the device.

Van Riper predicted that using a portable stuttering biofeedback computer to monitor your speech would cure stuttering in a month. My company's Desktop Fluency System monitors your speech on telephone calls. I leave it on my telephone, and over several years, my fluency off the telephone has gradually improved.

Some of my customers have reported similar results, but most seem to prefer DAF rather than the vocal tension monitor. They want a device that makes them talk fluently — the device telling them if they are using therapy techniques correctly is secondary.

The lesson I get is that stutterers want gradual change. Van Riper may have been right that stuttering can be cured in a month, but stutterers don't want to be cured that fast. Many stutterers say, "I'm not looking for a quick fix." Stuttering is a deeply-learned, complex, life-long condition. Stutterers are comfortable gradually improving their fluency over a few years. My customers like using my devices for immediate fluency, and then using fluency techniques with the devices, and gradually their speech without the device improves.

THIRD-PARTY PAYMENT

Most Americans can get help paying for an anti-stuttering device:

• If you're looking for a job, vocational rehabilitation programs are your best bet. Look in you telephone directory's blue government pages for your state's department of labor. Voc rehab will pay for whatever, therapy, device, or job training you need.

• If you already have a job, the Americans with Disabilities Act may help you. See the chapter "Stuttering and Employment."

• See the chapter "Telephone Advice" for state programs that may give you an anti-stuttering telephone device, or visit http://www.casafuturatech.com/Catalog/stedp.html.

• The Individuals with Disabilities Education Act (IDEA) helps children with disabilities. Ask your child's school principal or speech pathologist.

• The IRS allows you to deduct speech therapy equipment on Schedule A, if your total medical expenses exceed 7.5 percent of your adjusted gross income.

STUTTERING LAB DEVICES

For an extensive review of devices that measure aspects of stuttering, for research purposes, see "Instrumentation For The Assessment And Treatment Of Stuttering," by Klaas Bakker, in *Nature and Treatment of Stuttering: New Directions*, edited by R.F. Curlee and G.M. Siegel (Bakker, 1996).

COMPANY CONTACTS

Casa Futura Technologies
DAF, FAF, MAF, and stuttering biofeedback devices for clinical, home practice, telephone, and pocket use, $300-700.
P.O. Box 7551, Boulder, CO 80306-7551
(888) FLU-ENCY; fax (303) 417-9752
http://www.casafuturatech.com

Free DAF software for Macintosh computers, developed by Tom Morrow, available on the World Wide Web from:
http://www.concentric.net/~tmorrow/stuttering.html

Phonic Ear
Phonic Mirror DAF for clinical use, about $900
3880 Cypress Drive
Petaluma, CA 94954-7600
(707) 769-1110; fax (707) 769-9624

EZ-Speech, Inc. Sustained Phonation Unit DAF with transcutaneous electrical nerve stimulation (TENS), about $500
P.O. Box 31
Chester, VA 23831
(800) 758-8255; fax (804) 796-9332

Pacemaster hearing aid-size metronome, about $500.
Associated Hearing Instruments
6796 Market Street
Upper Darby, PA 19082
(800) 542-2923; Fax: (215) 352-2469

CAFET, about $4,000.
CAFET; 4208 Evergreen Lane, Suite 213; Annandale, VA 22003
(703) 941-8903; Fax: (703) 658-4529

Dr. Fluency, $995-$1,295:

United States
c/o SAI Consultants Ltd.
845 Third Avenue, 6th Floor
New York, NY 10022
Tel: 1-212-688-3480
Toll Free: 1-888-DFLUENC
Fax: 1-212-688-1327
usa@dfluency.com

Sweden
Mrs. Helena Waestlund
Sigillgatan 167, S-703 78
Orebro, Sweden
Phone/Fax: 46-19-2006-78
helena.waestlund@swipnet.se

Israel - Head Office
POB 7, Kalev Ben Yefune 1
Kiryat Arba, 90100, Israel
Phone: 972-2-9968002
Fax: 972-2-9968018
info@dfluency.com

Computation of Rate Exercises (CORE) trains you to talk slower. It

provides paragraphs to read, and times how fast you read them. Macintosh or PC, $60.
Fluency Management Program
2173 SE Morningside Blvd.
Port St. Lucie, FL 34952

Kay Elemetrics
Visi-Pitch II, computer-based DAF and pitch and volume biofeedback for clinical use. Includes video games. PC only. About $4,000
P.O. Box 2025
Pine Brook, NJ 07058-2025
(800) 289-5297; fax (201) 227-7760

Micro Video's Video Voice trains easy onset, increasing length of phonated intervals, and slowing rate of speech. Also includes pitch, intensity, rhythm, duration, and articulation. Includes video games. Macintosh or PC, about $3,000.
P.O. Box 7357
Ann Arbor, MI 48107
(800) 537-2182

Alternative Medicine Stuttering Therapies

GUIDED IMAGERY AND VISUALIZATION

Carl H. Scott, Ph.D., CCC-SLP, uses visualization in therapy to help stutterers "overcome the fears, repressed anger and helplessness that can hinder fluency" (Scott, 1998).

In guided imagery, the clinician guides the stutterer to "set up an internal scene." In the visualization, the stutterer does this with minimal prompting from the clinician. The internal scenes include pictures, feelings and sounds.

Dr. Scott incorporates visualization in three stages of his stuttering therapy:

1) Identifying obstacles to fluency, such as fear of certain speaking situations. The clinician and stutterer may go back to childhood events that left unresolved emotions or distorted beliefs. The stutterer may believe he is less intelligent, socially inept, or not capable of communicating effectively.

2) Initiating a healing process. The clinician helps the stutterer visualization his fear or anger, which may be a "large, black mass" or a dark tunnel. The clinician then urges the stutterer to "go into that mass [or tunnel] to see what it is, feel it, and experience their feelings as they go further."

3) Creating a positive belief system. This may include visualizing yourself talking fluently in front of a group or with a supervisor.

Visualization and guided imagery is not an overnight cure. It is an on-going process with repeated sessions. The visualizations must be done daily.

Dr. Scott con be contacted at 2000 Broadway St., Redwood City, CA 94063; (650) 369-5354; or chscott@earthlink.net. He recommends the books *Rituals of Healing: Using Imagery for Health and Wellness* (New York: Bantam Books, 1994); *Imagery in Healing* (Boston: Shambala, 1985); *Creative Visualization* (Berkeley: Whatever Publishing, 1978); and *Minding the Body, Mending the Mind* (Menlo Park: Addison-Wesley, 1987).

NEUROLINGUISTIC PROGRAMMING (NLP)

NLP connects our thought patterns to our choice of words. By changing our choice of words, we can change our behavior. The goal is greater awareness of the choices we have in responding to people and situations.

A recent issue of the British Stammering Association's newsletter featured an article about an NLP treatment of a stutterer (available on the BSA website). The NLP practitioner approached the problem with the fundamental view that

> stammering was neither a dysfunction nor a handicap…[the stutterer] had spent a great deal of her life mastering a very complex set of speaking skills…an actor would require very advanced speech skills to consistently produce a stammer…to change stammerers' speech towards a more "normal" pattern, further skills or beliefs might need to be added, rather than the original skills discarded…

The NLP practitioner worked with the stutterer met for about 15 hours over 5 months, in 2-hour sessions. They began with identifying "secondary gains" or hidden benefits from her stuttering. The stutterer

> discovered that the stammer provided her with the perfect excuse to limit personal interaction and gained her with the solitude she needed without causing obvious offence to others.

They worked on "limiting beliefs," or whether the stutterer believed that she could improve her speech.

They worked on reducing situational anxiety by focusing on other people, instead of paying attention to inner thoughts and feelings.

They worked on regressing to the age of four, when the stutterer began to stutter, and also when she learned to read out loud, and "rewriting the script."

Lastly, the NLP practitioner noticed that when the stutterer had trouble reading out loud, she looked up and to her right. She then tried "imagining the page high on her left hand side." She was then "able to read it faultlessly out loud…They speculated that somehow, at the time of learning to read, anxiety about her fluency had started a pattern of faulty use of her brain.

Six months after the completion of therapy, "her speech remains amazingly improved."

RELAXATION AND STRESS REDUCTION

Learning to relax specific muscles — your breathing, vocal folds, jaw, etc. — while talking is highly effective in reducing stuttering.

But learning general relaxation techniques, especially relaxation when you're not talking, is not effective in treating stuttering.

However, general relaxation and stress reduction may help some individuals, especially if fear of stuttering causes panic.

The "fight-or-flight" response to stress increases blood pressure, heart rate, breath rate, and blood flow to muscle. It is caused by release of a hormone called adrenaline, or epinephrine. The "fight-or-flight" response helps when you're being chased by a saber-toothed tiger. But when psychological stress causes the same response, a variety of diseases can result.

Stress reduction techniques reduce these physiological effects of psychological stress. These techniques include meditation, autogenic training, progressive muscle relaxation, and hypnosis.

Stress reduction techniques have been carefully studied in people with heart disease. In many cases, the effects are dramatic. In other cases, there is little or no effect. According to Herbert Benson, M.D. (Goleman, 1993),

> For some people with hypertension, stress is the main cause, and the relaxation response may solve the problem entirely. For others, stress is not a factor at all and medication may be the best approach to the problem. Hypertension has many causes, and the relaxation response should only be expected to help in cases when stress is at least a significant component.

Similarly, for some stutterers, stress is the main cause and relaxing may solve the problem. But for others, stress is not the cause of stuttering.

HYPNOSIS TREATMENT OF STUTTERING

Hypnosis was widely-used to treat stuttering in the nineteenth and early twentieth centuries. A study of 40 stutterers found that (Moore, 1946):

• 23% experienced no effect from hypnotherapy.

• 30% had improved speech during the hypnosis sessions, but not afterwards.

• 28% were able to speak fluently immediately after the session.

• 20% of the stutterers had improved speech for "two or three days following hypnotic sessions."

ACUPUNCTURE & CHINESE MEDICINE

An study of acupuncture therapy on two adult male stutterers found no effect on fluency (Craig, 1995).

Chinese medicine has never developed a acupuncture, herbal, or other treatment for stuttering. Chinese doctors don't see isolated diseases, or divide people into disease categories. In other words, you're not a stutterer, but rather a person with various imbalances in life energies. Stuttering may be the manifestation of these imbalances, but stuttering is the symptom, not the disease. No two stutterers will receive the same treatment, because they don't have the same disease.

While this holistic view may sound appealing, the Chinese also see stuttering as an embarrassment to one's family. Stutterers are expected to not talk, and to let their families take care of them instead of seeking employment in the public view.

AVOIDING MILK & DAIRY PRODUCTS

Milk has been blamed for just about everything, including stuttering. One stutterer put this myth to rest:

> I quit drinking milk and eating dairy products for several years. I can assure you that it had NO effect on my stuttering. A couple of years ago, I started using dairy products again, and still no effect on my stuttering.

Zen in the Art of Fluency

John Harrison, Program Director of the National Stuttering Project, opens his "Stuttering Hexagon" essay:

> People frequently ask me, "When did you stop stuttering?" I usually answer, "I stopped stuttering a long time before I stopped stuttering." This is not meant as a cryptic response, but simply to point out how the transformation took place.

Harrison explains that when he stuttered, he thought he had a speech problem. But then he worked on self-awareness:

> I moved to San Francisco [in 1967] and immersed myself in a plethora of personal growth programs that were just then being introduced in California.

Harrison found that he had a variety of interconnected problems, all touching stuttering in some way. He no longer thought of stuttering as a speech problem. Instead, he saw stuttering as imbalances in his behaviors, emotions, perceptions, beliefs, intentions, and physiological responses. He no longer thought of himself as a stutterer. Over time, his stuttering disappeared.

Asian martial arts also integrate physical training with psychological or spiritual growth. These martial arts have been practiced for thousands of years, and have a sense of refinement and history that stuttering therapies lack.

Eugen Herrigel was a German philosopher. He taught philosophy at the University of Tokyo in the 1920s and 1930s. He wanted to learn the Japanese philosophy of Zen Buddhism. In 1953 he published a book about his six years learning archery with a Zen master. The book is called *Zen in the Art of Archery** (New York: Random House).

Daisetz T. Suzuki writes in the introduction to Herrigel's book:

> Zen is the "everyday mind," as was proclaimed by Baso (died 788); this "everyday mind" is no more than "sleeping when tired, eating when hungry." As soon as we reflect, deliberate, and conceptualize, the original unconsciousness is lost and a thought interferes. We no longer eat while eating, we no longer sleep while sleeping. The arrow is off

---

* Not to be confused with Robert Pirsig's 1974 book *Zen and the Art of Motorcycle Maintenance*.

> the string but does not fly straight to the target…Calculation which is miscalculation sets in…The archer's confused mind betrays itself in every direction and every field of activity.

Wendell Johnson said, "Stuttering is what you do trying not to stutter again."

Malcolm Fraser (founder of NAPA Auto Parts and the Stuttering Foundation of America) said, "Stuttering is largely what the stutterer does trying not to stutter. In other words, it is an incredible trick you play on yourself."

The goal of stuttering therapy is spontaneous fluent speech. The goal of Zen is to do life activities without self-conscious calculating and thinking.

Non-stutterers often talk without self-conscious calculating and thinking. But often they are self-conscious about their speech. Fear of public speaking is common. And non-stutterers are self-conscious about asking the boss for a raise, or asking someone out on a date, or when discussing a difficult subject in a relationship. Speech pathologists call this *pragmatics* — the mental effort of calculating the listener's reaction to your speech. In the Zen framework, pragmatics is the calculation that is miscalculation.

The goal of stuttering therapy should be to become a "Zen master of speech," just as other Zen masters are archers or swordsmen or calligraphers. To make an analogy to Baso, you sleep when tired, eat when hungry, and talk when you need to communicate. You don't worry about the listener's reaction. You don't fear embarrassment. If the listener doesn't do what you want or expect, you don't get upset.

You also must talk fluently — but let's define fluency as if we're learning a foreign language. You need vocabulary to express your thoughts, grammar so your meaning isn't misconstrued, and accent and articulation to be understood. Mild stuttering may be OK, if your listener understands you, and you don't fear or avoid speaking. Van Riper called this "fluent stuttering," and a Zen master might call it "fluency which is not fluency."

As an example, Mel Tillis, the country singer, stutters in his performances, delighting his audiences. Another example would be a Certified Toastmaster (from the public speaking clubs), which takes years of training and practice, and many stutterers achieve.

Eugen Herrigel studied archery, under the guidance of a Zen master. Like speech, archery is a combination of motor skills. You tense and relax certain muscles, with split-second timing. Like fluency for a stutterer, these motor skills are not easy or obvious.

Like many stutterers working on their speech, Herrigel worked six years before he considered himself an archer.

Why did Herrigel study archery to learn Zen philosophy? Most Zen students read books, take classes, and talk with Zen masters. How could learning a set of motor skills teach you a philosophy? Herrigel was told that to learn Zen he must begin "by learning one of the Japanese arts associated with Zen."

Master Kenzo Awa's first lesson was drawing the bow, letting "only your two hands do the work, while your arm and shoulder muscles remain relaxed, as though they looked on impassively."

This step is like stuttering therapy, with the goal of speaking while keeping your speech-production muscles relaxed.

Herrigel couldn't do this first step. He would "start trembling after a few moments, and my breathing became more and more labored." Sounds like stuttering!

He was trying to draw a six-foot bow held above his head, which requires great strength. But somehow the Master did this effortlessly.

> ...he called out to me to "Relax! Relax!"...the day came when...I lost patience and brought myself to admit that I absolutely could not draw the bow in the manner prescribed.
>
> "You cannot do it," explained the Master, "because you do not breathe right."

Sounds like stuttering therapy! The Master continued,

> "Press your breath down gently after breathing in, so that the abdominal wall is tightly stretched, and hold it there for a while. Then breathe out as slowly and evenly as possible, and after a short pause, draw a quick breath of air again — out and in continually, in a rhythm, that will gradually settle itself. If it is done properly, you will feel the shooting becoming easier every day. For through this breathing you will not only discover the source of all spiritual strength but will also cause this source to flow more abundantly, and to pour more easily through your limbs the more relaxed you are."
>
> And as if to prove it, he drew his strong bow and invited me to step behind him and feel his arm muscles. They were indeed quite relaxed, as though they were doing no work at all.
>
> The new way of breathing was practiced, without bow and arrow at first, until it came naturally. The slight feeling of discomfort noticeable in the beginning was quickly overcome. The Master attached so much importance to breathing out as slowly and steadily as possible

> to the very end, that, for better practice and control, he made us combine it with a humming note.

First relaxed breathing, and now vocal fold vibration!

> I cannot think back to those days without recalling, over and over again, how difficult I found it, in the beginning, to get my breathing to work out right…
>
> When, to excuse myself, I once remarked that I was conscientiously making an effort to keep relaxed, he replied: "That's just the trouble, you make an effort to think about it. Concentrate entirely on your breathing, as if you had nothing else to do!"

Martin Schwartz says the same thing…

> It took me considerable time before I succeeded in doing what the Master wanted. But — I succeeded. I learned to lose myself so effortlessly in the breathing that I sometimes had the feeling that I myself was not breathing but — strange as this may sound — being breathed. And even when, in hours of thoughtful reflection, I struggled against this bold idea, I could no longer doubt that the breathing held out all that the Master had promised.

Learning to draw the bow took a year. Perhaps stuttering therapies are unsuccessful because we expect results too quickly. Stuttering therapy could start with a year of breathing exercises.

Then Herrigel started working on loosing the arrow. This was even more difficult than drawing the bow. Herrigel kept jerking his hand at the moment of release, resulting in "visible shaking of my whole body and affected the bow and arrow as well." This caused the arrow to "wobble."

The Master told Herrigel, "Don't think of what you have to do, don't consider how to carry it out! You mustn't open the right hand on purpose."

Herrigel told the Master that after drawing the bow, "unless the shot comes at once I shan't be able to endure the tension…I can't wait any longer."

The Master replied that Herrigel's inability to wait was because, "You do not wait for fulfillment, but brace yourself for failure."

Herrigel spent three years working on releasing the arrow. The Master kept saying to release the arrow without tension, like a bamboo leaf holding snow, bending lower and lower until the snow slips off. The bamboo leaf waits without effort until the snow falls off.

Martin Schwartz says that as you exhale, the first word of a phrase should similarly be produced without effort, rolling off your vocal folds like the snow sliding off the bamboo leaf. You shouldn't intend to say the first word, as the archer doesn't open his hand on purpose. The word should say itself, without your planning or calculating or trying.

Herrigel's three years practice releasing the arrow suggests that learning to release the first word of a phrase may also take three years, and be the hardest part of stuttering therapy.

Herrigel was dedicated to his practice, but he couldn't release the arrow smoothly. The Master kept telling Herrigel to become "truly egoless." Herrigel became dejected, and planned to discontinue the archery lessons, concluding that, "all my efforts of the last few years had become meaningless."

> Then, one day, after a shot, the Master made a deep bow and broke off the lesson. "Just then 'It' shot!" he cried.

"It" meant that Herrigel had loosed a shot without loosing the shot. "It" had loosed the shot, not Herrigel. The Master could not say anymore what "It" was, just that "It" can only be known through experience.

> Only after considerable time did more right shots occasionally come off, which the Master signalized by a deep bow. How it happened that they loosed themselves without my doing anything, how it came about that my tightly closed right hand suddenly flew back wide open, I could not explain then and I cannot explain today…I got to the point of being able to distinguish, on my own, the right shots from the failures. The qualitative difference is so great that it cannot be overlooked once it has been experienced.

In stuttering therapy, the difference between your relaxed, fluent voice and your tense, stuttering voice is as obvious as night and day.

Now the Master began training Herrigel to shoot at a target, adding, "He who has a hundred miles to walk should reckon ninety as half the journey."

The Master refused to teach Herrigel to aim, insisting that the target was not the goal, and the goal cannot be aimed at, and that the goal doesn't have a name, except maybe "enlightenment".

But even though the Master did not aim, all of his shots lodged in the black center of the target, from sixty feet away.

At first Herrigel tried to shoot without caring if the arrows hit the target. But he couldn't take this, and "I confessed to him that I was at the end of my tether."

The Master replied:

> You worry yourself unnecessarily. Put the thought of hitting right out of your mind! You can be a Master even if every shot does not hit.

You can be a Zen master of speech even if you still stutter. Mild disfluencies don't matter, if you communicate well.

When the Master said he sees "the goal as though I don't see it," Herrigel replied that the Master should then be able to shoot blindfolded. The Master then had Herrigel set up the target in darkness, except for one candle. Herrigel could not see the target at all, but the Master shot two arrows. When Herrigel turned on the lights, he saw that not only had both arrows hit the bulls-eye, but the second arrow had hit the first and splintered it!

Herrigel describes the following months as the hardest yet, of trying to hit the target yet not trying to hit the target. He gradually came to see the value of this training:

> It destroyed the last traces of any preoccupation with myself and the fluctuations of my mood.

In the fifth year of training, the Master had Herrigel shoot in front of spectators, and awarded him a diploma, "inscribed with the degree of mastery." Before Herrigel returned to Europe, the Master added,

> I must only warn you of one thing. You have become a different person in the course of these years. For this is what the art of archery means: a profound and far-reaching contest of the archer with himself. Perhaps you have hardly noticed it yet, but you will feel it very strongly when you meet your friends and acquaintances again...You will see with other eyes and measure with other measures.

Choosing A Speech Pathologist

First, read everything you can find about stuttering. Decide which therapy interests you. Many books cost over $40. Don't be penny-wise and pound-foolish — the most expensive book is cheaper than the cheapest therapy.

Next, call the Stuttering Foundation of America (800/992-9392) for a list of recommended speech pathologists in your area.

Then attend your local National Stuttering Project (800/364-1677) support group, and ask people to recommend a speech pathologist.

Choose a speech pathologist that specializes in stuttering, who understands a variety of stuttering therapies, and can help you choose the approach that fits your needs. Such speech pathologists are rare!

If you have a serious complaint against a speech pathologist, call the American Speech-Language Hearing Association at (301) 897-5700.

STUTTERING THERAPY COSTS

Expect to spend $2000-3000 on a stuttering therapy program. That doesn't include air travel, hotel costs, etc., if the program is not in your area.

Speech pathologists usually charge between $60 and $120 per hour. You may go two hours a week, for a few months, then one hour a week for a few more months, depending on your severity and progress. Your speech clinic may also have group therapy sessions, for about $25 for two hours. You usually do the group therapy for maintenance, after a few months of individual therapy. The total is again around $2500.

Few health insurance carriers pay for stuttering therapy. They may say that stuttering is a pre-existing condition, or that (as the American Speech-Language Hearing Association says) stuttering is not a medical condition.

Federal law requires that public schools provide speech therapy for children as young as three. In some states, this may continue up to 21, if you're in college.

If you are unemployed, you may get stuttering therapy paid by your state's vocational rehabilitation. If you are employed, your employer may pay for your stuttering therapy under the Americans with Disabilities Act (see the chapter "Stuttering and Employment").

Stuttering therapies maximize the money you pay to speech

pathologists. The therapies involve lots of speech clinic hours over many weeks or months. The stutterer does little away from the speech pathologist. The therapies keep you coming back for "refreshers" year after year. Speech pathologists won't suggest you read books about stuttering, or watch videos. Few suggest that you join a self-help group. To be fair, few stutterers want to read a book about stuttering, or join a self-help group. Too many stutterers want to go somewhere, have something done to them, and be cured of stuttering. This attitude is foolish, and "a fool and his money are soon parted."

What's Wrong With Speech Pathologists?

One of the sad things about stuttering, that sad disorder of the human race, is that its victims far too often find themselves in the hands of a naïve rather than incompetent therapist.
—Charles Van Riper

Speech pathologists are the nicest people in the world. Unfortunately, their professional organization, the American Speech-Language Hearing Association, sometimes puts the needs of speech pathologists ahead of the needs of stutterers. The Ph.D. speech pathologists that conduct research sometimes put their academic careers ahead of the needs of stutterers.

Eugene Cooper and other speech pathologists have recently tried to "alleviate some of the suspicion and adversarial attitudes people who stutter often have towards specialists, such as feeling the clinician is not doing enough to explain fluency" (Shoemaker, 1997).

WHAT'S WRONG WITH ASHA?

A 26-year-old woman got up the nerve to see a speech pathologist. It was the first stuttering treatment she'd ever had.

The speech pathologist had recently graduated with her masters degree. With the stutterer sitting in her office, the speech pathologist opened a book and started reading about how to treat stuttering.

After six weeks of sessions, at $60/hour, the woman had made no progress on her speech. She concluded that her stuttering was incurable, and discontinued the therapy. She was depressed and went to see a psychiatrist instead, who prescribed Prozac (which can increase stuttering).

A year later the woman called me. Stuttering was ruining her life. I suggested she join our National Stuttering Project chapter. We encouraged her not to give up on her speech, and introduced her to a speech pathologist that specializes in stuttering.

Until 1993, ASHA required that speech pathology students take a course in stuttering, and have 25 hours experience treating stuttering. This requirement was changed to a certain number of hours in speech, language, and hearing. The requirement doesn't specify specific disorders, such as articulation, voice, or stuttering. A student can take all her speech classes in one disorder — including swallowing, which arguably isn't speech — and never take a course in stuttering (Starkweather, 1999).

University courses on stuttering don't have to teach stuttering therapy. The required half-course on stuttering can present only etiology or "science" research. Many textbooks are long on science and short on therapy. Silverman's *Stuttering And Other Fluency Disorders* has 170 pages on science and 40 pages on therapy. Bloodstein's *A Handbook On Stuttering* has 400 pages on science and 50 pages on therapy. Starkweather's *Fluency And Stuttering* has 260 pages on science and nothing on therapy.

ASHA's Special Interest Division #4 (Fluency and Fluency Disorders) is working on certification standards for stuttering specialists. The proposed guidelines emphasize many hours of experience treating stuttering under the supervision of a qualified "mentor." This is a step in the right direction, but the guidelines lack any requirement that the speech pathologist understand more than one stuttering therapy. Stuttering is a complex disorder, with many approaches to therapy. SID4 could certify a speech pathologist as a stuttering specialist if she had a certain number of hours doing one type of therapy, but knew nothing about other stuttering therapies.

SPEECH PATHOLOGISTS DISLIKE STUTTERING

A few years ago ASHA asked speech pathologists to rank 20 speech disorders in order of preference. Childhood stuttering was ranked in the middle. Adult stuttering was at the bottom. Speech pathologists dislike adult stuttering because they know little about it. Their lack of training makes them uncomfortable in treating stuttering. You may be the first stutterer your speech pathologist has ever seen.

A speech pathology professor wrote on the Internet:

> One of my students came to me and asked if I was serious about wanting them to go out and stutter [for a day]. She didn't want to do that. Another said she was sweating it out too...I had difficulty getting students to fake stuttering to get the feeling people who stutter have every day.

In the past 20 years, speech pathologists have improved their knowledge and attitudes about stuttering. They have become less likely to believe that parents cause children to stutter, more likely to advocate early intervention for preschoolers who stutter, and less likely to believe that stutterers have certain personality flaws (Cooper, 1996). Hopefully ASHA will change its policies and continue this trend towards better knowledge about stuttering among speech pathologists.

WHAT'S WRONG WITH RESEARCHERS?

Speech clinicians complain that the research published in journals has no relevance to stuttering therapy. Why doesn't research provide new ideas to try with stutterers?

Over 90% of stuttering research is about etiology (the origin and nature of stuttering), and less than 10% about stuttering therapy.

There hasn't been a major advance in stuttering therapy in the last 25 years. New ideas in stuttering therapy are ignored (e.g., Craig's research on biofeedback, in the chapter "School-Age Stuttering Therapy"). New research that disproves old ideas is ignored (e.g., the research about changing parents' speech, in the chapter "More On Childhood Stuttering Therapy"). There is little interaction between stuttering researchers and other fields, such as genetics, neurology, or psychology.

Stuttering therapy is a *loosely-structured field.* Psychologist Mihaly Csikszentmihaly differentiates well-structured fields of knowledge from loosely-structured fields (Csikszentmihaly, 1996). Math and physics are well-structured fields:

> The symbolic system of mathematics is organized relatively tightly. The internal logic is strict; the system maximizes clarity and lack of redundancy. It is easy for a young person to assimilate the rules quickly and jump to the cutting edge of the domain in a few years…
>
> Hans Maier-Leibnitz tells the story of a small physics seminar he taught in Munich, which was interrupted one day by a graduate student who suggested a new way to represent on the blackboard the behavior of a subatomic particle. The professor agreed that the new formulation was an improvement and praised the student for having thought of it. By the end of the week, Maier-Leibnitz says, he started getting calls from physicists at other German universities…The next week, calls began to come in from American universities…The young student…was eventually awarded the Nobel Prize in physics…

The professor immediately saw that the new idea was worthwhile. Word spread quickly, because everyone saw the value of the new idea. The young man's creativity was rewarded with a great prize.

Csikszentmihaly adds that,

> This story could never have been told about my branch of psychology. If a student stood up in a psychology seminar...and uttered the most profound ideas, he or she would not create a ripple outside the walls of the classroom...psychology is so diffuse a system of thought that it takes years of intense [effort for an idea to be recognized] as new and important.

Csikszentmihaly continues, quoting Freeman Dyson that in physics "there is usually some particularly fascinating problem that everybody is working on and it tends to be sort of one thing at a time." This implies that physicists have excellent communication with each other, even back in 1948, when Dyson did the work that won a Nobel Prize.

A well-structured field has:

- Defined terms.
- Rules, e.g., the laws of physics.
- The ability to judge whether new ideas are worthwhile.
- Communication between researchers, and with other well-structured fields (e.g., physicists tend to also be good at math and computer science).

Stuttering etiology (the origin and nature of stuttering) is relatively well-structured. If a speech pathologist has a new idea for etiology research, a grant-providing agency can evaluate whether the idea is worthwhile. After the research is completed, speech pathology journals can evaluate whether the study is worth publishing. After publication, the research is likely to be cited in textbooks and other papers. Professors who want to get tenure concentrate on etiology.

Stuttering therapy is not well-structured. There's little agreement about what stuttering therapies should do. Some therapies make you talk fluently...although, perhaps, slowly, monotonously, and with great mental effort. Other therapies claim to improve your overall communication...although you might not talk fluently.

Some therapies focus on psychology, others on physical techniques. Some therapies encourage substituting sounds and words, others discourage substitutions (De Nil, 1996).

There's little agreement on how to measure the results of stuttering therapies. Should you only count disfluencies? Or should you include speaking rate and "speech naturalness"? What about covert stuttering, and fears and anxieties?

If someone gets an original idea for a new stuttering therapy, there's no way to judge if the idea is worthwhile. The new idea will be ignored. Grant-providing agencies won't fund research. Professors who want tenure avoid stuttering therapy research.

NARROW-MINDEDNESS

A young man stuttered severely, and went to a well-known intensive fluency shaping program. After three weeks, he still stuttered severely. The staff said he could go through the program again, at no extra charge. After another three weeks, he still had no improvement in fluency.

The speech pathologists then had him try a delayed auditory feedback (DAF) device, "to see if he has neurogenic stuttering." (Whether DAF can diagnose neurogenic stuttering is debatable.) Immediately he talked fluently, for the first time in his life. The speech pathologists said, "This proves that fluency shaping is the best therapy for you. We'll let you go through the program a third time at no extra charge."

The young man said no thanks, and asked where he could buy a DAF device. The speech pathologists refused to tell him. They insisted that fluency shaping therapy is better than DAF, even though that was obviously wrong in this case.

Some speech pathologists have a single view of the cause and treatment of stuttering, and ignore anything that challenges their view.

The most dogmatic speech pathologists are often ex-stutterers. They believe that whatever they did to overcome stuttering will work for everyone else, and that all other treatments are shams.

FALSE OPTIMISM AND FALSE PESSIMISM

When I was 22, I completed my third speech therapy program (Precision Fluency Shaping Program). It worked! I talked fluently, although abnormally slowly. My friends were amazed. I talked to everyone I met. This lasted three days. Then my stuttering returned as severely as before the therapy program.

I didn't call the speech clinic. The speech pathologist hadn't said anything about relapse. He'd given me the impression that once the therapy program was complete, I was cured and would have no reason to call him again. This false optimism caused me to think that my stuttering was both incurable and my fault. I didn't seek therapy again for another four years.

Speech pathologists see stutterers in speech clinics. They don't see what happens outside their speech clinics. Getting fluency in a speech clinic is easy. Don't trust therapy programs that send you a "before" and "after" promotional video in which you only see fluent speech in their speech clinic.

Martin Schwartz is sometimes accused of false optimism. The titles of his books are *Stuttering Solved* and *Stutter No More*. The subtitle of *Stutter No More* is "The Fast, Simple, Proven Technique with an Astonishing Long-Term Success Rate." The back cover states that the "astounding long-term success rate" is 93.4%. Like any other stuttering therapy program, some of Schwartz's clients experience relapse down the road. Schwartz's optimism can lead to disappointment and bitterness in some clients.

But false pessimism can be equally damaging. One speech pathologist started each session by asking what my speech goals were. Each session, I said that my goal was to be a great public speaker, better than non-stutterers. She then lectured me for the rest of the hour that severe adult stutterers can never talk fluently, no matter what. She never did anything other than tell me to accept my fate as a severe stutterer. After a dozen sessions I stopped seeing her and found another speech therapist.

According to an article in *Psychology Today* (December, 1998) by stutterer Barry Yeoman, "achieving fluency...is nearly impossible" and "stuttering is a physical impediment for which little can be done." Yeoman's false pessimism could cause thousands of parents reading *Psychology Today* (circulation 300,000) to pull their children out of speech therapy. In the chapter "More on Childhood Stuttering," I referenced studies showing better than 90% success rates, even "near-zero" stuttering years later, for childhood stuttering therapy programs. I was surprised to see praise for Yeoman's article in an e-mail stuttering support group. The same discussion group regularly features anger directed at Martin Schwartz for his optimistic views. Why are these stutterers so pessimistic? Perhaps the stutterers who are successful with therapy don't join support groups?

Eugene Cooper coined the term "chronic perseverative stuttering" in 1986, meaning that some stutterers are never going to overcome stuttering, no matter how many therapy treatments they complete. This idea is controversial.

The problem with "chronic perseverative stuttering" is that speech pathologists are unable to distinguish stutterers with CPS from stutterers who can overcome stuttering. If there were tests for CPS, or at least for certain therapy programs, stutterers could save money by finding out in advance whether a therapy will help. But if there's no test to diagnose a disease, the term is meaningless.

Physician Andrew Weil said about the pessimism of doctors, of their tendency to say,

> You have to live with this, you can't get better, there's nothing we can do for you, this is the only way, you'll have to take these drugs for the rest of your life...These are very powerful statements that have huge influence on people. Behind them is this deep pessimism about what the body is capable of.

Dr. Weil described several sources of this pessimism, including, (Weil, 1995)

> It may be more psychologically comfortable for doctors to predict negative outcomes, because then if the patient does get better, they can be pleasantly surprised and they can take credit for it. But if a patient doesn't get better, they've predicted it and so they still appear to be in control. This may be an unconscious motivation that leads doctors to make these statements. In any case, they're very destructive. Belief is a powerful influence on the body's healing system, and the pronouncements of medical doctors are one of the greatest influences on your own beliefs.

Becoming A Speech Clinician
by Barbara Dahm

Reprinted with permission.

My personal story about my experience with stuttering is filled with anxiety, frustration, fear, and that search for the elusive magic cure. It all started thirty years ago. No, that wasn't the first time I stuttered. You see, I don't stutter. It was the first time that I heard someone stutter.

I remember the moment well. My professor in "Introduction to Stuttering" had just introduced our undergrad class to one of his clients. The young man standing before me was handsome and personable and had a lot of courage. In spite of the blocks and repetitions in his speech, he tried to help us understand what it was like to be a stutterer.

It was probably then that I knew I had made the right choice of a major. I was going to learn how to treat stuttering and all those other speech disorders that could make communication and even living difficult. It seemed like a worthwhile career.

As the course progressed, I kept waiting for the day that I would learn how to give therapy to people who stutter. I waited and I waited and I waited. Our professor made the wait interesting. He told us anecdotes about his therapy sessions. He believed that people stuttered because they had disturbed interpersonal relationships and he treated clients through his own psychological approach that I could never grasp. The one thing I remember is that he said that the clinician is the single most important variable affecting success in therapy. That was very scary. He was dynamite, the kind of man who could really touch others, but who was I to take on such a task.

I finished the course with an A, but I still didn't have the foggiest idea how to treat a person who stutters. It didn't matter though. I hardly saw another person who stuttered until two years later, when I was hired as a speech therapist in an outpatient clinic.

I was thrilled to at last have the opportunity to be a real speech therapist. I have to confess though, I was not at all qualified for this job. You see, I couldn't speak the same language as my clients. After leaving college I had emigrated to Israel and by the time I had to either work, starve, or give up my dream of becoming an Israeli, my language level in Hebrew was that of a four-year-old.

Since there were no home-grown Israeli clinicians at the time, a very kind man, Jerry Reichstein, decided to invest in me. He hired me believing that I would learn how to speak Hebrew on the job. Fortunately, most of my clients were severely language-delayed, so I was able to learn the language while keeping two steps ahead of the children.

I did, however, have one twelve-year-old boy with a moderate stuttering problem. Needless to say, there was little I could do to help him as he chatted on too fluently for me to keep up with him.

In those therapy sessions, it was I who learned just how painful it is not to be able to communicate. Feeling frustrated and a total failure, I decided that the time was right for me to go back to the USA and enroll in a grad program in speech pathology.

I got my master's degree and returned to Israel to try again. My inner voice said, "So what if I can only understand half a conversation, I can always ask questions. Who cares if people think I'm stupid? So what if I make mistakes? Who's perfect?"

I think that experience helped me a lot to treat people who stutter because I realized a very important fact: the less I tried, the better I did. Amazingly, after not having spoken Hebrew for five years, I could communicate better than when I had left.

I soon became a public school speech therapist and for the first time had to treat people who stutter. What to do??? I dragged out my old books and ordered a few new ones and did my best. I read that stuttering was an iceberg and I was determined to help my clients melt into good communicators.

The only problem was that they wanted to speak fluently. Sure they'd work on shame, guilt, and avoidances if it would make them speak fluently, and some did work diligently, but they still were disfluent and disappointed. I felt very helpless.

One client was a high school student named Jane. She was a lovely girl who had so much potential that was hidden because she avoided communicating with her classmates. She suffered so from her stuttering, and I suffered too because she put her trust in me and I didn't know how to help her. All I could do was to guide her to accept herself as a person who stutters, and to learn more positive attitudes that would enable her to live a more satisfying life.

But who was I to do that? I had never stuttered. How could I have the gall to advise her how to cope? I decided that if I didn't really stutter, I would pretend. One Saturday night I went out and spoke disfluently to everyone. That was an experience I will never forget and never chose to repeat. Voluntary stuttering is not easy. I felt silly and embarrassed and imagined all sorts of negative thoughts in my listeners.

I did develop more empathy for people who really stutter, and I tried very hard to understand how Jane felt. She and I developed a warm relationship but I'm afraid I wasn't much help to her. Throughout the therapy, I found myself functioning more as a psychologist than a speech therapist. I accepted my lack of qualification as the reason for my failure. It was probably this experience more than any other that made me decide to devote the rest of my professional life to improving my ability to treat stuttering.

My first step was to become better qualified. If stuttering was a psychological problem as I had been taught, I had to improve my ability to give psychologically-oriented therapy. Israel is the land of miracles and so one happened. Just when I needed them, a couple from Canada arrived in Israel to give seminars in Gestalt Therapy and Stuttering. I listened to their ideas and thought they sounded logical. At last I would achieve the ability to really help my clients overcome their personal anxieties and fears.

My experience with Gestalt turned out to be a long and satisfying one. I grew both personally and professionally and I helped many people who stutter to grow as well. At last I had some "successes." Oh, none of my clients became fluent speakers, but I remember a glorious day when a soldier I had been treating for a few months took the courage to call a girl on the telephone and ask her out. She accepted and we shared the joy of his very first date.

As a therapist, I enjoyed the Gestalt approach. For the first time I felt that I had something to offer my clients. The only problem was that they were still interested in consistently being able to speak fluently. I knew I had made progress but I wasn't there yet.

I heard about the Precision Fluency Shaping Program, and that it was very successful. Well, it certainly was a 180-degree turn around, but I was willing to change direction if it would help my clients become fluent speakers.

Adrianna DiGrandi, who practiced PFSP in Boston, was kind enough to let me observe her group. I was favorably impressed. As far as fluency was concerned, the results certainly surpassed those of my clients. I decided that I needed to learn how to administer this program. In 1987 Dr. Ronald Webster gave me the opportunity to learn his program. I will always be grateful to him.

Many of you are familiar with PFSP. It is a controversial approach that leaves few clients and clinicians indifferent. Having practiced this therapy program from 1987-1992, I can understand why some praise it and others denounce it. Whatever one's experience is with PFSP, we have to recognize that PFSP gave stuttering therapy a giant step forward.

As a PFSP clinician, for the first time I *began* to understand what a person who stutters actually does when speaking. I learned to pay attention to vocal folds and articulators. I learned that there is a connection between the diaphragm and the vocal folds and I learned that there was something about targets that made some people fluent.

But I also had questions. Why did some people succeed and other not? Was I missing something? For five years I tried to follow the program to the letter so that I wouldn't overlook any important points. I tried to develop my skill in evaluating targets and I tried to give clear concise instructions. I observed my clients' behavior and attitudes and I listened to them when they described their achievements and their failures.

The most common complaint that I heard was, "But I can't do gentle onsets when I have to think about what I want to say!" That puzzled me because I could. It wasn't for a very long time that I realized that when people who stutter refer to "thinking about what they want to say," they are talking about a very different activity than people who speak fluently. Stuttering became a Rubic's cube for me, and thanks to my Gestalt training and Dr. Webster's approach, I began to make progress in putting all the squares in place.

Today I don't practice PFSP. I have developed Comprehensive Speech Processing Therapy (CSPT) as a result of my clinical experience. Although it touches on aspects of other therapy approaches, it is not eclectic.

The perspective of CSPT is that stuttering occurs when the speaker does not correctly integrate the language formulation, motoric, and cognitive processes involved in the production of speech. Although the aim of the therapy is to achieve normal-sounding fluent speech, none of the specific goals are either stuttering- or fluency-oriented.

Cognitively, clients learn that speaking is a motoric/linguistic activity, rather than an attempt to "get words out." Linguistically, they learn to formulate a speech plan automatically without monitoring the words or sounds in the plan. Motorically, they learn to renew the stimulation of the vocal folds while allowing the articulators to function automatically, without being controlled or monitored.

The end result is that speaking becomes a less controlled activity. My firm belief is that people stutter when they are exercising control over speech processes that are meant to function on an automatic mode. In trying to control speech or fluency, speakers use incorrect speech processes that cause breakdown in the system. Techniques and strategies that require more control really cause the speaker to be in less control. CSPT clients, therefore, learn how to process speech correctly in a less controlled way.

What about the psychological aspect? Our thoughts and feelings can interfere with the way we function. A goal of therapy is to develop positive attitudes that support the acquisition of new behaviors, coping with fear, and motivation to affect change.

From psychology to stuttering modification therapy to fluency shaping therapy to speech processing therapy, it's been a long journey. I know there are still miles to go before I sleep. However, it has been a worthwhile journey. When my clients tell me that they are able to speak normally without struggle and anxiety, I know that people who stutter can learn to speak fluently and even enjoy doing it.

Stuttering Aid Dogs

My April Fools Day (1995) Internet joke provoked strong reactions. One speech pathology professor asked permission to distribute it to her class. On the other hand, Miss E. F. K. Chadwick, of Leigh-On-Sea, Essex, England, found it to be in "deplorable taste...offensive...anti-tolerance to our condition... totally unacceptable and increasing abrasive...an insult" (Chadwick, 1997).

Have you ever wondered what happens to seeing-eye dogs, hearing-ear dogs, etc., that flunk out of training school? We buy them and train them as *stuttering aid dogs*.

When you stutter, the dog barks to distract you, to get you out of the block.

If barking doesn't help, the dog bites your leg until you get the word out.

The preferred breeds are yellow labs and German shepherds. These breeds are intelligent and dependable. Pit bulls have more sensitive hearing, and so can sense pre-stuttering tension inaudible to humans. However, the program no longer provides pit bulls, after a woman named Sally Thistlethwaite lost a leg introducing herself.

For persons who have completed speech therapy programs, we can provide a fluency shaping dog. These dogs wag their tails and nuzzle you whenever you breathe with your diaphragm, talk slower, continuously phonate, and relax your articulation muscles. However, when you stutter, the dog discreetly disappears, so it's not there when you most need it.

The program also provides stuttering modification dogs. They are scientifically trained as follows:

First, the dogs are trained to identify the core behaviors, secondary behaviors, and feelings and attitudes that characterize stuttering.

Next, the dogs are trained to help you confront your stuttering. Whenever you take the dog for a walk, it stops people and won't let you go on until you do a stuttering survey.

When you stutter, the dog bites you and doesn't let go until you've frozen whatever speech behavior you're doing for several seconds. E.g., if you prolong a sound, you then have to continue prolonging that sound.

You then have to pause several seconds, and say the word again, using easy or fluent stuttering.

When you talk fluently, the dog bites you until do voluntary easy or fluent stuttering.

Customers complain that they can't remember exactly what "fluent stuttering" is, but the dogs are carefully trained to recognize fluent stuttering and will bite you if you do anything else.

Ted Peters has been trying to use two stuttering aid dogs, one fluency shaping dog and one stuttering modification dog. Unfortunately his two dogs keep chasing and biting each other.

The astounding long-term success rate is 93.4%. If you don't believe us, we'll send you a videotape of several people talking fluently in our offices, like you get from other therapy programs.

Our Chief Scientist, John Swaney, D.A.W.G. (Doctorate in Animal Welfare Graduate studies), has a new program with a 100% success rate: if early indicators suggest failure is likely, the offending party (either the dog or the person who stutters) is taken out and shot.

This has two beneficial effects upon the published success rate:

1) It removes from the population those individuals likely to fail.

2) Those remaining in the population feel extremely motivated to work harder at the therapy.

In compliance with ASHA's ethics policy, we GUARANTEE that we'll keep your money whether you're cured or not!

AND THE PUNCHLINE IS…

A speech pathologist thought this was real. She wrote to me asking for the video.

Please Help, by Mike Wlosek

Reprinted with permission.

Hello all,

My name is Michael and I am a 25-year-old male that has stuttered for as long as I can remember. I still remember being made fun of as a child. In 2nd grade my school tested me for speech, but nothing ever came of it.

It didn't really kick in until high school though. I remember being horrified to death of going around the room and introducing myself. One time a priest came into our class and wanted to get to know who we all were. I knew all of these students for a couple of years already, but I was scared to death. When we were halfway through the room I raised my hand to be excused, I went straight to the vice-principal's office, who I had become friends with and he was also a guidance counselor in the past.

I never did go back to class that morning. I also remember a time when I was called on in English class, I had the correct answer right in front of me and it started with a "b." I was blocking so bad that I looked up at the teacher and said I didn't get that one.

In college I used to get sick on the way to class for fear of any public speaking or especially the first week of school when we would go around the room and introduce ourselves. I could never ever say my name, without stuttering. My heart would go crazy and I would lose track of time and even get numb sometimes. I would look at the syllabus and make sure there were no oral reports that semester, if there were I dropped the class. That did happen a couple of times.

I took public speaking in high school and I didn't stutter but was always nervous the first minute or so, but I was at the point in college that I could not take public speaking again. My first semester was at Seton Hall University. It was a requirement, for that reason among others I dreaded it. I then transferred to the University of Florida. There it was pretty easy, the classes were very large and I never had to worry about the go around the class thing.

After two years there I decided to move back home in Orlando and I finished my bachelor's degree in liberal studies at the University of Central Florida.

After college I was stuck working in a warehouse job that paid nothing, because of fear I think. Now I have worked for GE Capital/Total Audio and Visual Services. I work AV and also in their business centers. These two different jobs are based in hotels and I have to speak with the guests and clients doing meetings and conventions all day long. I stutter a lot and it drives me crazy. I went to a speech pathologist about 4 years ago but it was too expensive to keep going to, so I only saw her twice.

I really do not know what to do, it has been holding me back all my life and I am trying to push forward. I just hate when I am talking on the phone, at work or home and I sound like a nervous idiot. At work you can see kind of a panic in my eyes I am sure. People still make fun of me too, which makes me feel like I am an inch tall. Luckily it doesn't happen too much it still does happen. You would think adults would know better.

I could probably talk about this subject all day. I wish it would get out of my head, but I am constantly reminded every time I say a sentence.

I do speak clearly a lot of the time, but it always happens when I want to look smooth and important.

I would love to hear from all of you about this subject. It is great to read all of your postings. My e-mail address is pinola@aol.com.

I would appreciate any suggestions or just people saying hi.

Thanks,

Mike

My Life As A Stutterer, by Asim Khan

Reprinted with permission.

A couple of years ago, someone asked me what is the one thing I want most in life. I did not say it aloud, but to me the answer was crystal clear. Something you all take for granted - fluent speech. I do not want to be a stutterer! So even though there was a lot more to me than just being a stutterer, it sure was a big big part of my life. Last month when I read John Ahlbach's comment on the lack of therapy experiences type articles in *Letting GO*, it prompted me to put it all down on paper. It went from just being the therapy experiences to encompass all the other stages of my life, in fact my whole life, as it was affected by my stuttering. It ended being a lot longer than I intended, but I had to do it. This was like a catharsis for me and hopefully someone else might gain something from my experiences. What I went through in my life may be a lot less frustrating and painful than what many of you have endured. For me it hurt the most because this was MY pain. I lived it every day. This was my life — my life as a stutterer.

I was born 25 years ago in Pakistan. From what my mother tells me, I started to stutter around 4 or so. My father used to stutter too, so it was probably hereditary, but looking back at it now, my stuttering might have been triggered by some traumatic experiences I went thorough at that time.

There was no concept of speech therapy in Pakistan, at least when I was growing up. Actually, I don't really remember stuttering all that severely in those early years. There were quite a few occasions when I forgot that I stutter and did not stutter until the realization came back. Of course there was the childhood teasing and all but that was OK. What was not OK was, when once in fifth grade my teacher imitated my stuttering in responding to my question.

Grown-ups around me usually ignored my stuttering but felt it their duty to reprimand me on my fast rate all the time. Distinctly remember running to an adult all pumped up about something, telling them excitedly what had happened and getting the response "Why can't you just slow down. Gosh, what's the rush. You sound like a record set at a wrong speed." It got to a point, when I got so frustrated with these comments that I decided that I would not speak at all, unless I had to. All in all, I was an unhappy child. Low self-esteem, full of inferiority complexes. I was too thin, too tall, too dark and on top of everything I could not even speak properly! The saving grace was my academic record. I was always among the top students in my classes.

Most people at NSP tell me about the feeling of alienation they felt growing up as the only stutterer around. I knew at least 4 other people who stuttered but we never ever talked about it. As a matter of fact, in all of my 19 years in Pakistan, stuttering was something I never talked to anyone about — not friends, not family, nobody. It was all inside of me and other than wishing and praying that the next morning I would wake up completely fluent, there was nothing I could do about it.

Around the age of 12, I vividly remember telling myself that I can't go on like this. I have a lot of potential, which I won't ever be able to realize, if I keep myself shut off like that. To desensitize myself, I just tried to speak in almost every situation. It helped that my teachers always gave me a lot of prominence in the class. I was the star pupil and I had to speak, if I wanted to live up to my image. My mother used to encourage me a lot to participate in extracurricular activities. So I started participating in debates, speeches and other such activities. That definitely helped me in overcoming my fear of speaking and just becoming more social and outgoing. However the fluctuations were still mind boggling. I could pass off as a fluent speaker with strangers by word substitutions and other crutches but stuttered a lot with friends and family. That perhaps was the most frustrating part. Since I had the luxury of being fluent at some times, the dysfluency in others bothered me all the more. It was still however a completely personal battle. A sorrow which remained unspoken.

> Give sorrow words. The grief that does not speak, whispers the over-burdened heart and bids it break.
>
> — Macbeth

In August 1988, I came to the states and started my bachelors in Electrical Engineering at the University of Texas at Austin.

Once I was studying in the library, it was the summer of 1989, and accidentally came across some books on stuttering. One of them was *Self-Therapy For The Stutterer.* Therapy? Hmm, that was a totally novel idea to me. So there was something which can be done about IT. There is a cure after all! I was totally excited by this discovery. The book recommended seeking professional help, if possible. This is how I landed at UT speech and hearing clinic in the fall of 1989 and was characterized as a mild to moderate stutterer.

That was like the opening of a whole new world to me. Finally I could talk to someone about my frustrations, my problems - my stuttering life. They started the therapy with block correction techniques. Cancellation (Post Block correction) where you say the word again, fluently, after you have stuttered on it, was the most difficult one. Once I had struggled through a word and managed to get it out finally, there was no way I was going back and saying it again! Pull out (in-block corrections, where you take control of the repetitions by doing a few voluntary repetitions and ease out of the block) and Pre-block correction (where you use try to relax your speech mechanism on anticipating a block before saying the word) came more easily. We also worked on a lot of problem-solving for difficult situations and relaxation techniques.

They all worked fine but the problem was that I did not stutter much in the clinic atmosphere anyway. So there was not an opportunity for me to test or practice the techniques in actual difficult situations, and in real life they did not work all that well. My clinician had to rely on my reporting my successes in real world, and I had this big idea that once therapy is over, all my problems are over, so I was reporting a lot more successes than I was actually seeing. To cut a long story short, I was released from therapy in fall of 90 with the understanding that I have completed my therapy successfully and now I could go out and conquer the world!

The next year was the realization of the cruel reality that things had not really changed all that much. I still was helpless in many situations; in fact I had started to stutter a lot more in some situations than I did earlier. What made things worse was that now I would analyze each and every stuttering episode to death and come out blaming myself entirely for the failure of not using my techniques. I was just overly self-critical. I had techniques that were supposed to make me fluent. Why could I not use them effectively now, when they were so easy in the clinic? One positive aspect of therapy was that now I could at least share my stuttering with some close friends. I just could not bring myself to advertise it as much as my clinician wanted me to, but, at least, now there were some people I could talk to about stuttering

After a long period of repeated failures and inconsistent fluency, I went back to therapy in January of 1992 at the UT speech center once again. This time I was being completely honest in reporting my successes or rather my failures in transferring my techniques to the real world. We went back to slow rate, block correction techniques, and all the other stuff we had done before. But nothing really helped. My fluency was still very sporadic. The problem with block correction technique was they only applied when I started having a block and by that time it was just too late for me to exercise any sort of control, and just like the waterfall effect, once the blocks started, it was downhill from there on. I did get a lot better in advertising my stuttering, but the funny thing was even though it made me more relaxed with my audience, my stuttering intensified once the cat was out of the bag.

Something was just not right. I needed a different approach. In fall of 1992, my speech pathologist, Ann Thomas, came to the conclusion that the focus had to be shift away from stuttering and towards maintaining my fluency. It might sound like the same thing, but for me it was a big shift. For the next couple of months, we worked on the BRAT program by Gronhovd, where the emphasis was to focus towards relaxation and using passive air flow by achieving a state of relaxation in the respiratory pathway. During the same time I read Dr. Martin Schwartz's book *Stutter No More*. I also had a phone evaluation with Dr. Schwartz and thought about attending his two day workshop on passive air flow very seriously, but at $1800, it was way beyond my meager student budget. To set the record straight I don't agree with Dr. Schwartz's claims that his is the be all and end all ultimate "CURE" for stuttering. Nevertheless for me it was the perfect technique as it could be used all the time (and not just when I started having disfluencies). It would slow down my rate (a known effective strategy for me), and it would shift the focus of therapy away from my over-analysis of my stuttering episodes.

Even though it sounds like that this was the perfect technique for me, it took me 2 semesters to get to the point where I could actually go out into the real world and use passive airflow consistently even for 10 minutes. The whole passive air flow approach was something new that our university clinic was trying and, to put it bluntly, the clinicians were moving on the learning curve at the same time as me. One drawback with a university clinic is that you have a different student clinician each semester. Even though I had the advantage of having a great speech pathologist like Ann as the supervisor, trying to develop good rapport with a new clinician each semester hindered the progress to a certain extent. With the shift in focus, one good thing was that even though I did not stutter in the clinic atmosphere, now the challenge was not just being fluent but consistently using passive air flow for the full hour. In a nutshell what my technique entailed was: Breathe in. Let some air out in a passive way. Start the first word in a slow, slightly prolonged manner. Continue the easy onset throughout. Don't scan ahead or preform the word. If you do come to a block, pause, reinitiate your technique on that word or sound. Do not rush!

So now I knew my technique, knew exactly what I was supposed to do. However transferring it to the real world effectively was another story. I had started my job search, graduated and job interviews and all had a big stress level associated with them. It was still very hard to be able to use passive air flow in tough situations but in easier situations there sure was a good progress. One thing, which really helped me there, was sharing my technique, and not just the stuttering, with people around me. Telling and demonstrating to them that I had a technique that could make me fluent, if used properly, made me all the more motivated to use it. I also made up a hierarchy of situations based on the level of difficulty of using my technique, and failure to be effective in a higher up situation on the hierarchy made it easier not be so hard on myself. Ann had always told me to be less self critical and that if I could turn the feeling of frustration and dismay with my speech to motivation to practice harder, it can do wonders for me, and as always Ann was right. Around that time, the NSP chapter of Austin was also taking off and that provided me with an excellent opportunity to practice and share. I practiced with friends, by myself, in the car - actually I practiced quite a bit.

In February 1994, I landed a job in Sunnyvale, California. My speech was much better, but still everything was not all together. In March, I attended a workshop with Dr. Ted Peters at NSP San Francisco. I did not realize it then, but now in retrospect, this was like a big milestone in my life. Coming back from this workshop I started to do something new. I did not beat up on myself for using passive air flow all the time. What I started to do now was, I would start off with passive air flow, slide into spontaneous fluency naturally, and slide back to controlled passive airflow at the slightest inkling of trouble. The slow rate of the controlled speech and the easy onset carried on quite a bit during the spontaneous phase too. But I must warn that I could only do it after having some intense practice with passive air flow. Doing it on a premature stage can be dangerous.

It is about time I came to the present. I have been back in Austin since June. My speech in the last 6 or 7 months is the greatest it has ever been this consistently all through my life. What's more is that I would like to think that my life as a stutterer is over. I still stutter every now and then (when I am "laxing" on my technique), but my level of fluency is very acceptable to me. I try to go to our NSP meetings quite regularly, as they provide me with a good opportunity to practice and rebrush my technique. Also, I try to maintain the same spontaneous and controlled fluency balance I have described earlier.

Sometimes in difficult situations, it is not smooth sailing all along, but then who is looking for perfection!?

It just feels so heavenly to be able to say that in the past 6, 7 months there has not been a single day that went bad because my speech was bad. I can pick up the phone and call up anybody, any time I want to. My friends, people who have known me for a while, come up to me and comment on the tremendous improvement they are seeing in my speech and it ... it just feels great! I have the "If you stutter you are not alone" NSP button on my office wall. I have just come a long long way! I may have a relapse, my speech may go back to what it was before. Call me overconfident, but I would like to believe that having done it once, I can always do it again.

I don't think I hate my stuttering any more. It is a part of me, just as so many other things are. My fiancée made an interesting comment. She said, "You are the person you are today because you went through all these experiences in your life. The stuttering, the frustrations, the struggles, the triumphs." Not to sound corny, but most of the time I like the person I am today.

Self-Help Is The Best, by Ratan Punjabi

Reprinted with permission.

Dear Friends,

I live in Taiwan. I am 37 years old. I do export business. Here are the facts on my stuttering:

1. I used to stutter very badly during my early teens and early 20s.
2. My stuttering has considerably improved in the past 6-7 years.

I underwent many speech therapies. Some worked (for short time) and others simply didn't. From my own personal experience, I would like to contribute the following to all of my friends who stutter.

1. Every morning, take out 10-15 minutes and sit quietly and just breathe normally. Don't think or negate any thoughts. Just observe your thoughts. That's all, do nothing. This sort of meditation will surely reduce the normal anxiety that we all suffer from and which makes our stuttering worse.

2. Have a positive attitude towards yourself. Don't indulge in self-hatred. We stutter, so WHAT? Many unfortunate people suffer from fatal diseases, physical handicaps that are irreversible, AIDS, cancer, etc.

Would you trade-in your stuttering for any of the above? NO. MAN, NO WAY.

3. Develop self-love. Accept your stutter as part of life. Facts are 1 percent of the world population stutters. So we belong to an elite group (take this lightly please).

4. Don't be shy of your stutter. The more you try to hide it or substitute certain words the more this problem goes inside the subconscious mind, where it is difficult to eradicate.

5. Every night, before sleeping, auto-suggest to yourself that "My stutter is going away slowly but surely. I will stutter less tomorrow. But in case I stutter more, then it will not bother me."

Now, the above suggestions are just psychological.

Get ready for some concrete ways, if you follow these, you are on your way to being an ex-stutterer or less-stutterer.

1. Make a fun-thing out of your stutter: If while buying a theater, train, cinema ticket etc., you feel you are going to stutter, pause. Relax. Taking a few normal breaths will be good. If you stutter, then wait there immediately, and if your feel other person is getting irritated (let him be, it's his blood pressure!) or impatient, then LAUGH. Yes, I repeat LAUGH. Laugh at your own stutter, laugh at the other person's irritation. (Don't laugh so hard that someone kicks you...). Laughing will relax you completely and the word that you could not say, will come out naturally, either in the course of your laughter or

immediately after it.

2. GOLDEN RULE: Before beginning any conversation, tell the other person/s LOOK, I STUTTER, SO IN THE COURSE OF CONVERSATION IF I STUTTER, THEN PLEASE BEAR WITH ME. This will immediately relax you and you will stutter much less. Chances are people will tell you that you were lying when you said you stutter!

3. If you are sure to stutter in certain situations like talking to your boss, girlfriend, audience, parents, etc., then try to look away at a different thing rather than their faces. Looking away or focusing on something else, while talking, will take your mind away from the anxiety that the other person will be angry if you stuttered.

4. Try to adopt a sort of singing style when you speak (particularly on alphabets or words where you are sure you will stutter). I could not say Hello when answering the phone. So after I adopted a sort of singing style, then Hello came out naturally (remember, it is impossible for us to stutter when singing.

5. Stuttering usually happens when we are speaking to a person or group of people, who we feel are superior to us, maybe bosses, parents, teachers, etc. When speaking to these people, imagine that they are all inferior to you, because stutterers are fast thinkers and more creative and artistic than normally speaking people. Stutterers are wonderful crossword solvers because of their ability to substitute words that are weak for them. Imagine that all these people are inferior to you. This should cool you down and reduce the stutter.

6. Remember, there is nothing physically wrong with us. We are as normal as the next door neighbour. Count your blessings rather than having a negative attitude.

7. Try to speak louder than usual.

8. Do these only when desperate: Try to imitate anyone you know, maybe a movie star, politician, teacher, friend, anyone. and speak.

9. Tell stuttering jokes to people around you. This should lighten the atmosphere and relax you. You will be surprised how people react positively to this.

10. Finally (at least until now) if you have a nice speech therapist nearby, try using this option also. Thousands have improved by undergoing therapy. But for friends who cannot go to a therapist, either due to economic or business etc. reasons, then it will not harm to consider my options listed above. Please trust me I was a good stutterer and now I have improved quite a lot.

Drop me a line, punjabi@pristine.com.tw.

Conclusion — Adult Stuttering Therapy

This "Therapy" section presented a wide range of adult stuttering therapies. Some of these therapies contradict each other. The little research into therapy effectiveness has shown that few therapies are effective for more than 70% of stutterers.

This may lead a reader to conclude that nothing can be done about stuttering. The purpose of this book is to tell stutterers that much can be done to improve their speech. This chapter presents my views on the best approach to stuttering therapy.

LATERAL VS. MEDIAL

Goldberg (1985) described two cerebral systems for speech and language production.

• The *lateral* system produces and understands language. This area produces speech under closed-loop motor control. We have conscious awareness and control of lateral system speech and language production.

• The *medial* system produces speech via open-loop motor control, or the retrieval of motor programs from long-term memory. We have no awareness or control of medial system speech production.

Stuttering is produced in the medial system: environmental cues cause the medial system to retrieve stuttering motor programs (learned in early childhood) from long-term memory rather than retrieve fluent speech motor programs. Stuttering has two key components:

• The stuttering motor programs, or the memories of *how* to stutter.

• The environmental cues, or the memories of *when* to stutter.

Too many stuttering therapy are ineffective because they focus on the lateral system. Too many stuttering therapies train consciously-controlled therapy techniques, which only work when you pay attention.

For example, Russell J. Humphries developed the "Lift and Drive" stuttering therapy. He writes,

> The method works, and we can prove it, "if" the stutterer makes a genuine effort to exert his own self-control and self-discipline to use LIFT AND DRIVE in every speaking situation.
>
> Fluency can be accomplished, but not without honest effort on the

part of the disfluent. It takes determination and motivation…"Make the mind command the body, never permit the body to command the mind." — General George S. Patton, Jr. [Patton overcame dyslexia to become a four-star general in World War Two.] (Humphries, 1998)

Patton was a great general, but the mind/body split isn't so clear-cut. There are some things the brain evolved to handle automatically, without conscious control by your mind. Speech motor control is one of these areas. Your mind decides what to say, and your brain's medial system takes care of the details. Humphries is right that overcoming stuttering requires determination and motivation, but the goal should be automatic, effortless fluency, not the use of consciously-controlled speech in every conversation.

MEDIAL SYSTEM THERAPY

A stuttering therapy that focuses on the medial system would strengthen fluent speech motor programs in your long-term memory, and recondition environmental cues to retrieve these fluent speech motor programs in situations that now cause you to stutter. You would learn *how* to talk fluently, and *when* to talk fluently. The therapy would make fluent speech production automatic and effortless.

Gymnastics coaches teach this way. Zen masters teach archery this way. Typing is taught this way. Speech is not fundamentally different from gymnastics or archery or typing — there's no reason that fluent speech can't be taught.

The major difference is that stutterers already know how to talk, but know the wrong way to talk. Novice gymnasts and archers and typists are a "blank slate" with no deeply-learned maladaptive motor programs. Stuttering therapy must teach the stutterer to forget old memories as well as to learn new memories.

Speech is learned at an early age, and speech motor skills become "hard-wired" in the brain. So are athletic skills, which is why parents start their children in gymnastics and other activities when the children are 3 or 4. An adult stutterer can learn to speak fluently as easily as he can learn to be a gymnast — you can become good at it, but don't expect to make the Olympic team.

Also, gymnasts and archers practice many hours daily for years, when stutterers think they can learn everything in a 2-week stuttering therapy program.

On the positive side, stutterers have two tools that athletes lack:

drugs and electronic devices. (OK, athletes also have drugs!)

A medial system therapy would start with drugs and/or electronic devices for immediate fluency. Then the stutterer would do use traditional stuttering therapy to reduce dependence on the drugs and/or electronic device. But unlike other therapies, practice would be based on motor learning theory to develop automatic, effortless fluent speech.

The second stage is to train fluent speech motor skills. These skills include relaxed breathing, vocal fold control such as gentle onsets, integrated breathing and vocal fold control (letting a little air out before tensing your vocal folds), stretched vowels and continuous phonation, reduced articulatory pressure, phrasing, and other skills. These skills are best taught with a DAF device and a biofeedback system, such as the CAFET. The result should be mastery of slow, relaxed fluent speech, although it may sound abnormally slow or relaxed.

The fourth stage is to practice these skills, but increase the utterance complexity (from sounds to words to sentences to conversations), to increase the speed of execution or speaking rate, and to increase the intensity or volume of practice. This should result in fast, fluent, automatic fluency.

Mastering these skills requires daily practice and using the motor skills in real conversations. A biofeedback computer monitors the stutterer's speech. The computer alerts him when his speech is "off-target" (Van Riper, 1974). Leaving a Desktop Fluency System plugged into your telephone is an easy way to do this.

After mastering fluent speech motor skills, the stutterer is ready to recondition environmental cues to stutter. The emphasis shifts from *how* to talk fluently, to *when* to talk fluently.

The stutterer identifies the situations that make him stutter. He also identifies the situations in which he is fluent. A checklist of speaking situations can be used, with columns to check if the situation causes stuttering or fluency. The situations include speaking on telephones, telling jokes, if the listener is not paying attention, reading out loud, etc.

The stutterer then chooses one stuttering cue to work on. He identifies all the fluency-enhancing conditions he could use in the stuttering situation. For example, the stuttering cue may be calling answering machines. His fluency-enhancing conditions may include talking to his speech pathologist, using DAF, using therapy techniques, and planning what he'll say in advance.

The stutterer calls his speech pathologist's answering machine every day, using his DAF device and fluency techniques, and planning his message in advance. This should be easy (if not, he should go back to the earlier stages). When he feels that this exercise is too easy, he removes one fluency technique. He calls other people's answering machines, or he doesn't use DAF, or he doesn't use fluency techniques, or he doesn't plan his message in advance. Eventually this exercise should be easy. He then goes to using two fluency-enhancing techniques, then one technique, and eventually he should be able to call any answering machine and leave a fluent message.

The stutterer then chooses another stuttering cue, and goes through the exercise again. Reconditioning every stuttering cue into a fluency cue will take months, if not years. Other therapy programs encourage the stutterer to use his fluency techniques in every conversation. This leads to tenuous fluency, and then relapse. This therapy program slowly builds from a solid foundation of fluency, and so avoids relapse.

The stutterer should alter his work and social habits to talk more. This might include making customers calls, or joining a club devoted to a hobby. The stutterer should also consider joining a public speaking club, such as Toastmasters or a National Stuttering Project "speaking circle."

At this point, the stutterer should be off of any drugs. If he has a stuttering biofeedback computer system, it should be saying that is speech is on-target all of the time. If he has an anti-stuttering device, he should only need it for difficult conversations. He's not cured of stuttering, but he is well along the road to recovery. He should be in control of his speech, know what to do when he feels a relapse of stuttering, and should find his speech gradually improving and his time and effort on therapy diminishing.

THE VICTIM ARCHETYPE

In the path of personal growth, recognizing one's wounds is an important stage. Each of us is a victim in some way. At first we deny it, but when we recognize our wounds we can connect with other people who have the same wound. Support groups help you realize that you are not alone. The Stuttering Science & Therapy Website has a penpals page (http://www.casafuturatech.com/penpals.html) and pointers to e-mail stuttering support groups. If you prefer a face-to-face support group, call the National Stuttering Project at (800) 364-1677.

After recognizing your victimhood and connecting with other victims, you need to move on with your life. Some people get stuck in the victim mode. They see racism, sexism or another -ism at every turn. Author Carolyn Myss writes about 50-year-old women who were childhood incest victims, whose lives revolve around incest survivor support groups and newsletters and conventions. One of the stuttering e-mail groups is dominated by a handful of "career stutterers." They don't want to overcome stuttering because then they couldn't get the psychical benefits of victimhood (e.g., blaming others for your problems, avoiding responsibility, not growing).

Psychologist Carol Pearson writes about moving from the victim archetype to the warrior (strength), caregiver (helping others), and other archetypes of the hero's journey. Her books include *Awakening The Heroes Within* (ISBN 0-06-250678-1).

PRACTICE

Organizations for Stutterers

A study of people with cancer found that those who attended a support group lived longer than patients without a support group. Joining a support group increased their survival more than surgery, chemotherapy, or any other cancer treatment. Joining a stuttering support group is an important part of overcoming stuttering.

When traveling , contact the stuttering organization in the city or country you plan to visit. They'll invite you to a support group meeting, and maybe someone will want to show you around their city.

SUPPORT GROUPS WITH AND WITHOUT SPEECH PATHOLOGISTS

Some stuttering support groups are run by a speech pathologist. These groups focus on using techniques and improving your speech. There is a sense of progress. The downside is that all activities center on the speech pathologist.

Stutterers run other support groups. These have more variety of activities. Some groups invite guest speakers. Typically a different person "facilitates" each meeting, so each meeting is different. The downside is that chapter members may not be experts on stuttering, so there isn't much information to share. People share experiences, but without a feeling of progress people stop attending the meetings.

ORGANIZATIONS IN THE U.S. & CANADA

• The National Stuttering Project is a non-profit membership organization for stutterers (and speech pathologists treating stuttering). The NSP has about 1000 members. There is a bi-monthly newsletter, about 75 local self-help groups, weekend workshops in various cities, and an annual convention.

Annual dues are $35. Join by calling (800) 364-1677 or write to 5100 E. La Palma, Suite 208; Anaheim Hills, CA 92807; or NSPmail@aol.com. The website is at http://members.aol.com/nsphome.

The annual conventions are fun — you meet lots of people, and there are workshops and social events.

The NSP does weekend "youth day" workshops for children and teenagers who stutter, and their families. These are run by speech pathologists specializing in childhood stuttering.

The NSP's orientation is towards sharing experiences and emotions. The motto is "If you stutter you're not alone."

When traveling, visit an NSP chapter. You'll be sure to make friends, and possibly have a native offer to show you his city.

• The Stuttering Foundation of America is a non-profit publisher of books and videos about stuttering. It does not have members. See the chapter "Books and Journals About Stuttering." The SFA maintains a list of speech pathologists that treat stuttering, organized by state. The SFA also sponsors an annual workshop for training speech pathologists. Contact the Stuttering Foundation of America at (800) 992-9392, P.O. Box 11749, Memphis, TN 38111-0749. The website is at http://www.stuttersfa.org/.

• The American Speech-Language Hearing Association is the professional organization for speech pathologists and audiologists. The Special Interest Division on Fluency Disorders (SID4) is developing certification standards for fluency specialists.

Non-speech pathologists are allowed to subscribe to the scientific journals. The annual convention (or your state convention) may be worth attending. The National Stuttering Project usually has a booth, and volunteers get to meet the experts on stuttering.

Contact ASHA at (301) 897-5700; 10801 Rockville Pike, Rockville, MD 20852.

• Speak Easy is a non-profit organization with 180 members. They have support groups in New Jersey, New York and Connecticut. They have a quarterly newsletter and an annual retreat each fall and an annual symposium in early summer. Call Bob Gathman at (201) 262-0895; 233 Concord Drive, Paramus, NJ 07652.

• National Council on Stuttering hosts an annual convention in Chicago every October. Call Constance L. Dugan at (312) 996-3132 or e-mail cdugan@uic.edu.

• Toastmasters is for public speaking, not stuttering, but many stutterers find the experience valuable. See the chapter "Public Speaking For Stutterers." There are thousands of local chapters. Toastmasters International, P.O. Box 9052, Mission Viejo, CA

92690-9052, (714) 858-TALK.

• The Canadian Association for People who Stutter (CAPS) is a non-profit organization with local self-help groups, a quarterly newsletter, and conventions in odd-numbered years. CAPS memberships are $20 per year. Contact: Jaan Pill, 2269 Lakeshore Blvd. West, Suite 709, Etobicoke ON M5V 3X6, tel: (888) STU-TTER or (416) 252-0855, fax: (416) 252-0720, E-mail: jaan_pill@sbe.scarborough.on.ca or rinomata@dgs.dnd.ca. The website is at
http://chat.carleton.ca/~dblock/caps.html.

INTERNATIONAL ORGANIZATIONS

• The International Fluency Association is a small membership organization composed mostly of Ph.D. speech pathologists. Stutterers are encouraged to join. The IFA publishes the *Journal of Fluency Disorders*, which is the only scientific journal devoted to stuttering research. Annual dues are $60 ($40 for students). (205) 348-7131; Box 870242, Tuscaloosa, AL 35487-0242. The IFA has a convention every two years.

• The International Stuttering Association (ISA) is an umbrella Association of 25 national stuttering associations.
The website is at http://www.xs4all.nl/~edorlow/isa.html

• European League of Stuttering Associations (ELSA) is a non-profit umbrella organization of Europe's national stuttering charities and self-help associations. Contact: ELSA, c/o BV Stotterer-Selbsthilfe, Gereonswall 112, D-50670 Köln, Germany; tel: +49-221-139-1106; fax: +49-221-139-1370. The website is at
http://www.hugur.is/~benedikt/elsa

• There are associations for stutterers in almost every European country, plus Australia, New Zealand, and South Africa. If you're traveling and wish to make some friends, the Open Directory Project has links to these organizations:
http://dmoz.org/Health/Conditions_and_Diseases/S/Stuttering/

Internet Resources for Stuttering

Netscape's Open Directory project has thousands of volunteer experts link the best Internet resources in their fields. I was appointed editor of the "Stuttering" area. The URL is http://dmoz.org/Health/Conditions_and_Diseases/S/Stuttering/.

I've listed over 50 websites in the Open Directory Project. These are, in my opinion, the best websites about stuttering. The websites are grouped into the following subcategories:

- General Information About Stuttering (2 websites)
- Childhood Stuttering (3 websites)
- Stuttering Science and Research (7 websites)
- Stuttering Therapies and Treatments (14 websites)
- Organizations For Stutterers
  - Africa (1 website)
  - Asia (1 website)
  - Australia (4 websites)
  - Canada (2 websites)
  - Europe (8 websites)
  - United States (5 websites)
- E-mail Discussion and Support Groups (10 websites)
- Stuttering Penpals Webpages (2 websites)
- Books About Stuttering (3 websites)
- Other Stuttering Websites (6 websites)

I've also included the Stuttering FAQ file, with answers to 25 questions.

Books and Journals about Stuttering

RECOMMENDED BOOKS

• *Stuttering: A Life Bound Up In Words*, by Marty Jezer ($23, New York: BasicBooks, 1997). Jezer is a talented and entertaining writer, and author of biographies of Abbie Hoffman, Rachel Carson, and other books. This book is Jezer's autobiography, and stuttering affected everything in his life. You learn much about stuttering and especially stuttering therapies, because Jezer has gone through just about every therapy program (and still stutters).

• *Knotted Tongues*, by Benson Bobrick ($22, Simon & Schuster, 1995). The book has a thirty-page overview of stuttering science, and a twenty-page overview of stuttering therapies. Bobrick is a historian, and the bulk of the book (110 pages) is about historical and literary persons who stuttered. These include Moses, Charles I, Lewis Carroll, Henry James, W. Somerset Maugham, Winston Churchill, and Marilyn Monroe. Bobrick also covers the history of stuttering treatments. Written for non-professionals.

• *A Handbook On Stuttering*, by Oliver Bloodstein, Ph.D. ($45, 1995, San Diego: Singular Publishing). Covers all research on stuttering. It is 90% "science," and 10% therapy. The book can be dense reading, and too often focuses on older research at the expense of current thinking. For example, there's a long section on metronomes, but nothing about the CAFET biofeedback system. But if you have a serious interest in stuttering, you need this book.

Bloodstein also wrote *Stuttering: The Search for a Cause and Cure* (Allyn & Bacon, 1995, about $40). This book covers the same material as his *Handbook*, but is written for non-professional readers. It is less than 200 pages long and easy to read. This book is about two-thirds therapy and one-third scientific research. It is structured as a history of stuttering therapies, but, because most stuttering therapies of the past are still practiced, the book is a good overview of the therapies now available.

• *Self-Therapy For The Stutterer*, by Malcolm Fraser (1993, Stuttering Foundation of America, $3). This is the most widely-published book on stuttering. Your local library probably has it. The book is short and extremely easy to read. The book is a stuttering modification therapy program that you can do without a speech therapist. You work on your feelings and emotions, on relaxation, speaking slowly, stuttering easily, eliminating secondary behaviors and avoidances, listening to your voice, and talking more. You also do voluntary stuttering, cancellations and pull-outs. I met a stutterer who bought the book, did the exercises, and was cured. I bought the book, tried to do the exercises, and wasn't helped a bit. Hopefully you'll have better luck.

• *I, Claudius*, by Robert Graves (1934). A fictional autobiography of the Roman emperor Claudius, who lived from 10 B.C. to 54 A.D. Claudius survived the violent and treacherous reigns of his relatives Augustus, Tiberius, and Caligula because he stuttered and was thought to be feeble-minded. Claudius maintains a positive attitude in the face of ridicule and cruel insults, because of early advice from a wise mentor that his disabilities would cause others to not take him seriously, and he would outlive his tormentors and become a much-loved emperor.

• *Stuttering And Related Disorders Of Fluency,* edited by Richard F. Curlee, Ph.D. (1993, about $50, New York: Thieme Medical Publishers). A good collection of articles for speech pathologists. It is 100% about stuttering treatments — not etiology. Articles cover preschool, school-age, adult stuttering, cluttering, and neurogenic stuttering.

• *Living and Learning with a Child who Stutters — From a Parent's Point of View* by Lise G. Cloutier-Steele, 1995, NC Press Ltd,, 120 pages, ISBN 1-55021-094-7, $16.95. Written by the mother of a disfluent teen who has stuttered since the age of 3. The book also contains a chapter on scientific research by David Forster of Carleton University. To order, write to: University of Toronto Press 5201 Dufferin Street Downsview, Ontario Canada M3H 5T8 or call: (800) 565-9523; fax: (416) 667-7832

PUBLISHERS & DISTRIBUTORS

• The Stuttering Foundation of America (P.O. Box 11749, Memphis, TN 38111-0749, 800/992-9392) publishes books about stuttering. They are all easy to read and inexpensive. The books are "originated in conference setting and are group edited by experts in the field"...which means that sometimes a book sounds like it was written by a committee. You won't find anything new or radical here, but it's all "tried and true" trustworthy advice. You can get the whole set of

16 books for $25. Several books available in Spanish and French translations.

Books for non-professionals:
Self-Therapy For The Stutterer ($3, 192 pages)
To The Stutterer ($2, 116 pages)
If Your Child Stutters: A Guide For Parents ($1, 56 pages, also in Spanish and French)
Do You Stutter: A Guide For Teens ($1, 80 pages)
Stuttering and Your Child: Questions and Answers ($1, 64 pages)
A Stutterer's Story (autobiography of a speech pathologist who stutters), by Fred Murray ($5, 176 pages)

Books for professionals:
Stuttering Words (glossary) ($1, 64 pages)
Therapy For Stutterers ($2, 120 pages)
Treating the School-Age Stutterer ($2, 112 pages)
Stuttering: An Integration of Contemporary Therapies ($2, 80 pages)
Counseling Stutterers ($2, 80 pages)
Stuttering Therapy: Transfer and Maintenance ($2, 112 pages)
Stuttering Therapy: Prevention and Intervention with Children ($2, 152 pages)
The Child Who Stutters: To The Pediatrician ($1, 16 pages)
The Child Who Stutters: To The Family Physician ($1, 16 pages)
Treatment of the Young Stutterer in the School ($2)
Stuttering: Successes and Failures in Therapy ($2)

Video tapes:
Stuttering and Your Child: A Videotape for Parents ($10, 30 minutes)
Do You Stutter: Straight Talk for Teens ($10, 35 minutes)
Therapy In Action (Eight one-hour sessions of Charles Van Riper treating a stutterer with his stuttering modification therapy, $50)

• The National Stuttering Project (5100 E. La Palma, Suite 208; Anaheim Hills, CA 92807, 800/364-1677, NSPmail@aol.com) sells the following books:
Knotted Tongues, by Benson Bobrick ($22)
Self-Help Workbook for People Who Stutter, by Michael Sugarman ($10)
To Say What Is Ours: The Best of 13 Years of Letting GO (articles from the NSP newsletter, $10)
Understanding and Controlling Stuttering, by Bill Parry ($15)

How To Conquer Your Fears of Speaking Before People (public speaking skills for persons who stutter), by John Harrison ($12)
A Stutterer's Story (autobiography of a speech pathologist who stutters), by Fred Murray ($7)
Tangled Tongue: Living With A Stutter, by Jock Carlisle ($13)
Self-Therapy for the Stutterer, by Malcolm Fraser ($3)
Living and Learning with a Child Who Stutters, From a Parent's Point of View, by Lise Cloutier-Steele ($15)
The Adventures of Phil Carrot: The Forest of Discord (children's book about stuttering), by Michael Sugarman and Kim C. Swain ($8)
Dead Languages (short stories about growing up stuttering), by David Shields ($19)
Not Good At Talking (funny and inspiring), by Tim Newark ($11)
The NSP also has pamphlets and posters.

• Communication Skill Builders is a publisher of materials for speech pathologists (555 Academic Court, San Antonio, TX 78204-2498; (800) 228-0752). They have games, videos and lesson plans related to childhood stuttering.

• Pro-Ed is a publisher of materials for speech pathologists. Contact them at 8700 Shoal Creek Blvd., Austin, TX 78757-6897, (512) 451-3246. Their fluency materials include test instruments for diagnosing stuttering, and therapy manuals and games for childhood stuttering.

JOURNALS & NEWSLETTERS

• See the chapter "Organizations For Stutterers" — all have newsletters.

• *ADVANCE For Speech-Language Pathologists* is a free weekly newspaper for speech pathologists and audiologists. It prints articles on stuttering fairly often, and devotes the second issue in May entirely to stuttering. Merion Publications, 650 Park Ave. West, King of Prussia, PA, 19406, (800) 355-5627.

• *The Journal of Fluency Disorders* is the only journal exclusively about stuttering. It is 90% science and 10% therapy. It is written by and for Ph.D. speech pathologists. Published by the International Fluency Association. About $60/year for four issues.

• The American Speech-Language Hearing Association (ASHA)

publishes the following periodicals for speech pathologists:

The Journal of Speech and Hearing Research covers "science" research. There are lots of articles about stuttering.

American Journal of Speech-Language Pathology covers "therapy" research. There are few articles about stuttering.

Language, Speech and Hearing in Schools has articles about treating children who stutter. There are relatively few articles about stuttering.

The Special Interest Division on Fluency Disorders newsletter focuses on professional issues for speech pathologists treating stuttering.

Famous People Who Stutter

Stuttering is a difficult and demoralizing disability, but with hard work and persistence, many stutterers overcome the disorder and go on to successful lives.

Singer/songwriter Carly Simon started stuttering severely when she was eight years old. She blames her stuttering on her then 44-year-old mother's long affair with their 20-year-old live-in tennis instructor. The affair caused jealousy, anger, "lies and a train of deception" in the Simon household.

Simon's mother sent her to a psychiatrist who unsuccessfully tried to cure her stuttering. Instead, Simon turned to singing and songwriting. "I felt so strangulated talking that I did the natural thing, which is to write songs, because I could sing without stammering, as all stammerers can" (Brenner, 1995).

Simon wrote some of the most-loved songs of the 1970s, including "Anticipation" and "You're So Vain," and won an Oscar and a Grammy. She was married to James Taylor for 9 years, and they have two children. Her recent presidential performance "delighted" Bill Clinton (Carlin, 1997).

Mel Tillis, 1976 Country Music Entertainer of the Year, wrote (Nefsky, 1997) that as a child, he was laughed at because he stuttered. He said to himself, "Well, if they're gonna laugh at me, then I'll give them something to laugh about." In 1957 he arrived in Nashville and started working as a singer for Minnie Pearl, the great country comedienne. Pearl encouraged Tillis to talk on stage, but he refused, afraid that he'd be laughed at. Pearl replied, "Let 'em laugh. Goodness gracious, laughs are hard to get and I'm sure that they're laughing with you and not against you, Melvin."

Little by little, Tillis increased his speaking on-stage, and developed humorous routines about his stuttering. Then "word began to circulate around Nashville about this young singer from Florida who could write songs and sing, but stuttered like hell when he tried to talk. The next thing I knew I was being asked to be on every major television show in America." Tillis' career took off.

But before Nashville and fame and fortune, Tillis was looking for a job in Florida. No one would hire him. At the last place he applied, the owner said that he had once stuttered. He wouldn't hire Tillis, but gave him a piece of paper to read every night, saying that it had changed his life.

On the paper was a prayer: "Oh Lord, Grant me the Courage to change the things I can change, the Serenity to accept those I cannot change, and the Wisdom to know the difference. And God, Grant me the Courage to not give up on what I think is right, even though I think it is hopeless."

Tillis concludes his story, "For the first time in a long time, I slept well that night. I woke the next morning with a different outlook on life. I told myself that if I couldn't quit stuttering, then the world was going to have to take me like I was. What you see is what you get. From that day on, things started looking up for Mel Tillis. Soon after, I headed for Nashville in a '49 Mercury with a wife and a four month old baby girl — her name was Pam."

Other stutterers with successful singing careers include Metropolitan Opera singer Robert Merrill, and jazz vocalist "Scatman" John Larkin.

In 1965, Roger Daltry of The Who used stuttering in the song "My Generation": "The stutter was introduced because the 'My Generation' character was supposed to be a mod blocked on pills — and amphetamine abusers stammered like mad" (Marsh, 1983; I've never seen an amphetamine abuser stutter, nor have I seen research showing amphetamines to cause stuttering).

Also in 1965, stutterer Ian Whitcomb recorded the hit "You Turn Me On." According to radio host Dr. Demento, "Whitcomb stutters quite a bit in conversation, but very rarely when he's on mike.." Whitcomb had a popular public radio show in Los Angeles for many years (Hansen, 1999).

In 1975, stutterer Gary Bachman was managing his brother Randy's band, Bachman-Turner Overdrive. The song "You Ain't Seen Nothing Yet" was written as an inside joke, and the band didn't intend it to be heard by anyone else. But a label executive heard the song and insisted that it be included on an album. The song went to #1 on the Billboard charts (Morthland, 1993).

The most in-demand voice in Hollywood — James Earl Jones — is a stutterer. In his autobiography *Voice and Silences*, Jones wrote that he was "virtually mute" as a child. With the help of his high school English teacher, Jones gradually overcame stuttering by reading Shakespeare "aloud in the fields to myself," and then reading to audiences, debating, and finally acting.

Jones is proudest of his roles as Shakespeare's *Othello*, but is best-known as the voice of Darth Vader in *Star Wars*. He recently portrayed a stutterer in the movie *A Family Thing*.

Other stutterers who found fluency in acting include Peggy Lipton (*The Mod Squad*, *Twin Peaks*) and Bruce Willis (*Die Hard*). Sculptor and theater director Robert Wilson overcame stuttering at 17 with the help of his dance teacher. (Hutchings, 1988; Carlson, 1990; Kaylin, 1996; Wilson, 1996.

Peter Bonerz — Jerry the dentist on *The Bob Newhart Show*, and director of *Friends*, *Murphy Brown*, and *Home Improvement* — said about his stuttering: "I'm 58 years old, and if I stutter while giving Candice Bergen a direction, who cares? If (the stuttering) is really difficult, I exaggerate it and get everyone on the set to laugh with me. A stutter can really be quite charming. We are human and not perfect." (Drew, 1997)

Some stutterers make up for their inability to speak by excelling at sports.

Bob Love was a 3-time NBA All-Star and led the Chicago Bulls in scoring for seven consecutive seasons, but reporters rarely interviewed him. "I would score 45 points, go into the locker room, and all the reporters would come down," Love recalls. "Everybody would pass me by."

Love retired in 1977. Because of his stuttering he went from one dead-end job to another. The low point was in 1985, at the age of 42, when he was hired at Nordstrom's as a $4.45/hour busboy. Love had tried speech therapy twice before without success. He tried again. After a year of stuttering therapy, Love began public speaking. As a boy he had a dream of standing on a podium, speaking to thousands of people. Love gave motivational speeches to churches, high school students, and other groups. Love is now director of community relations and spokesman for the Bulls. "It's hard to believe I make a living speaking. It's a dream come true. I held onto my dreams, and I tell kids they have to hold on to theirs." (Lawrence, 1993)

Other athletes who stutter include

• Olympic diver Greg Louganis. In 1994, Louganis announced that he is gay and HIV-positive (Louganis, 1995).

• Basketball star Bill Walton was an NBA All-Star and is now in the Hall of Fame (Walton, 1996).

• Golfer Ken Venturi won 1961 U.S. Open, and is now a commentator for CBS Sports (Venturi, 1994).

• Sprinter Ben Johnson ran the fastest 100-meters ever, but then tested positive for steroids. "He speaks with a heavy Jamaican accent made at times incomprehensible by a stutter" (Kram, 1998).

• Baseball pitcher Tommy John was a four-time All-Star, and was the winning pitcher in two World Series games (Gathman, 1998).

• Baseball and football pro Bo Jackson wrote (Ghostwriter, 1993):

> My teachers thought I couldn't read. I could read, but I'd never read aloud because I stuttered. The other kids would laugh at me, and I became a recluse. I was angry at myself and at them, and it often resulted in my beating someone up after school. I had to live with it for eight or nine years, but I finally decided to pay it no attention and forced myself to do everything from reading in class to making speeches. Eventually, I learned to relax and take my time."

Writers who stutter include Lewis Carroll (*Alice's Adventures in Wonderland*), Somerset Maugham (*Of Human Bondage*), Margaret Drabble (*The Witch of Exmoor*), and John Updike (the *Rabbit* series, *Brazil*). (Bobrick, 1995)

Thomas Carlyle wrote of stutterer Henry James (*Portrait of a Lady*, *Turn of the Screw*): "A stammering man is never a worthless one...It is an excess of delicacy, excess of sensibility to the presence of his fellow-creature, that makes him stammer." (Bobrick, 1995)

John Updike, espousing Joseph Sheehan, believes that his stuttering is precipitated when "I feel myself in a false position," such as guilt of being "in the wrong." (Bobrick, 1995)

Publishers who stutter include Henry Luce, founder of *Time* magazine and *Sports Illustrated*; and Walter Annenberg, founder of *TV Guide* and *Seventeen.* Annenberg recently donated $500 million to improve American schools. (Wallichenski, 1995; Fonzi, 1969; Toch, 1993)

Photographers who stutter include P.F. Bentley, who photographed Bill Clinton's 1992 campaign, and Howard Bingham, friend of Muhammed Ali and O.J. Simpson, who stuttered as a witness in Simpson's trial. Growing up, Bingham "endured the usual teasing from schoolmates because of his stuttering. In high school...he hid behind his stuttering and didn't volunteer for anything." His friendship with Muhammed Ali began in 1962, continued through photographing the Black Panther Party and "virtually every significant urban uprising" in the 1960s, and later working as Bill Cosby's photographer. He wrote the book *Muhammed Ali: A Thirty Year Journey* (Simon and Schuster, 1993), and worked for years to get his friend the honor of lighting the Olympic flame that started the 1996 Atlanta Games. Ironically, Bingham now sometimes has to talk for Ali, due to Ali having

Parkinson's disease (Zimmerman, 1998).

Representative Dennis Kucinich (D-Ohio) overcame stuttering as a child. Rep. Kucinich was elected mayor of Cleveland at the age of 31. As a state senator, he won the 1996 National Association for Social Workers Outstanding Senator of the Year Award. He also won an Emmy for his political analysis on WJW-TV (ASHA Leader).

Which *20/20* reporter stutters? No, not Barbara Walters! John Stossel overcame stuttering with therapy from the Hollins College speech clinic, in Roanoke, Virginia (Stossel, 1997).

In the business world, John Sculley's stuttering "has taken him many years to overcome. He was also painfully shy." Sculley wrote in his autobiography, "I was determined to build a strength out of what was originally a weakness. I went to the theater to watch how performers positioned themselves on stage. I'd practice for hours. I became obsessed with the idea that I was going to become better than anyone else as a business communicator." (Sculley, 1987) Sculley rose to president of Pepsi-Cola (succeeding in overtaking Coca-Cola as the #1 soft drink), and then changed coasts and cultures to become president of Apple Computer for ten years. Sculley became a great public speaker, gaining "renown for his ability to deliver rousing speeches in front of thousands, sometimes without notes." (Carlton, 1997)

Stutterer and CEO Jack Welch has led General Electric to become one of the largest and most profitable corporations in the United States.

Several British royals stuttered. Charles I was king from 1625 until 1649, during the English Civil War. His inability to speak to Parliament "had an unfavorable influence on his affairs." Charles lost the war and was executed. It didn't help that he proclaimed that he was above the law: "a king and a subject are two plain different things." His father, James I, was described as "having a tongue too big for his mouth" — possibly an articulation disorder (Fraser, 1974).

George VI was king from 1937 until 1952. He was father of Queen Elizabeth II. His annual live Christmas broadcasts were "always an ordeal" (Bobrick, 1995). Robert Graves' novel *I, Claudius* is ostensibly about the Roman emperor Claudius, who stuttered. But the personality and life of Graves' Claudius were taken from the shy George VI. George survived the scandals of his brother Edward's abdication, was thrust into a role to which he was thought unsuited, and surprised everyone by becoming one of the most capable and loved modern kings.

More recently, Bruce Oldfield outgrew childhood stuttering and designed gowns for Princess Diana (Johnson, 1987).

After examining a series of killings near San Francisco-area hiking trails in 1979, FBI psychological profiler John Douglas concluded that the Trailside Killer was a stutterer. Most serial killers approach their victims in a social situation and talk the victims into getting in a car, such as picking up hitchhikers. But the Trailside Killer attacked women hiking alone. The Trailside Killer used a "blitz" attack to overpower and dominate his victims, suggesting that he was "someone with some condition he felt ackward or ashamed about" who overpowered and controlled women as "his way of overcoming this handicap." But the power of the attack ruled out a physically-disabled killer. A "very homely" or disfigured individual would have been remembered by witnesses. Douglas concluded that stuttering can make a strong man feel powerless, and was something the killer "could easily feel ashamed of or uncomfortable with...yet wouldn't 'stand out' in a crowd. No one would know about it until he opened his mouth."

One victim was a high school student working part-time at a bank. She had been "kind and sweet...to a regular customer with a severe stutter" — who had an incarceration record for sex crimes. 50-year-old industrial arts teacher David Carpenter was investigated and convicted of murdering eight women.

In 1983, a seventeen-year-old prostitute in Anchorage, Alaska told a fantastic story to police. A man had handcuffed her, taken her home, and raped and brutalized her. Then he took her to his private airplane, telling her they were going to his remote cabin. She escaped and ran to the police.

Robert Hansen was in his mid-forties, married with two children, and managed a successful bakery. He owned an expensive home, as well as an airplane and mountain cabin. He was "short and slight, heavily pockmarked, and spoke with a severe stutter. [The FBI profiler] surmised that he had had severe skin problems as a teenager and, between that and the speech impediment, was probably teased or shunned by his [childhood] peers, particularly girls. So his self-esteem would have been low. That might have [explained] why he moved to Alaska [from Iowa, when he was 25] — the idea of a new start in a new frontier."

Hansen was also a "proficient hunter" with a "well-outfitted trophy room where he watched television, full of animal heads, walrus tusks, horns and antlers, mounted birds, and skins on the floor." Under attic floorboards was another "trophy room": a hunting rifle matching bullets that had killed four prostitutes, as well as "various items of cheap jewelry belonging to the victims...a drivers license and other ID cards from some of the dead women...[and] an aviation map marked with where he had left various bodies." Other jewelry "trophies" he had given to his wife and daughter (Douglas, 1995).

Two murder/suicides strangely echoed each other. In 1993, John O'Brien asked members of his stuttering self-help group where the heart is located in a person's chest. The next day he brought a handgun to the New York subway equipment facility where he worked. He shot a co-worker in the head, killing him instantly, and then shot his supervisor in the chest, leg, abdomen, and back. The supervisor lived. O'Brien then killed himself with a shot to his heart (Laboy, 1993).

O'Brien stuttered severely. He had been denied a promotion because of his speech, but co-workers didn't know whether his victims had ridiculed him. Friends described O'Brien as "an unbelievably-nice guy," "quiet," who "never bothered anyone."

In 1999, Pierre Lebrun brought a high-powered hunting rifle to the Ottawa, Canada, city bus transit complex machine shop where he worked. He killed four co-workers and then killed himself. A suicide note listed many more co-workers that he disliked, and his pockets were full of live ammunition, leading police to speculate that his gun jammed and prevented more killings.

Lebrun stuttered mildly. Lebrun's mother reported, "He said a group of people were harassing him — not only one person, but a group of people. That's why he killed, that's why he went there — to kill the people who harassed him."

Lebrun's cousin recalled teasing in school. "That was the only thing that bothered him. It didn't bother him that he had the stutter; it bothered him that people would bug him about it." (Ottawa Citizen, May 3, 1999)

Lebrun had completed a four-month speech therapy program two years earlier. He was described as "a really nice guy," "friendly," and "quiet and well-mannered." (Reuters, Sun Media; April 7-9, 1999)

The man who brought us LSD was "a lifelong stutterer." Sidney Gottlieb, described by friends as "a kind of genius," had a Ph.D. in biochemistry from Caltech. He joined the CIA in 1951. In 1953 he founded the MKUltra program, which gave LSD to thousands of CIA agents, military officers, college students, prisoners, and mental patients. Many of the study participants were unknowingly dosed with the drug. Gottlieb took LSD hundreds of times.

Gottlieb's later work at the CIA included developing "a poison handkerchief to kill an Iraqi colonel, an array of toxic gifts to be delivered to Fidel Castro, and a poison dart to kill a leftist leader in the Congo. None of the plans succeeded."

After leaving the CIA, Gottlieb studied to be a speech pathologist, and raised goats on a commune in Virginia (Weiner, 1999).

Stuttering is one of the few disorders that generally gets better over time. Most children who stutter outgrow it. Even adults who stutter severely in their teens and 20s often overcome stuttering — via speech therapy or on their own — in their 30s or 40s. At the time when other people have the dreams of their youth crash down, stutterers realize they can do accomplish anything they want, regardless of their speech. Stutterers are less likely to be famous in their youth, and more likely to be famous five hundred years later.

Or five thousand years later. Moses stuttered (Exodus, 4:10-12):

> Moses, however, said to the Lord, "If you please, Lord, I have never been eloquent, neither in the past, nor recently, nor now that you have spoken to your servant; but I am slow of speech and tongue."
>
> The Lord said to him, "Who gives one man speech and makes another deaf and dumb? Or who gives sight to one and makes another blind? Is it not I, the Lord? Go, then! It is I who will assist you in speaking and will teach you what you are to say."

Demosthenes, the greatest orator of ancient Greece, overcame stuttering by speaking with pebbles in his mouth to improve articulation, shouting above the ocean waves to improve his volume, and working with an actor in reciting Sophocles and Euripedes to coordinate his voice and gestures. (Bobrick, 1995)

Aesop was born a slave and "most deformed" and "he coulde not speke." One day he fell asleep under a shady tree. The Goddess of Hospitality appeared to him in a dream and gave him the gift of speech. His life changed and he became a master storyteller. (Bobrick, 1995)

Claudius, the crippled Roman emperor who used his disabilities to make murderous rivals think he wasn't a political threat. (Graves, 1937)

In the sixteenth century, Dekanawida convinced the fifty leaders of the Iroquois nation to sit as "a brother among brothers" at a grand council to work out problems peacefully, and created the world's first representative government. Benjamin Franklin studied the Iroquois and proposed that the new United States adopt a similar system. Because Dekanawida stuttered, his assistant Hiawatha spoke for him. (Kehoe, 1992)

Cotton Mather found that fasting and prayers failed to affect his stuttering, but speaking in a "drawling...little short of Singing" enabled him to become a Puritan preacher, and prosecutor of the Salem witch trials. (Bobrick, 1995)

Other stutterers included nurse Clara Barton, the Civil War "angel of the battlefield" and founder of the American Red Cross; and naturalist Charles Darwin and his grandfather Erasmus Darwin, who was personal physician for King George III of England. (Bobrick, 1995)

60 years ago the best orators of the British Parliament were both stutterers. Aneurin Bevan, leader of the Labour Party and architect of the National Health Service, forced himself to do public speaking as often as possible. He spoke fluently when his passions were aroused, so he spoke passionately for British workers in the 1930s. Bevan developed an extraordinary vocabulary by substituting words to avoid stuttering. (Bobrick, 1995).

Winston Churchill, leader of the Conservative Party, could speak fluently only by preparing his remarks in advance. He studied issues weeks in advance, and wrote out responses to any possible objection. This extra effort made Churchill more knowledgeable than other leaders. (Bobrick, 1995)

Each man found a way to overcome stuttering, and this way became the basis of his success. In this way they were like Carly Simon, whose songs connected with listeners emotionally because she couldn't express her feelings through speech; like James Earl Jones, who wouldn't have dedicated himself to acting if it hadn't been his only way to communicate; and like Bob Love, whose drive to be the best basketball player was fueled in part by his feelings of inadequacy due to his speech. For each, their disability became their strength — and perhaps each looks back and sees stuttering as a gift.

AND MORE FAMOUS STUTTERERS

From *Knotted Tongues*, by Benson Bobrick, New York: Simon&Schuster, 1995:

Vergil — Roman poet.

Robert Boyle — British chemist, known for his experiments on the properties of gases.

Moses Mendelsohn — Born 1729, grandfather of the composer. Advocated assimilation for German Jews.

Charles Lamb — British writer. He was not allowed to pursue a scholarly education because of his stuttering, but worked as an accountant and wrote on the side. Lamb advocated smoking heavily to loosen your tongue.

Leigh Hunt — British writer, founded the liberal *Examiner* newspaper.

Charles Canon Kingsley — British orator, writer, and chaplain to Queen Victoria. He recommended treating stuttering with a "manly" diet of beef and beer.

Arnold Bennett — British novelist and playwright (1867-1931).

Marilyn Monroe — Actress, who used a breathy way of speaking to avoid stuttering.

Kim Philby — British spy. Stuttering once saved his life, by confounding a fast-paced interrogator.

Nevil Shute — British novelist and aeronautical engineer.

Elizabeth Bowen — Anglo-Irish novelist.

Edward Hoagland — American writer.

Patrick Campbell — British humorist.

From other sources:

John Slaughter — Elected Cochise County, Arizona sheriff in 1886 with a mandate to clean up crime in Tombstone, after Wyatt Earp's 1881 shoot-out. "Slaughter, with penetrating black eyes, was only 5 feet 6 and often stuttered. But he wore a pearl-handled .44 and carried a 10-gauge, double-barreled, sawed-off shotgun, 'which was an equalizer.'" That's one way to get equal rights for stutterers! (UPI news story)

Lord David Cecil — Professor of English literature at Oxford in the 1950s. "Lord David's stutter was thought of as a mark of high-bred diffidence...As an Oxford undergraduate in the fifties, I expected my tutors to stutter; it was their way of not *insisting*, I thought, and very Oxford." (Ian Hamilton, "An Oxford Union," *The New Yorker*, February 19, 1996. Hamilton adds that John Bailey, husband of novelist Iris Murdoch and another student of Lord David Cecil, also stutters.)

How Gracie Allen met George Burns: "She was looking for [vaudeville performer] Billy Lorraine who was a terrible stammerer. He was shy about his stammering. Gracie approached him and asked him if he was Billy Lorraine. Billy said he wasn't and pointed at George Burns. George Burns pretended he was Billy Lorraine for a while." (*George Burns: And the Hundred Year Dash*, by Martin Gottfried)

Paul Johnson — Detective novelist, author of *Killing The Blues*. (Interviewed on National Public Radio's *All Things Considered*.)

Annie Glenn — Wife of astronaut and Senator John Glenn. Tom Wolfe's book *The Right Stuff* says that Mrs. Glenn once refused to talk to President Johnson because of her stuttering.

Berkeley Free Speech leader Mario Savio. (Reference from Richard Benyo.)

Frank Wolf — Virginia congressman. (SFA)

Marilyn Monroe — actress. (SFA)

Antonio Bassolino — Mayor of Naples "stuttered in childhood, and still at present sometimes has minor disfluencies." (Roberto De Simone, personal correspondence)

Nino Salvatore — Past president of the Medical University of Naples. "He is a very successful professor of General Pathology. He is also a very clever and eloquent speaker, and his stuttering is, for listeners, just a fascinating style of speaking." (Roberto De Simone, personal correspondence)

Marion Davies — Actress. "Fifty-two-year-old publishing magnate William Randolph Hearst was smitten the first time he saw eighteen-year-old Marion Davies in a chorus line. A year later, when she was given one speaking line in Ziegfeld's Follies, she botched it. Hearst, determined to make her a star, provided coaches to work day and night on her stammer. She improved, and starred in a number of films." (From *The Book of Lists*, by David Wallechinski; and *The New Yorker*, March 23, 1998, p. 70)

Ty Cobb — Baseball player. (*Cobb: A Biography*, by Al Stump).

Jake Steinfeld — Bodybuilder, television fitness trainer. (New York Daily News, November 12, 1997).

Successful Stuttering Stories

DEKANAWIDA — FATHER OF REPRESENTATIVE GOVERNMENT

Dekanawida invented representative government. He united the Iroquois nation in what is now New York state. This was in the sixteenth century, before the Iroquois encountered Europeans.

Dekanawida's ideas influenced English philosopher Thomas Moore, and American Benjamin Franklin. The Iroquois model of representative government inspired the Americans and French to create representative democracies.

Before Dekanawida was born, a messenger from the holy spirit told Dekanawida's grandmother that the child would become a great leader. Perhaps Dekanawida's mother and grandmother had high expectations for the child to speak well and be an overachiever, and their high expectations caused the child to stutter.

Anthropologist Alice B. Kehoe writes,

> The League of the Five Nations of the Iroquois was established, according to eighteenth-century sources, in the late sixteenth century. Iroquois tradition tells of constant warfare...One bereaved by this warfare was a Mohawk man, Hiawatha ('He Who Makes Rivers').
>
> Crazed by grief for his murdered family, Hiawatha fled into the forests, living like a cannibal monster in the Iroquois myths. One day, Hiawatha met Dekanawida. The charismatic goodness of this man, said to have been a Huron miraculously born of a virgin, reawakened in Hiawatha his humanity.
>
> Dekanawida confided to Hiawatha plans to free their peoples from the horrors of war by allying all the Iroquois in a grand league, a longhouse...in which [the leader of] each Iroquois nation would sit as a brother with brothers.
>
> The visionary felt himself unequal to the task of forming the league because he suffered a speech impediment. Hiawatha, however, was an imposing man with a fluent tongue. Together, in the time-honored fashion of a wise leader who relies on his executive assistant to make his speeches (as among the Cherokee and Creek), Dekanawida and Hiawatha might be effective in restoring sanity and peace to their nations.
>
> Hiawatha was inspired. Tirelessly, the two men traveled up and down the land...Hiawatha fervently preaching the alliance outlined by Dekanawida.
>
> Most Iroquois were at first hesitant to trust a plan that contained their enemies. Thadodaho, an Onondaga leader, relentlessly opposed

Hiawatha. In a dramatic showdown, Hiawatha's superior spiritual power overcame the evil Thadodaho. Hiawatha combed out of Thadodaho's hair the snakes that had marked him as a fearful sorcerer.

Then the five nations — Mohawk, Oneida, Onondaga, Cayuga, and Seneca — came together, fifty great chiefs meeting in a grand council at the principal town, in the center of the alliance territory. (Kehoe, 1992)

BILL WALTON — "A WIN OVER STUTTERING"

Bill Walton led UCLA to two NCAA titles, and the Portland Trailblazers and Boston Celtics to NBA championships, but his stuttering was so severe that he couldn't say simple phrases like "thank you."

Today, Walton has overcome his stuttering and works as a sports commentator for NBC Sports.

As Walton was battling stuttering through childhood, college, and his professional career, he used basketball as a sanctuary, a place where he didn't have to think about his speech. The challenges in his personal life pushed him to be one of the best players on the court. Amazingly, on the court, he could not only play ball, he could speak, too. Or at least yell. "I never had any trouble yelling at the refs," Walton said. "In the heat of the game...when it was just totally spontaneous, I could get out there and really scream and yell at the refs. But it was only in basketball, and it was only at the refs."

When each game ended, Walton stuttered again.

"During college, the teasing was tough," he said. "I had a speech class one year, and they laughed me out of the class." It didn't matter to his classmates that he was the college basketball Player Of The Year. "I was trying to make it in school, and they just laughed me out of the class."

At awards ceremonies and media events, Walton shied away from microphones. He even had other people speak on his behalf. "When I had to actually formulate words and make a statement, I could not do it at all," he recalls.

In the NBA, he faced some of the toughest and most legendary players in the history of the game. Playing basketball with Kareem Abdul-Jabbar and Larry Bird came naturally. Speaking, still, did not.

After he retired from basketball, the sanctuary was gone. The hiding place that had protected him for 28 years could shelter him no longer. But his love for the game helped him with stuttering.

According to Walton, long-time friend and Hall of Fame broadcaster Marty Glickman pulled him aside at a social event and said, "You've got to learn how to talk." "He gave me some very basic tips, and I applied those tips to the learning techniques I learned from my coach at UCLA John Wooden about how to develop as a basketball player," Walton explained. "I thought about fundamentals and how to start with the basics like the ability to mechanically duplicate moves on the basketball court. And I just applied that to speaking."

So Walton learned to speak, just as he had learned basketball years before. Not only did he stop stuttering, he found a way back — through sports commentating — to the game he loved so much.

When he began broadcasting for NBC Sports, all of his fears resurfaced. Off the court, he was still afraid to talk. He describes his first broadcast as "painful" but knows now that the worst is over. "I used to be really embarrassed about stuttering. But now I realize that it's something that is a part of me...something that I have to deal with and work on every day. If I don't work on it, I'm not going to be able to do my job. It's always a challenge," Walton said. He doesn't mind the challenge — that's what makes him strive to do his best.

Walton challenges others to get on top of stuttering too. "It's important to know that help is out there. The ability to learn how to talk is easily the greatest thing I've ever done. Winning two NCAA championships and two NBA titles was nice, but I knew it was going to happen. But learning how to speak has given me a whole new life. I have been set free."

(Reprinted with permission from the Stuttering Foundation of America newsletter Spring/Summer 1996.)

COLLEEN WILCOX — "IF I'M SPECIAL, IT'S BECAUSE I STUTTER"

This is about a woman who stuttered severely. She used a variety of compensatory strategies to overcome her inability to communicate. The result was that she not only overcame stuttering, but also became successful in many endeavors.

Colleen Wilcox is Superintendent of the Santa Clara County Office of Education. She is responsible for 33 school districts, 7 community colleges, and other education programs.

Dr. Wilcox is a speech pathologist. She is on the board of directors of the American Speech-Language Hearing Association Foundation. She has written and illustrated two children's books. She plays piano, guitar, banjo, and mandolin.

She says that all that is a result of stuttering.

Growing up in Moline, Illinois, she was an hour from the University of Iowa's famous stuttering clinic. At age seven, Wendell Johnson treated her. Johnson believed that stuttering is caused by parents' negative reactions to a child's normal disfluencies.

Wendell Johnson's therapy didn't help, and Dr. Wilcox no longer agrees with Johnson's views on stuttering. But she decided to be a speech pathologist when she grew up.

Unable to talk, Dr. Wilcox developed her talents as an artist and a musician. Stuttering also made her sensitive to other people's needs. She worked harder at everything she did. She concludes, "If I'm special, it's because I stutter."

Dr. Wilcox also realized that communication is essential in every area of life, both professional and personal. She married for the first time a year ago, at age 44, because she felt unable to form close relationships at an earlier age.

Dr. Wilcox's speech sounds fluent now. She developed fluency through laryngeal awareness and control. She believes that stuttering is a dysfunction in the area of the brain that controls the larynx.

She explained that your vocal folds vibrate when they catch air flowing past. To phonate, the vocal folds must be neither too relaxed (allowing air to flow past without catching), nor too tense (blocking air flow). Sounds can be voiceless, such as /s/ and /p/, which are produced by the lips and tongue; or voiced, such as vowels, which also require vocal fold vibration (phonation).

Because most words have both voiced and voiceless sounds, your vocal folds start and stop vibrating many times each second as you talk. Stuttering occurs at the transitions from voiceless to voiced sounds. If you say "c-c-c-c-cat," you're saying the /c/ fine. Your problem is getting your vocal folds to relax to say the /a/.

Dr. Wilcox explained that all stuttering therapies ultimately do one thing: continuous phonation. If you keep your vocal folds vibrating, you won't stutter.

There are many ways to do this. Speaking slower with prolonged vowels, maintaining steady air flow, using voiced starter sounds, even speaking in a Southern drawl or singing enables continuous phonation.

Dr. Wilcox uses a unique technique to speak fluently: she substitutes voiced for voiceless sounds! For example, her stepmother Patty is now "Baddy." Because she speaks quickly and emphasizes vowels, no one notices the change.

While there is no one technique that works for everyone, Dr. Wilcox believes that everyone can and should find a technique that works for them. Communication is so important in every aspect of life that you should do everything you can to improve your communication skills.

Dr. Wilcox explained that the larynx is one of the first muscles tensed when experiencing fear or anxiety. When you fear a speaking situation, you tense your vocal folds, and are unable to speak. While learning to reduce your fear of speaking is important, Dr. Wilcox believes that stuttering is ultimately neurological, and people who stutter must learn compensatory behaviors to produce normal phonation and speech.

BILL PARRY — AN ATTORNEY WHO STUTTERS

Bill Parry, who is on the National Stuttering Project Board of Directors, wrote the following about himself. More of his writing is available at his website, http://members.aol.com/wdparry/index.htm.

–

I am an attorney and a PWS, although I'm much more fluent now than I used to be. I graduated from an Ivy League law school where I was on the Law Review, but was openly rejected by a number of law firms because of my stuttering. While stuttering was a indeed a handicap, it was not nearly as bad as my own negative attitude toward stuttering and myself, my belief that it was a sign of psychoneurosis, and my tendency to struggle against stuttering and to blame myself for my disfluency.

For several years I edited a legal magazine, until I decided I had to take another plunge into the real practice of law, stutter or not. I started working at low wages for a trial lawyer who appreciated my intellectual skills and research and writing ability. Before long I myself was in court handling motions and even trying jury cases, regardless of the stuttering. Eventually I developed my own approach to handling my stuttering, and I improved my fluency to the extent that it was no longer a problem. Subsequently, when I moved on to other firms, stuttering has been a non-issue.

Unless it is very severe, stuttering need not prevent one from communicating effectively. If you have a positive and accepting attitude toward yourself and your speech, as well as the necessary intellectual, research, and writing ability, and if you like communicating with and trying to persuade people, stuttering need not stop you from being a lawyer.

Stuttering in the Movies

Items by Ira Zimmerman reprinted with permission.

IRA ZIMMERMAN, PORKY PIG, & THE MEDIA

Ira Zimmerman has changed the portrayal of stutterers in movies and other media. His accomplishments include convincing film producer Gerald Rafshoon to have Ben Kingsley portray Moses as a stutterer. Zimmerman also consulted for a *Quantum Leap* television series episode in which Scott Bukala portrayed a stutterer.

Zimmerman's latest success is persuading Warner Brothers to use Porky Pig on a poster promoting tolerance. The poster, which can be downloaded from

http://wbanimation.com/cmp/kidspstr.htm

shows cartoons and children, some with handicaps, above the caption, "Everyone's Unique & Th-Th-That's Good Folks!"

Newspapers have provided his views on the Porkster to 30 million readers. In 1996 *NBC Nightly News* interviewed Zimmerman on a variety of stuttering issues, and then edited out everything he said except his remarks on Porky Pig. His comments were then followed up on "pundit" talk shows, with conservative pundits such as Rush Limbaugh calling Ira too "politically-correct."

Zimmerman even became a question on the game show *Jeopardy*, the second-highest-rated syndicated TV show in the United States. Oliver North choose the category "Politically Incorrect" for $500, but didn't know that Zimmerman had led a protest of the mocking of Michael Palin's character's stuttering in the 1988 movie *A Fish Called Wanda* (Zimmerman, 1997).

DISCOMFORT WATCHING STUTTERING

Of the 60 chapters in this book, the least-requested chapter (from the Stuttering Science & Therapy Website) is "Stuttering In The Movies". One stutterer explained why:

> I usually have a very uncomfortable feeling whenever I see a [movie/TV] character stuttering. It doesn't matter whether it is a "good" or "bad" portrayal of stuttering. It is worse when I am with others, especially family. I feel uneasy about it, and I guess I hope they will not mention anything. I suppose I am afraid of what they think.

Another stutterer added:

I used to feel that way, when I was little and didn't want to draw attention to my stutter. Anyone remember the crummy TV show "Small Wonder"? Well I was about 10, and I knew that an episode was going to be coming on where there was a girl who stuttered badly. I DID NOT want to watch this show, either by myself or with others, so I conveniently left the house for that half hour. I guess I didn't want a discussion to develop about my problem.

But now that I'm 21, I don't think it's so unnerving. I find the more I talk openly about my stutter, the less anxious I feel about it. If you fear it and allow it to become a thing of anxiety, then you'll always feel uncomfortable about it. Far better to confront it and get the mental advantage over 'it'.

TELEVISION/VIDEO

• My favorite video is about Bob Love, former Chicago Bulls NBA basketball star. The video was produced by John Stossel for ABC's "20/20" program.

• *Speaking of Courage* and *Voices to Remember* are each one-hour videos, both from the Canadian producer Vladimir Bondarenko. *Speaking of Courage* is about children, and *Voices to Remember* is about adults. The videos interview children and adults who stutter, parents, spouses, teachers, and speech pathologists. Available in the United States from Suncoast Media, P.O. Box 990, Largo, Florida 34649; (800) 211-2954; fax: 813-392-2559. Cost is US$39 for home use only, US$89 for public performance. In Canada, the distributor is: Magic Lantern Communications #38, 775 Pacific Road, Oakville, ON L6L 6M4 (800)263-1717 (Eastern Canada); (800) 263-1818 (Western Canada).

• Robert Graves' book *I, Claudius*, about the Roman emperor who stuttered, was made into a BBC television series. Some public libraries have the video. You can buy the entire 14 hours for $130 from Fusion Video, 17311 Fusion way, Country Club Hills, IL 60478, 800/959-0061.

• Two episodes of the television series *Quantum Leap* (1993) had Scott Bukala portray a stutterer.

• Garry Hancock writes, "On a show called 'Here Come The Brides' in the late 60s, Bobby Sherman portrayed a PWS very well. It was one of the first times that it really dawned on me that maybe I wasn't alone in this." He adds also "one 'MASH' episode in which Charles was dealing with a young soldier who stuttered. It also was well done." Ira Zimmerman adds an episode of "Little House on the Prairie" where Laura's Swedish girl friend stuttered and the other little girls were cruel to her.

• *Moses*, starring Ben Kingsley (Turner Network Television, 1996). Ira Zimmerman wrote the following review:

Academy Award-winner Ben Kingsley stars as one of the most beloved and inspiring heroes of the Bible.

Moses film director Roger Young said, "Knowing what we do of the time, we can surmise that this adopted Hebrew child might not have been entirely accepted in the court of Ramses II. The Bible talks about Moses being slow of tongue, shy and humble. That's the Moses we've chosen to portray: a small man, an outsider, flawed, a stutterer who is, in fact, a very large man."

Kingsley gives a riveting portrayal of Moses as a person tormented by not knowing his place in his world and laughed at in pharaoh's court because of his stutter and questionable background — born to a Hebrew mother but raised by the daughter of an Egyptian pharaoh.

Kingsley considered Moses to be "a survivor of the Holocaust," displaying "what I recognize in Simon Wiesenthal as the 'guilt of the survivor.' Moses as a child survived the killing of contemporaries by being put in a basket in the river," Kingsley related. "He was then adopted by the very people who killed his peers. If you can imagine this in World War II parallels, it would be like a Jew being adopted by the SS." Is it any wonder that Moses stuttered, Kingsley asked.

Kingsley's Moses does not stutter severely because the filmmakers believe that frequent stuttering will test the audience's patience and distract them from the story.

Moses' deliverance of Jews from slavery in Egypt, which is recorded in the biblical book Exodus, is celebrated during Passover. While the holiday is usually a time of rejoicing for Jews, I always faced Passover with much trepidation as a child because I stuttered quite severely.

Our family gathered at the beginning of the eight-day Passover holiday for the Seder meal. During the Seder, it is traditional for the youngest child — which was me — to ask the four questions about the uniqueness of Passover. My grandfather answered the questions in the telling of the Passover story from a Haggadah. I remember every year having much difficulty asking the questions and felt a great deal of shame because of my stuttering.

I wish I had been told — as part of the story contained in the Passover Haggadah — that the Lord had chosen as his messenger someone who was "slow of speech and slow of tongue." Many Biblical scholars have interpreted this passage to mean that Moses was a stutterer. I believe this would have greatly comforted me as a child who stuttered and helped with my self-esteem.

A review in *TV Guide*, in which reviewer Susan Stewart called Moses a "stuttering nerd," brought letters of protest from readers, including the following from Pastor Dan Lozer, Tabor, Iowa:

> Susan Stewart is entitled to her opinion, but her implication that portraying Moses as a "stuttering nerd" renders him not so inspiring requires some challenge. Scripture cites Moses as being "slow of speech," and many believe that to be a specific idiom for "stuttering" (Exodus 4:10). It is extremely consistent with both Scripture and life that God chooses some very unlikely people (i.e., those "we" wouldn't choose) as bearers of the message.

FEATURE FILMS

Ira Zimmerman writes that there have been many minor film roles that portrayed stutterers in an unfavorable light:

The incompetent public defender in *My Cousin Vinny.*

The boxing champion in *Harlem Nights.*

The murderers in *Primal Fear* and *Dead Again.*

Oscar had a stool pigeon as a stutterer.

A weirdo in *Do the Right Thing.*

The driver for a drug dealer in *New Jack City.*

The head crook in *Die Hard With a Vengeance.*

The shy guy in *One Flew Over the Cuckoo's Nest.*

In *Smoky and the Bandit*, Mel Tillis did a cameo appearance as an amusement park employee. "He stuttered badly and was made to look like an idiot by the main characters."

These following are positive portrayals:

The story about Annie Glenn in *The Right Stuff.*

The sexually confused teenager who fought back when someone made fun of his stuttering in *Color of Night.*

A black young man in *Glory*.
Gabriel Byrne's character in *Smilla's Sense of Snow*.

• Stephen King's horror movie *It* features a stutterer in the leading role. The character, Bill is portrayed as a teenager and as an adult. The teenager's stuttering is mild, but his fluency deteriorates badly under periods of stress. Thirty years later, the adult Bill has lost his stutter. But when the antagonist returns to terrorize the small Maine town, Bill's stuttering returns too.

• The British comedy *A Fish Called Wanda* (1988) features Michael Palin as a severe stutterer. Palin's father stuttered, and Palin wanted to show how difficult and painful stuttering can be. Palin founded the Michael Palin Centre for Stammering Children in London.

Like many severe stutterers, Palin's character is sometimes too eager to please people, even people who treat him poorly.

The character played by Jamie Lee Curtis is able to look beyond Palin's stuttering to see his inner qualities. The antagonist, played by Kevin Klein, can't get past Palin's stuttering. He bullies Palin, emotionally and physically.

• Michael Shamberg, the producer for *A Fish Called Wanda*, has learned how to portray a stutterer in a positive way. In the film *Leaving Minnesota* (1996), there is a police detective who stutters and who by the end of the film brings law and order to the crazy society portrayed in this wacky film which I enjoyed. (Review by Ira Zimmerman)

• *A Family Thing* (1996). Ira Zimmerman wrote the following review:

During the years that I lobbied Hollywood for a more balanced portrayal of stutterers, I always hoped that one day moviemakers would produce a film with a powerful story and interesting characters — one of whom happened to stutter.

The United Artists' film, *A Family Thing*, starring Academy Award-winner Robert Duvall and multiple Emmy and Tony winner James Earl Jones, is such a film. It is filmmaking at its best, with wonderful character development, casting, and direction — a compelling story that tests what binds blood relations together.

Jones' role of Ray Murdoch, a Marine-turned-Chicago-policeman, posed a challenge to both actor and director regarding how to convey the character's vulnerability. They discovered a way, almost by accident, during one of the first read-through rehearsals.

"I'm a stutterer," Jones revealed, "and it inadvertently came out at that moment. Dick [Pearce, director] noticed and suggested I let Ray be a stutterer to make him more vulnerable. I agreed, as long as it wouldn't be played to make fun of the stutterer. It helped us reach this character who — although he's been a Marine and a cop and has gone through the [rural] Arkansas and urban Chicago experience — feels things very deeply.

"All the hurts that have happened to him in life are still sitting deep inside him," he stated, "so they crop out once in a while."

In the film, producer Randa Haines noted, "James gets to show a side of himself that we haven't seen before. He has such an incredible presence, you think of him as being so powerful. Here he's much gentler, humbler. It's a nice change for him."

Duvall portrays Earl Pilcher, Jr., a man who has lived all of his life in the same house in the same town in rural Arkansas. Pilcher's life starts to unravel when his mother dies. She leaves behind a letter that reveals she was not his real mother. The woman who died giving birth to him was black and had been raped by his father. The dying wish of the woman who Pilcher knew as his mother is that he seek out his half-brother, Murdoch.

When Pilcher and Murdoch meet, both men have issues of mistrust, anger and prejudice. Their personal odyssey spotlights the strengths and weaknesses of family ties.

For those of us who stutter and are fighting for a fair deal from the Hollywood film industry, this film has historic significance.

James Earl Jones almost didn't portray the policeman with a stutter. James' agent was dead set against it because he thought that if he voluntarily stuttered for a part he would have a relapse that would destroy his career. He got some advice from some fluency disorder specialists that voluntary stuttering is a good thing and might even help his real stuttering. So he agreed and went ahead with the portray a tough policeman who just happens to stutter.

Employment and Stuttering

WHAT DO I DO?

The following letter appeared in a stuttering support group newsletter (Giret, 1996):

I am 21 years old. Recently, I graduated from my third college course and still no job. Interviews come by the dozens but job offers are none! I am a Pharmacy Assistant Health Care Aide plus a medical transcriptionist, but after all the years in school and all the money spent on education, I am still unable to find work! Am I to live in poverty because people only see me at my worst?

Interviews for me are a horrid experience. I've had people pick up a newspaper and start reading it, waiting for me to get out of a block. All the interviewers act as if I'm wasting their time. It's more like they're wasting mine.

If people could only see me when I am fluent I'm sure I would have a job. On interviews I find myself apologizing for my speech...but why do I?

Is there anyone out there who is experiencing the same problems? I need help to cope.

A stutterer wrote on an Internet support group:

I am a embedded software engineer, and today I was faced with a situation that I have not ran into yet in my pursuit of employment. Like many of you I have had the phone hung up on me by recruiters, or they rudely and quickly end the phone conversation. I had a personal phone interview with Motorola. First, the interview was designed to be very high stress. Second, the questions were given to me in advance which only made the situation worse. Of course it being a phone interview made it worst. I was unable to form sentences and completely locked up on the interview and was eliminated from the running for this software engineering position. Can I do anything? According to the recruiter I'm a great fit for the position, god this frustrating.

A speech pathologist described his experience as a witness in a case of employment discrimination (Starkweather, 1993):

A weather forecaster for the National Weather Service, based in Washington, D.C., was denied promotion to a higher position, where he would have had to make rapid decisions about forecasts, on the grounds that he was 'indecisive'. He sued the government, claiming discrimination against him based on his speech. The supervisor, who made the judgment, had no other evidence that he was indecisive, except his speech, and of course hesitancy in speech does not in any way imply hesitancy in decision making.

I was asked to supply expert testimony and did so by reviewing the scientific literature showing a cleat tendency for listeners to make false judgments about stutterers, and employers in particular. A telling piece of evidence for this case came from a study in which it was shown that the personality characteristics that non-stutterers attribute to people who stutter are based on the feeling that the non-stutterers feel when they are hesitant, or stumble, in their speech — nervousness and uncertainty primarily. We were able to argue that, in the case of the weatherman seeking promotion, the supervisor had made just such an error concluding from his speech pattern that he was uncertain because she (the supervisor) stumbled in her speech when she felt uncertain. Upon presentation of this testimony, the case was settled and the man promoted.

THREE STUDIES OF EMPLOYMENT AND STUTTERING

Francis Freeman (1993) wrote:

> Graduate students in my stuttering class [surveyed employers, who] indicated that they would prefer to hire someone who was deaf or someone with moderate cerebral palsy rather than someone who stuttered. Interestingly, several of the employers who said they would not hire a stutterer had one or more stutterers already working for them.
>
> When we probed to understand the WHY behind the employers' responses, we learned that essentially they thought they "understood" deafness and cerebral palsy, but stuttering was strange — and they assumed that persons who stutter were strange.

An Australian study found that in the ten months after completing a "smooth speech" (fluency shaping) program, 44% of employed stutterers had received a promotion. 40% had changed jobs, 36% reporting that the change was for the better. Combining these, about 60% had improved employment after stuttering therapy. The study also found that 88% of the stutterers had maintained their fluency.

The same authors report a study of the employers of 38 stutterers who completed the "smooth speech" program, and 20 stutterers on the waiting list for the program. The employers completed a survey before therapy, and then two months after therapy. The employers reported about a 20% improvement in "communication effectiveness" for the stutterers completing therapy, and no change for the stutterers who didn't do therapy. (Craig, 1991)

Research found that stutterers earn approximately $7200 less per year than non-stutterers. Two groups of 25 persons were examined. The groups were matched for age, sex, IQ, race, education, and socioeconomic background. The subjects were contacted 10 years after graduating from college. They were asked a number of questions relating to levels of achievement. The difference did not appear to be the result of employer discrimination. Rather, the stutterers were reluctant to accept promotions that involved making presentations to groups of people (Schwartz, 1996b).

A stutterer sent me the following e-mail:

> I have refused (or went "kicking") different projects at my job, which may/may not lead to promotions. Most recently, I went kicking on co-facilitating a corporate-wide quality workshop initiative. My partner in facilitation, after much coaxing by me, took the majority of the speaking sections, while I became her assistant. (Please be aware that I have not discussed my disorder with my co-workers, I am a mild stutter that can usually "pass" for a fluent speaker.) I am now interested in changing careers and am looking for careers that focus on "behind the scenes" work…i.e., technical writing. I have considered such careers as Law, but have veered away from them.

TALK ABOUT YOUR STUTTERING

> Another interview lasted about two minutes. The interviewer (another personnel director — they seem to be the worst problem) found an excuse to say I was not qualified for the job — so good-bye. I protested, asked for the technical interview and was asked to leave. As his excuse was plainly made up — this was also probably a case of discrimination. (David Bertollo)

Whether you're looking for a job or already have a job, talk about your stuttering. Many people feel uncomfortable talking to a person who stutters. Educate them about stuttering to make them feel comfortable.

Some people make incorrect assumptions about individuals who stutter. For example, some people think that individuals who stutter are mentally retarded — even if you have a Ph.D.!

"Excellent communication skills" is the #1 qualification employers look for. Regardless of whether the help-wanted ad included this, you should say that you have excellent communication skills, despite stuttering. Give concrete examples:

- If you're in a speech therapy program, discuss your progress and the techniques or strategies you use.
- If you learned nonavoidance skills in speech therapy, explain that although you stutter, you've overcome your fears of talking to strangers, etc.
- If you use an electronic fluency aid, explain how your device works.
- "Although I stutter, I've developed my public speaking skills through membership in Toastmasters." Toastmasters gives out lots of ribbons and prizes and titles, so be sure to mention if you are a Certified Toast Master or that you won a blue ribbon for best speech.
- "When making presentations, I can't say as much as fluent persons, so I prepare my remarks in advance and get right to the main points, unlike some people who ramble on for half an hour."
- "I can say a phrase fluently if I say it a lot. In my last job, I pretty much said the same things to customers all day, and my speech was fine." This should be acceptable for retail jobs, etc.
- Communication is a two-way street. Say that you may not speak as well as other people, but you listen more carefully, such as not interrupting people before they finish. Ask the manager whether listening well or speaking well is more important in the job — they'll say that listening is more important.

> The interview for the job that I currently have was one of the few interviews in which I discussed in depth the nature of my stuttering problem. I spent about a half-hour discussing my speech, and I think that it was very helpful for the interviewer in understanding how well I could work around my handicap. (Tom Morrow)

VOCATIONAL REHABILITATION

If you're looking for a job, make an appointment with a vocational rehabilitation counselor. Look in your telephone directory's blue (government) pages under your state's department of labor.

Voc rehab counselors want you to succeed. They will get you whatever therapy, devices, or job training you need. I have heard many good reports from stutterers about voc rehab counselors.

One stutterer complained that, after paying for stuttering therapy and an electronic device, the counselor also tried to pay for his CPA certification — but the stutterer insisted he would pay for his own certification.

There are many other government programs and organization assisting persons with disabilities. See the *Americans With Disabilities Act Resource Directory* and the *Pocket Guide to Federal Help for Individuals with Disabilities* (available from the U.S. Government Printing Office, Pueblo, CO 81009).

THE AMERICANS WITH DISABILITIES ACT

The Americans with Disabilities Act (ADA) prohibits employment discrimination against qualified individuals with disabilities. The definition of an "individual with a disability" includes "a physical or mental impairment that substantially limits one or more major life activities." Speaking is one such major life activity. You are also protected if you are not substantially limited in a major life activity but are perceived to have such a limitation. For example, you may be capable of communicating, but your employer thinks that you can't communicate.

The ADA applies to private employers, state and local governments, employment agencies, and labor unions. The ADA does not apply to the federal government, including the military services.

ADA protects individuals with disabilities who are qualified for jobs. ADA defines two steps in determining qualification for a job:

- Education, work experience, training, skills, licenses, certificates, etc.
- Whether the individual can perform essential functions of the job, with or without reasonable accommodation.

An essential function is a task that the employees in the position actually do. To remove that task would fundamentally change the job.

The Americans with Disabilities Act requires that if an employee with a disability asks for a *reasonable accommodation*, the employer must provide the accommodation. The employee must ask for the reasonable accommodation. The employee could ask for different job responsibilities, such as having someone else make telephone calls. Or the employee could ask the employer to pay for stuttering therapy or an electronic anti-stuttering device.

In the few cases I've heard of in which a stutterer asked for help from an employer, the employer gladly paid for what the employee asked for, because the employee's increased capabilities made him more valuable. However, I've talked to far more stutterers who say they would never discuss stuttering with their employer. Several stutterers have insisted to me that stuttering is not a disability, and that the ADA should not protect stutterers!

Employers are not "...obligated to provide personal use items, such as glasses or hearing aids..." (EEOC, 1990). You will have to prove that stuttering does not affect your life outside of work, and that you don't need the fluency aid or speech therapy outside of work.

A reasonable accommodation need not be the best accommodation available, as long as it is effective. If a $400 electronic fluency aid enables you to talk fluently, your employer does not have to pay $2500 for speech therapy.

A employee with a disability has the right to refuse an accommodation. I've gotten calls from human resources managers wanting to promote a stutterer to a management position. The positions required talking to clients, and the human resources manager asked me about electronic anti-stuttering devices. In each case the stutterer refused the promotion (in one case turning down a $23,000 raise!) because he didn't want to talk to clients.

Two federal programs help employers pay for "reasonable accommodations":

• The Tax Credit for Small Business (Section 44 of the Internal Revenue Code) credits smaller employers for half the cost of "eligible access expenditures."

• The Targeted Jobs Tax Credit Program gives tax credits to employers who hire individuals with disabilities. The IRS will give your employer up to $2400 for hiring you.

WHO CAN YOU CALL?

I have completed a Ph.D. in Electrical Engineering. I have been applying to several places for jobs. Fortunately, I did get three interviews. It is sad to say that, despite my excellent qualification and technical abilities, after the interviews, they are suddenly not interested in education and obviously do not want to extend any hopes (after finding out my stuttering problem). During the last interview, the vice-president of the division asked me if I have any speech problem. I honestly explained my stuttering and told him about my ongoing speech therapy. Needless to say that my confrontation immediately turned him off and I never heard back anything from that company. Please note that it does not seem to be open discrimination but I feel that had I been fluent, I could have had a possible job offer since it was directly in field of my research work. (Name withheld by request)

Employers may not make any pre-employment inquiries regarding disability, but may ask questions about the ability to perform specific job functions. In other words, an interviewer may not ask you about your stuttering. An interviewer may ask if you have experience making telephone calls to customers, or about your experiences in public speaking, if these are essential job functions.

If you feel you have been discriminated against, call your local office of the Equal Employment Opportunity Commission and file a complaint. You can also call the EEOC at (800) 669-4000.

You must file a charge of discrimination within 180 days of the alleged discriminatory act.

After you file a charge of discrimination, the EEOC notifies the charged entity. The EEOC then investigates, and attempts to resolve the charge through conciliation. If conciliation fails, the EEOC files suit or issues a "right to sue" letter.

For publications about ADA, call the EEOC ADA Helpline at (800) 669-EEOC. Request the publication *A Technical Assistance Manual on the Employment Provisions (Title I) of the Americans with Disabilities Act.*

Also request the accompanying *Resource Directory*, which lists assistance programs and organizations.

If you're in a vocational rehab program, ask interviewers to fill out a form for your voc rehab counselor, explaining why you weren't hired. This could help you prove discrimination.

ADA covers only employment discrimination. If you experience discrimination or harassment outside of work, you will have to rely on other federal or state laws.

Telephone Advice For Stutterers

> ...when working at my local library...I answered the phone and a man asked for the director. I hesitated for a second or two and the man then started ranting on about how I have a terrible problem — so terrible that I should not be allowed to live with other people or hold down a job of any kind. (Hurwitz, 1997)

A recent study listed previous research on stuttering and telephones use (Zimmerman, 1997 — references are in the article):

> The use of the telephone has been acknowledged subjectively by individuals who stutter and their therapists as one of the most stressful situations encountered in daily living.
>
> • Brutten's (1975) analysis of self ratings by individuals who stutter on the "Fear Survey Schedule" indicate that speaking on the telephone was said to elicit "much fear."
>
> • Georgieva (1994) found that talking on the telephone was listed by stuttering participants as the most stressful and with the most stuttering-inducing potential of all situations examined.
>
> • Leith and Timmons (1983a) indicate that 72% of their sample found calling people on the telephone among the top three stressful situations of daily living, with severe stutterers rating calling directory assistance, calling the operator, and calling a store with questions as the top three stressful telephone situations.
>
> • Employing a lie detection device to assess stress reactions to speaking situations, Leith and Timmons (1983b) found that stuttering and non-stuttering participants were heterogeneous: "...the stutterers reported feeling stress and manifested overt stress-related behaviors while the non-stuttering group reported no stress associated with telephone calls and manifested no stress-related behaviors."
>
> • A study assessing objective measures of the stuttering-evoking potential of telephone calls (Ladoucer, Leblond, and Bouchard, 1982) noted that "subjects stuttered significantly more during telephone conversations than during [face-to-face] interviews."
>
> • Many therapies have telephone use as one of their explicit goals (e.g., Perkins, 1973a, 1973b; Ryan & Van Kirk, 1974). Clearly, the telephone is an area of significant communicative concern for those who stutter.

Many persons who stutter experience anxiety regarding telephones. This is unnecessary. You can use telephones to your advantage:

1) Plan what you will say. Stutterers are usually more fluent on pre-planned speech than on spontaneous speech. Assume you'll get an answering machine. On the rare occasions when a real person answers, you'll know what to say.

2) When leaving a message on an answering machine, use your stuttering therapy techniques. No one is going to interrupt you and tell you to talk faster.

3) Use a mirror when talking on the telephone. Watch your mouth as you talk, and exaggerate your movements. E.g., open your mouth wide, and move your lips, tongue, and jaw slowly and deliberately. This is a form of "closed loop" motor control, which reduces stuttering (see the chapter "Motor Learning Theory"). Ira Zimmerman adds,

> I think visual feedback on what I do when I stutter has been helpful. Looking at a mirror while I talked on the phone helped me get rid of many of my severe physical tics and secondaries associated with my severe stuttering.

4) Some people find that using a cordless telephone and walking around helps fluency. Walking alters your brain's cerebral activity and may improve fluency in some people. If walking doesn't help — crawl! A 1935 study found that stutterers could talk fluently while crawling on all fours. Just tell your boss you lost your earring.

5) If you have a phrase you say often (such as answering the telephone at work), buy a micro digital recorder (Radio Shack #63-945, $15) Record yourself saying the phrase fluently. When you pick up the telephone, hold the recorder to your other ear, push the button, and speak in chorus with your fluent recording.

6) Use a Casa Futura Technologies anti-stuttering telephone device. About 20 states have said they may provide anti-stuttering telephone devices to stutterers. For more information on these "special telephone equipment distribution" programs, visit http://www.casafuturatech.com/Catalog/stedp.html.

7) If you stutter severely, use a Telecommunications Device for the Deaf (TDD). This device lets you type over a telephone line instead of talking. You can call non-TDD users through a free operator-

assisted relay service. Speech-impaired residents in many states can get a free TDD from their telephone company.

8) Torment listeners! See the subsection "Be Mean To Telemarketers" in the chapter "Psychological Self-Therapy."

DO TELEPHONE COMPANIES GIVE DISCOUNTS FOR STUTTERING?

California's "TDD Toll Discount" gives a discount on intrastate long-distance tolls. If you stutter severely, your telephone company will give you a free TDD. They can't differentiate TDD and voice calls, so you get the same discount whether you use the TDD or choose to stutter. This sounds fair to me!

Suggestions For Listeners

Stuttering can make fluent speakers uncomfortable — more uncomfortable than other disabilities such as blindness or deafness.

Charles Van Riper wrote (Van Riper, 1971):

> Stuttering…dramatically exposes many of the unpleasant sides of social living. It is the dark mirror of speech, reflecting man's frustrations in communicating with his fellows. It portrays his fears of social penalties, it reveals his shame for deviancy, it is the hallmark of man's inability to communicate with his fellows.

Stutterers look like anybody else. We're not visibly disabled, like a paraplegic, for example. Stuttering has no apparent cause, and can come and go for no apparent reason. People think they understand visible disabilities, but this uncertainty about stuttering makes listeners uncomfortable.

Everybody has disfluencies, and at times is unable to talk. Non-stutterers experience disfluencies when they are nervous or anxious, or indecisive or lying. Some non-stutterers think that stutterers are just nervous. They think that if stutterers would "get a hold of themselves" they wouldn't stutter.

Be patient when listening to a stutterer — as you are patient when walking with a person who has a mobility impairment. Do not fill in words or finish sentences for a stutterer, unless you ask for permission first. Stutterers can talk, but getting a sentence out may take a while. Stutterers have pride in their ability to talk despite their disability.

If you saw a person walking slowly with a cane, it would be rude to force the person into a wheelchair, then push them along at a jogging pace. You'd be showing off how much stronger and faster you are.

Similarly, by finishing a sentence for a stutterer, you are showing that your speech is better, and making the stutterer feel incapable. The stutterer may be perfectly capable of finishing the sentence, if you'd give him or her a chance.

Don't tell a stutterer to "slow down," "take a breath," "relax," or "think about what you're going to say." This advice is simplistic, useless, and patronizing. If you saw an overweight person eating lunch, would you tell him or her to eat less or get more exercise?

When talking to a stutterer, slow down and relax your speech. People tend to imitate each other's speech (called "convergence"). For example, if you talk fast, the people you talk to will try to talk fast. If you interrupt people, they will interrupt you.

If you relax and talk slowly, let the other person finish what he is saying, and count to ten before you start talking, you will remove the time pressure stutterers often feel, which makes stuttering worse. But you probably can't talk slowly for more than one sentence — and this will show you how difficult changing your speech is.

A teenage girl went into a hardware store with her younger brother. She tried to ask the clerk for something, but couldn't say the word. The clerk laughed at the girl, then turned away and rang up another customer. The girl struggled to ask her question. The clerk than asked the younger brother what the girl wanted. After five minutes of this, the girl left in tears.

Laughing at stuttering or making jokes like "Must be cold out there!" isn't funny.

When listening to a stutterer, maintain eye contact and listen patiently. My dad always listens to me and is interested in everything I say. I hardly stutter around him.

My aunt starts talking whenever I talk (she does this to everyone). When I talk to my cousin, he wanders away, plays his guitar, makes telephone calls, etc. He may be listening, but he doesn't give the appearance of listening. I stutter more with my aunt and cousin.

If you want to ask a stutterer about his speech, try to frame it positively. For example, you could say, "My neighbor stutters too, but your speech is much better than his. Do you have a suggestion I could give to my neighbor?"

Directly asking a stutterer about his speech can make the stutterer upset. Stuttering shouldn't be a taboo subject, but too often the person is so sensitive about his speech that he doesn't want to talk about it.

If you can't understand something a stutterer said, don't be afraid to ask the person to repeat it. Or if you have some idea what the person tried to say, ask "Did you say such-and-such?" Don't nod and pretend that you understand. That is acting like an immigrant who doesn't speak English and says, "Yes, sir" to everything you say.

Use active listening. Repeat back what the person said. This gives the best impression that you were listening, that you value what the other person is telling you, and insures that you understand what the person said.

Stuttering In The Military

One young stutterer in the Marine Corps Reserve told me that, in three months of boot camp, his officers never found out that he stuttered. Recruits never talk to officers — recruits scream everything, in an emotional style of speech not used anywhere else. Yelling, especially with emotional arousal, is one of the ways stutterers can communicate fluently. The young man was 100% fluent when yelling back at officers.

His friends soon figured out that he stuttered, and word got to the officers. One day when the recruits were lined up outside, the stutterer was called out and ordered to recite the twelve rules of the Marine Corps. Reciting memorized material is another fluency-enhancing condition. He stepped right up and screamed the rules, rapidly and fluently. The officers concluded that he didn't stutter, and never bothered him again!

19 YEARS IN THE MILITARY

By Yancel Campbell, Jr.

There are many people in the military that stutter. What the exact number is I have no idea. However, most military regional medical centers have speech clinics. An example is the clinic at the Army's Tripler Regional Medical Center, Honolulu, Hawaii.

All my life I have stuttered. Upon entering the Marine Corps I was made an intelligence specialist. After seven years as an enlisted person, I was commissioned a Warrant Officer and later promoted to Captain. During this time, I stuttered through many briefs. Most of the senior officer level and to many generals. Most of my superiors understood I could not control my speech at times. However, because I knew my job and the subject, often I was picked to brief.

During 19 years of service only two senior officers took offense at my speech. Only once did a senior mention my speech in my permanent record book. So the bottom line, it really has not hurt my career.

I once met a Marine Major who flew F-18 fighter aircraft. He stuttered so badly that it was very hard for him to speak a single sentence. As far I know he is still flying. So, as far as the Marine Corps goes, stuttering will not end a career. The only time I have seen stuttering mentioned in Marine Corps orders, was that a drill instructor or a recruiter could not have a speech problem, because of the high visibility.

Having worked in the joint world with all services, the senior commands, create briefing teams, with talking heads. We prepare the briefs, and the polished talking heads give the briefs to senior government officials.

Giving briefs is a problem for everybody, i.e. public speaking, I have watched the best get up and stutter. So if everybody were fired for stuttering I think the whole armed services would be fired. Most seniors find their best talking heads and appoint them to brief and the rest becomes the people behind the scenes, just like the normal corporate world.

REJECTION TO ACCEPTANCE

By Matthew Benson

I've been a stutterer for about 20 years, and I now realize that I will always be a stutterer. I knew I would have to learn to deal with my problem myself. When I turned 18, I enlisted in the US Navy, mostly to get money for college, but partly to prove to myself and everyone else that I could do it.

I still remember riding that bus from the airport to boot camp. I was so terrified. What would they do when they found out I stuttered? What would I do when they told me to leave? It wasn't until the next day that I even had to talk to anyone.

After one hour of sleep my CCs, or Company Commanders, switched the lights on and started yelling at us to form two lines and count off. Luckily my number was thirty something and very easy to say. I dodged the bullet this time, but for the next 8 weeks I was number 2. Every morning the count seemed to stop after number 1, but I pretended not to hear the laughing and snickering from down the line.

For 4 weeks, I passed all my inspections, and excelled in all my classes. I was terrified to stand watches, fearing that I would have to sound off when a CC walked through the door, but I never made a fuss about standing watches. By this time our company had slimmed down from 85 down to 75 people.

I signed up for the nuclear propulsion field when I enlisted and really had my heart set on it. All us "nukes" had to go through rigorous medical examinations for the first 4 weeks. On one of my last medical examinations, I had to fill out a questionnaire and one of the questions was "Do you stutter or stammer?" This wasn't the first time I answered the question and so I thought nothing of it as I checked yes. An hour later the doctor called me into his office.

"This is the hardest part of my job, son. But I have to reject you from the nuke field. In fact, I can't accept you into the military. I'm going to recommend you be discharged."

My world crashed down before me. It finally happened. What would I do now? If I couldn't make it here, how could I make it anywhere in the outside world? That was one of the worst days of my life. I was so afraid of the future, tears began to well up in my eyes. I couldn't let the guys see me cry; after all what kind of a man was I? I found the nearest bathroom and sat down to think alone for almost an hour.

When I regained my composure, I found the rest of my company and marched back to the barracks compartment. I had the next watch and stood there by my post in a perfect military manner. I stared straight ahead, showing no emotion, as my insides twisted and turned. The guys would walk by me and say hi or jokingly comment at my statue-like stance not knowing what was going on in my mind. Eventually they figured out something was bothering me and one of the guys took it upon himself to find out. I couldn't take it any more, and I broke down again telling them what happened.

They told my CC, and she brought me into her office and asked me to explain what happened. She then asked me if I wanted to stay in or get out. Of course I told her I wanted to stay in. So she said "then you will." They swept the discharge recommendations under the rug and I never heard about it again. From that day on I was a new man.

All my life I had been rejected because of my speech, and for the first time I was accepted. That was only the first of many battles. By the way, I was still rejected from the nuclear propulsion field, and the job they gave was Weapons Technician. I served two years in Guam and was awarded a few commendations and awards, including the Navy Achievement Medal. I'm 22 years old now and serving in Strike Fighter Squadron 151 as an Aviation Ordnanceman (another story in itself). I've made four or five cruises including a six-month WestPac cruise aboard the *USS Constellation*.

I have seven more months left on my enlistment and then I'll finally go to college.

Cultural and Ethnic Differences in Stuttering

Stuttering should vary between cultural and ethnic groups, for two main reasons:

1) Children are raised differently in different cultures.

2) Different cultures react differently to stuttering and other disabilities.

Speech plays different roles in different cultures. In some cultures, people only speak when they have something to say, and silence is acceptable. In other cultures, skillful use of language is a source of recognition and power.

Stuttering therapy may vary between cultures as well. For example, in "machismo" Mediterranean cultures men may not be willing to talk about their fears and anxieties. In Japanese or Korean cultures, "losing face" is such a concern that people may not want to admit that they stutter (Leith, 1986).

A study found that foreign-born Americans have different attitudes towards stuttering than at least second-generation Americans. On the question whether stutterers "could try harder" to speak fluently, Americans and Canadians, generally didn't think so (scores of about 1.8 on a scale of 1 to 4). Persons from Southeast Asia, China, and Hong Kong were clear that stutterers "could try harder" (scores above 3). Latin Americans were in the middle. Similar, but less dramatic differences were found on other questions, such as whether stutterers are "emotionally disturbed," "less intelligent," or are being "punished by God." (Bebout, 1992)

ANTHROPOLOGY OF STUTTERING

There was a controversy for several decades about whether stuttering exists in certain American Indian tribes.

In the 1940s, a student of Wendell Johnson studied the Bannock-Shoshone Indians of Idaho, and found that stuttering was unknown in the tribe. This tribe was characterized as allowing children freedom, not demanding conformity of adherence to standards of behavior, and not expecting adults to talk if they chose not to. A similar lack of stuttering was reported among the Navaho Indians — except among Navaho children attending white schools.

Another anthropologist reported numerous stutterers among the Salish, Kwakiutl, and Nootka tribes of the Northwest Coast. These tribes have the "potlatch" culture, characterized by a need to impress neighboring groups, and demands that individuals not embarrass their families.

Yet another anthropologist found a high incidence of stuttering among the Ibo and Idoma tribes of West Africa. These cultures place a high value on public speaking, and people "make speeches on any pretext." These cultures are more competitive and demanding of their children than other cultures.

The idea developed that cultural demands cause stuttering. This view fit Wendell Johnson's "diagnostogenic" theory of stuttering.

Later studies found stuttering in the Bannock-Shoshone Indians in Idaho, and that their language had a word for stuttering. The Indians had been so embarrassed about stuttering that they insisted to the original researchers that no one in their tribe stuttered.

Stuttering has been found in every culture studied. Stuttering prevalence seems to vary between cultures, but measuring stuttering is difficult, so comparing data between cultures is difficult. Currently, most authorities believe that cultural demands have little effect on stuttering.

BILINGUALISM AND STUTTERING

A 1932 study found that bilingual children are more likely to stutter than monolingual children.

A Los Angeles speech pathologist studied bilingual children who stutter. These children spoke Spanish at home, as their first language, and English in school. She found that the older children stuttered more severely in Spanish. English had become their dominant language, and they were losing their ability to express themselves in Spanish. This suggests that stuttering is affected by the process of translating thoughts into sentences, called encoding. This fits with the "capacities and demands" model of stuttering, in this case the children have lower capacity to encode their thoughts into Spanish sentences, and so they stutter more (Weliky, 1994). These results confirm earlier studies reported by Oliver Bloodstein in *A Handbook On Stuttering*.

If your school's speech pathologist only speaks English, you speak another language at home, and your child stutters at home, don't assume that your child's speech with the school speech pathologist is anything like what you hear at home.

MINORITIES AND STUTTERING

Some speech pathologists have speculated that stuttering is more common among higher socioeconomic classes, because of more language and conformity demands. In other words, rich children are more likely to stutter than poor children. Different socio-economic studies have found different results, but there appears to be no correlation between income and stuttering.

Many studies have found stuttering to be more common among African-Americans. A few studies have found the opposite, but the balance of evidence indicates that stuttering is two to four times more prevalent among African-Americans than among European-Americans. The male-to-female ratio among African-American stutterers is about 2:1 or 2.5:1. In contrast, the male-to-female ratio among European-American stutterers is about 4:1. In other words, black women are about five times more likely to stutter than white women.

A New Jersey school speech pathologist working in a school that is 98% African-American reported having 19 children who stutter in her caseload. Suburban school speech pathologists typically have only one child who stutters. This speech pathologist specializes in stuttering, so she gets cases from other speech pathologists, but she believes that stuttering is about five times more prevalent among African-American children.

No explanation has been presented why stuttering is more prevalent among African-Americans. Some studies have found unusually high stuttering prevalence in Nigeria and Senegal, in addition to the studies noted above, suggesting that West Africans and their American descendants may have genetic predisposition to stuttering.

Hispanic and Asian cultures appear to have stuttering prevalences similar to Europeans and European-Americans.

Cultural differences in stuttering therapy appear to be minor. There are some reports that African-American culture frowns upon voluntary stuttering, or abnormal-sounding fluency shaping speech. Some Arab cultures object to a speech pathologist touching a client. Some sounds in Spanish, German, and French may interfere with certain fluency shaping speech targets.

For more information on this topic, see *Communication Disorders In Multicultural Populations*, by Delores E. Battle (1993, Boston: Andover Medical Publishers).

Stuttering Self-Help Group Activities

I was leader of the San Jose chapter of the National Stuttering Project for two years. The best meetings had guest speakers, usually doubling our attendance to 15-20 people. Guest speakers included:

• Colleen Wilcox, Santa Clara County schools superintendent, speech pathologist, ASHA trustee, and a PWS. Dr. Wilcox talked about growing up stuttering severely, how she overcame stuttering, and the effects of stuttering on her life. (See the chapter "Successful Stuttering Stories."

• Jeff Shames, a New York filmmaker and PWS, showed a roughcut of his documentary about stuttering, filmed at the 1995 NSP convention. He talked about his experiences stuttering.

• Brendan Webster and Ellen Golden, speech pathologists with the Los Altos Center for Speech and Language, discussed their approach to stuttering therapy.

• Carl Scott, Ph.D. psychologist, speech pathologist, and hypnotherapist, discussed his mind-body-spirit approach to stuttering therapy.

• Michael Smith, Ph.D. psychologist and PWS, who specializes in marital counseling, conducted a workshop on improving communication in relationships. See the chapter "Improving Communication in Relationships."

• John Harrison, PWS and NSP board member, discussed "Zen and Stuttering."

• Joan Holland, speech pathologist and PWS, discussed her experiences stuttering and her approach to stuttering therapy.

• Twice we invited Toastmasters clubs to join us to discuss "Overcoming Fear of Speaking." They are the easiest guest speakers to get — you call, and a half-dozen loquacious people show up at your next meeting!

Other activities included:

• Watching a video about Tourette's syndrome ("Twitch and Shout"), and discussing similarities to and differences from stuttering.

• Watching videos about stuttering — the "Marilu" show, the Bob Love video, etc.

• A summer picnic.

• I presented my workshops to the local group before doing presentations at the NSP conventions.

• Various short activities, such as 2-minute speeches about "What I

Like About Summer."

We had several fun meetings:

• Reading children's books. Especially fun is two people reading Dr. Seuss together.

• Some of the games I describe at the end of the chapter on "School-Age Stuttering Therapies" were games I invented for our adult stuttering support group.

• The funnest meeting was the Speech Disorders Game. I passed out large cards, each with a speech disorder: stuttering, lisping, aphasia (forgetting simple words), speaking in a high voice, speaking in a low voice, speaking fast, speaking slow, unusual accents, switching the first sounds of words, spastic dysphonia, etc. Each person introduced himself using his speech disorder, explaining what it was. Then the speech disorders became hearing disorders. In other words, the "lisp" person could only hear people who lisped, the "accent" person could only hear people who spoke in a funny accent. To carry on a conversation with several people, you had to constantly change your speech! People talked and talked and talked, for an hour, saying inane things to each other in funny voices. Or else they were laughing at other people. No one stuttered! Several people were astoundingly good at hilarious accents and difficult speech disorders. We also learned that there are worse speech disorders than stuttering.

We met twice a month, and usually alternated an "important" meeting (with a guest speaker or activity) with a "sharing" support meeting.

Improving Communication in Relationships by Michael Smith, Ph.D.

Michael Smith, Ph.D. is a person who stutters, and a transpersonal psychologist specializing in marital counseling. He conducted this workshop for the San Jose chapter of the National Stuttering Project.

We're going to talk about communication, and what are the essential items in good communication. The trick is, they're actually very simple. They're so simple we don't even think of it. And they're simple, but they're not so easy to do.

A friend of mine did her doctoral work on couples. She studied all these different things they could do — psychotherapy, exercises, all these various things, to find out what was needed to have a good relationship. The thing that worked better than anything else was regular time together, simply saying whatever you needed to say.

The first part is that you have to have regular time to sit and talk. We do it over eating, or driving a car, or we avoid it, or whatever. What she found was that if you have half an hour a day where the two of you can sit and talk, and whoever wants to goes first, and the other person listens, and the second person goes, and the first person listens.

If you're like me, when I heard this, I heard it but I didn't really let it in. It's like, oh yeah, we need to sit regularly and talk. But I didn't quite get it. What it means is you really do have to make the time to get together and sit and talk, and not be doing a lot of other stuff. Because if there are difficult issues to talk about, and we're doing other things, we'll find ways to avoid the items we really need to be saying.

So the first one is just a regular time, a format, to hang out and talk with somebody. It sounds so simple, but most people don't do it.

The next one is really listening to somebody. Which, again, it sounds very simple. Oh yeah, I listen. Or, oh yeah, I naturally listen to what people say.

As a stutterer, I have found that really listening is a challenge for me, has been a real challenge, because often I'm thinking about what I'm going to say, and the words I'm going to stutter on. Or if it's a party I miss half the people's names because I'm worried about saying my name. I'm not there.

Communications get stuck when one person is not having the

experience of being heard. Usually what happens is that two people are talking, or they get into arguing, or whatever, and one person doesn't feel heard. Until somebody feels heard, it stays just like this. And if we're so tied up with our anxiety, that we can't listen, it makes it even more difficult.

The third very simple item, and probably the hardest of all, is to tell the truth. The whole truth. I am more apt to stutter when I am not quite telling the whole truth, like there was a word that I wanted to use, but I didn't. I substituted something a little nicer, or a little more vague, or a little more acceptable. When I would do that I would more likely stutter.

But a lot of the arguments happen because something's not being said. That's when things don't get completed. That's when arguments happen, is if I'm being vague, or I'm telling you how you feel, or I'm out and out lying.

So all these things sound very, very simple, and I suggest they're incredibly difficult to do.

In our case, maybe we don't tell the truth because we can't say the word we want to say, and we avoid the anxiety and embarrassment. Somebody that is fluent may be anxious for another reason, the feedback they'll get, or having to own up to something. Something doesn't fit.

For an exercise, choose who will go first. For 30 seconds, the person gets to talk about anything they want to. The listener's job is to listen to them, because at the end of the 30 seconds, you're going to repeat back to them what you heard them say. At the end, you say something like, "What I heard you saying was..." and you repeat it to them, in your own words. After you have reflected it back to them, ask them, "Is that what you said?" or, "Do you feel satisfied," or "Is there anything that I left out?" If there is, they fill it in, again you reflect it back to them, until they are satisfied and let you know that they are.

If someone is repeating something, you can bet that it's because they don't feel heard. They will go over it and over it and over it until they finally get the feedback that you got it.

Or what often happens is we begin to read into things, and instead of feeding back to them what we heard, we say, "You are insecure," which is not what I said and not what I felt.

When we interpret, assume, etc., and we tell them that's what they said, we get into trouble. It breaks down. Part of the trick is to listen carefully, and repeat back to them what they said, and give them the chance to give us feedback, "Is this what you said, or not?," until they actually get the experience of feeling heard.

What often works best is to give one of them a chance to talk, for 3 minutes, 5 minutes, whatever, and just sort of let them talk, and the other person just listens. If you try to start interrupting, then you start arguing. What usually works best is letting one person talk for awhile, feeding back to them, and then switching roles. So it's a bit unnatural perhaps, but it works well, and it requires a lot of effort on our part to attend.

Spouses of People Who Stutter
by Julia Boberg

Julia Boberg's late husband Einer was director of the Institute for Stuttering Treatment And Research (ISTAR), in Edmonton, Alberta, Canada. The following is reprinted with permission.

I met my husband Einer in January 1960, when he was taking violin lessons from a member of the Vienna Symphony Orchestra. We saw each other every day for three months and never once did I see Einer stutter. He spoke slowly and with an occasional very slight hesitation, but nothing that I would have recognized as stuttering.

However, on several occasions he spoke about his stuttering; about not being able to speak to anyone without extreme struggling and blocking throughout his childhood; about his trip to Minneapolis for a new stuttering therapy course one summer in his early 20s; about his brief period of fluency followed by a complete relapse; and about a second summer session in Minneapolis which produced a more lasting effect which I was now seeing. I found all of this fascinating and was full of admiration for the determination and courage it must have taken to persevere to this point.

We decided to get engaged and we set the wedding date for the following July. In the meantime, in April, I returned to my job in London. I began to worry when his letters cam describing fears of speaking, a resurgence of his old speech difficulties, and worries about meeting my family and getting through the wedding ceremony. Naïvely, I thought these would all disappear when we could be together again. I was wrong.

When Einer met me in London a month before the wedding date, he could not speak to any stranger at all, and would write out notes if he had to buy a railway ticket, for instance. Even talking to me he experienced blocks, facial contortions, tremors, and so forth. The calm and gentle man I had met seemed to have been taken over by some malevolent demon that wreaked havoc with any attempt to communicate verbally. My expectations of happy meetings with colleagues, friends, and family were dashed to the ground.

Three episodes stand out as illustrations of how devastating it was.

The first I'll call the "very sick young man" episode. It occurred before the wedding, when my mother took Einer to see our family doctor. The doctor took my mother aside and told her that this was a very sick man and she should do everything in her power to prevent her daughter from marrying him. The doctor said that the marriage was sure to be a disaster. I was very shaken by this and especially upset making my parents and family unhappy about me. Only my faith in Einer, my memory of the fluency he had demonstrated earlier, and my belief that eventually we would find a way to overcome stuttering kept me going on with the wedding plans.

The second episode I'll call the "super pill" episode. A psychiatrist had some pills he thought might help. Einer was to take one per day during the week remaining before the great day, and one extra big super pill on the morning of the wedding. The pills made him feel somewhat relaxed but had no noticeable effect on his speech. The wedding arrived, Einer took his super pill, and went off to London on the train to meet his relatives who had come for the ceremony.

An hour before the wedding Einer had still not returned. I kept the smiling calm that I had learned to assume in the face of all our difficulties and began dressing. Half and hour later I stood in white satin complete with veil and bouquet, looking out of the bedroom window towards the railway station, wondering what could have happened and preparing myself mentally for a last minute cancellation of the wedding. Had he thrown himself under a train, unable to continue life as a stutterer? Had he run back to Canada as a supreme act of avoidance? The minutes ticked by. Finally another train pulled in, and up the hill walked Einer, a lazy smile on his face, apparently unaware of the panic that he had caused. He had forgotten to take pencil and paper and so was unable to ask for guidance and had become hopelessly lost. However, the super pill had kept him smiling. I am glad to say that thanks to the kindly vicar in reading along with Einer, the wedding vows were the first and only fluent words my family heard Einer speak that summer.

The third I'll call the "walk out." This episode occurred a couple of weeks after the wedding. I had invited one very close, easy-going friend for dinner to meet Einer. I had acquiesced in his wishes to avoid all other social events, but hoped he could cope with just this one. She came back on the train with me after work. When we reached home my mother said Einer had been out all afternoon and had not returned. When I went up to our bedroom I found a note on the dressing table saying, "I can't go on like this. I have gone away and will not return until I can talk again. Don't try to find me. If you want to contact me, write to Canada House."

I was so upset I could not even tell my friend what had happened and merely pretended Einer had been delayed by a chance meeting with someone is London and would not be able to join us. I felt cruelly abandoned. If he had discussed this with me, I could have understood what he was doing and why, but this way I had no idea where he was, what he was doing, how long he would be gone or indeed if he would ever return. It began to look as though the doctor's prediction of disaster might be correct.

I did write to Canada House and Einer wrote back arranging a meeting at a certain bench in St. James' Park. He had decided to leave for the United States as soon as possible and quit music in order to become a speech pathologist specializing in stuttering. Instead of spending a year in a baroque apartment in Vienna, attending nightly concerts and meeting musicians from all over the world, we end up in Iowa, and I felt thousands of miles from anywhere.

These three episodes had profound effects of my emotional state, my relations with family and friends, and the course of my life. They give a good idea of how any spouse's life can be affected by a partner's stuttering. In 1990, one of the professional journals, *Seminars in Speech and Language*, invited us to write an article about the spouses of people who stutter. In the interviews I conducted I found the same themes in other couples' lives: social life being restricted to occasional very small groups or avoided completely; lack of communication about problems; anxiety and difficulties associated with the wedding ceremony; job choices being determined by the stuttering problem; not knowing where to turn for help and advice; and being too inhibited to discuss the problem with others.

In addition, some couples mentioned delaying having children because the person who stuttered did not feel able to cope with the speech demands of disciplining children, and was afraid of not being able to call for help in an emergency. Spouses often took over much of the contact with the outside world. Several mentioned the pain they felt as they shared the partner's anxiety and struggles.

The most striking finding in these interviews was the lack of communication about stuttering. Many couples never mentioned stuttering to one another. Some wives reported that they were astounded when their partner announced his decision to enter a speech therapy course. The partner had concealed his stuttering so cleverly that the spouse was not aware how much it affected him. Some of the most moving comments were from people who described the enormous relief to both of them when they could finally talk about the forbidden topic.

One man said, "Stuttering was something we never discussed.

She didn't want to hurt me by asking, and I 'ignored' it and never asked what she thought and felt about it."

The most important way spouses can help their disfluent partners is through communication. Let the person who stutters say what is helpful, describe the tensions and difficulties, express the pent-up emotions of a lifetime of disfluency, explain why he does or does not want to take speech therapy, and so on. It can be equally helpful to open up communication with others outside the marriage to broaden their understanding about stuttering.

Another important way spouses can help their disfluent partners is to encourage them and support them in getting professional help. If a therapy program can be found that includes spousal involvement, spouses should do their utmost to attend. These sessions increase understanding of stuttering, the aims and techniques of therapy, the problems and ways to help in maintenance, and so forth. Most importantly, they give the spouse a great respect for the hard work and perseverance that their partners put into therapy. Spouses who have attended such sessions consistently recommend them to others.

I'd like to close with a quotation from Jock Carlisle's book, *Tangled Tongue — Living With A Stutter*.

> Most married people I know who stutter severely have been fortunate in their marriage partners. This is not surprising, because any person taking on as a marriage partner someone who can hardly speak must have considerable courage, as well as the more than usual insight it takes to see beyond the tense, disfluent façade and love the person within.

Public Speaking for Stutterers

For most stutterers, speaking to an audience is a psychological cue to stutter. This cue can be reconditioned by doing public speaking while using therapy techniques.

By joining a public speaking club, you'll discover that non-stutterers have speech-related fears and anxieties too. Their speech isn't perfect. They work for years to improve their speech skills, and never expect to have perfect speech. Stutterers should adopt the same view.

Stutterers need motivation to work on their speech. Toastmasters public speaking clubs motivate you to attend every week. You get ribbons and recognition for speech competitions. You have a course of speeches your work through over a year or two, with constructive feedback from a mentor who's been through the course. At the end you get a "Competent Toastmaster" certificate. Then you can compete against other Toastmasters groups in tournaments and win ribbons for your local club.

Stuttering therapy, on the other hand, is usually done alone, or in a group too small to develop critical mass. You don't get ribbons or recognition. Your speech therapist probably never stuttered. When you're finished, there's nothing to continue. Stuttering support groups are important in their own way, but too often don't focus on improving your speech, and people stop attending.

Toastmasters is a non-profit organization with dozens of clubs in most cities. To find a club near you, call (714) 858-8255.

Perhaps someday there will be a special Toastmasters course for stutterers. For the moment, you can do your own "(Un)Certified Fluent Toastmaster" course. Join any local Toastmasters club, and work through the Competent Toastmaster course, doing the same speeches as everyone else. Also do a series of speeches related to stuttering, which are described below. First, here's how Toastmasters describes the Competent Toastmasters course:

You get a manual called "Communication and Leadership." Each project calls on you to prepare a speech using certain speaking principles.

At the end of the meeting, your evaluator will rise to give oral commentary on what you're doing well, as well as what you need to work on.

There are ten speech projects:

1. Icebreaker (4 to 6 minutes). Getting over nervousness by introducing yourself to the club.

2. Be In Earnest (5 to 7 minutes). Continue to get over nervousness by speaking about something you believe deeply in.

3. Organize Your Speech (5 to 7 minutes). Work on giving a well-organized speech.

4. Show What You Mean (5 to 7 minutes). This project calls on you to work with gestures and body language during your speech. Unfortunately, many members confuse the issue and show up with a bag full of props that they use in a "Show and Tell" style speech. Don't do that.

5. Vocal Variety (5 to 7 minutes). Work on rate of delivery, volume, speed, pitch, emphasis, etc.

6. Work with Words (5 to 7 minutes). Work on proper word choice, avoiding jargon and generalizations, etc.

7. Apply Your Skills (5 to 7 minutes). Go back and practice everything you've learned up to this point.

8. Be Persuasive (6 to 8 minutes). Give a persuasive speech on a controversial issue.

9. Speak With Knowledge (7 minutes, plus or minus 30 seconds). Research an issue, and write a speech.

10. Inspire Your Audience (8 to 10 minutes). Move your audience in a well-presented and well-prepared speech.

In addition to the above speeches, Toastmasters clubs have contests on the following speeches:

- Tall Tales (3 to 5 minutes). A tall tale, which must be original.
- Table Topics (1 to 2 minutes). Impromptu speaking.
- Evaluation (2 to 3 minutes). A target speaker gives a speech which all the contestants are to evaluate.
- Humorous speech (5 to 7 minutes). Year after year, people stand up and present Bill Cosby routines and then act puzzled when they're disqualified. It's supposed to be a *speech*, not a monologue, and it MUST be original.
- International Speech (5 to 7 minutes). Any topic at all, so long as it's original.

(UN)CERTIFIED FLUENT TOASTMASTER

For the "(Un)Certified Fluent Toastmaster" course, add in the following special speeches to the above ten speeches.

1. A speech about your stuttering. Explain what stuttering is, how

stuttering has impacted your life both negatively and positively, and what you are doing to overcome stuttering.

2. A speech using a fluency-enhancer. This could be stuttering therapy techniques, or an electronic device. Explain what you are using.

3. Another speech using a *different* fluency-enhancer. Explain the differences between the two approaches, and the advantages and disadvantages of each/

4. Have your fluency evaluated on four of your speeches. This shows your progress towards fluency, and motivates you to improve your speech. Don't worry if the evaluator isn't trained to scientifically measure stuttering — accuracy isn't critical.

5. Find an aspect of public speaking that you excel at, that you are better at than the non-stutterers in your club. Do one speech that showcases this aspect of public speaking.

SPEAKING CIRCLES

John Harrison, National Stuttering Project Program Director, has written a book entitled *How To Conquer Your Fears of Speaking Before People*. The book of available from the National Stuttering Project for $12.

Harrison facilitates something unlike a Toastmasters club and unlike a stuttering support group. He calls these "speaking circles." Each person has an opportunity to make a timed speech to the group. Each speaker then receives applause and positive feedback from the audience. There is no set course of speeches.

Harrison writes that speaking circles are intended to provide a "real," risky speaking experience "that helps to push the speaker out of his safety zone." Secondly, "the situation is made totally safe by the particular ways the audience supports the speaker." Harrison continues:

The speaking circle format is quite different [from Toastmasters]. It's not about how to make an effective talk, but how to get over stage fright by learning to feel comfortable connecting with people. It's also about learning to trust your spontaneous self by and allowing yourself to "stand in the void" and discover what comes up. What makes the speaking circle so appropriate for stutterers is that the program shifts the focus away from performance and onto self-assertion and self-acceptance -- precisely those areas where many of us are weak.

Chairs and couches are set up theater style in someone's living room. At the front of the room is a small platform, and a microphone. There's also a floodlight on the speaker… There's also a camcorder, so your talk can be videotaped…

During the program, you get to speak twice, the first time for three minutes and the second time for five. After each talk, you receive a strong round of applause, and you are encouraged to stand there and accept your applause. Then the facilitator asks what the experience was like for you. After the five minute talk, the floor is opened up to ONLY positive feedback — not on the subject matter of the talk but on the positive ways that your listeners were impacted by you as a speaker…

THE POWER POSITION…Most of us have grown up with fears and confusion about power, and about being in the spotlight. We also have issues about speaking from our truth, and instead, try to second-guess what others want us to be and say. The speaking circle gives you the chance to be in the power spot, but to show up *as yourself*.

CONNECTING WITH THE AUDIENCE….You are encouraged to look at someone for 4 or 5 seconds. Then look at someone else for the same amount of time...even if you're saying nothing at the moment…When you're a member of the audience, you are encouraged to totally support the speaker, to focus your attention on them and be there for them.

STANDING IN THE VOID. Most people, especially those who stutter, have a deathly fear of standing up and not being able to say anything or think of anything to say. People fear silences. In the speaking circle, if nothing comes to mind, you are encouraged to simply be there and connect with the audience…

SPEAKING YOUR TRUTH. We all grew up believing that a good speaker is one who performs well...someone who has the right technique, the right voice modulation, the right organization to the talk, and who delivers it flawlessly. As a member of the audience in a speaking circle, you soon learn that perfection is the booby prize. A perfect talk is no guarantee that the speaker will be interesting. What does seem to guarantee an interesting speaker is the individual's ability to show up "in his truth." It shows up in his ability to talk from a "real" place, without pretense…the experience is not about doing it right, it's about being there, having fun and connecting.

SUPPORT NO MATTER WHAT. If you were like me, you were constantly sensing what people wanted so you could modify yourself to be accepted and liked. [Speaking circles are always supportive, so you take risks.]

...stand in front of the group and take their applause. You'd be surprised how difficult it can be to simply stand in front of a group of people and accept recognition without wanting to get cute or awkward or rush from the stage. That, in and of itself, it a growth experience.

...videotape...can be transformational...I had a friend who ran a community TV interview program, and he invited John [Ahlbach] and I to be on the show to talk about stuttering. After the show, [we watched] the show in the control room...I remember how impressed John was with how he came off, even though he stuttered. It seemed to have a profound effect on him...we always tell newcomers to a speaking circle to watch their first tape three times. The first time, they'll pick up all the things they don't like. The second time, they'll begin to see past the imperfections. And the third time, they'll begin to see at least a few things they like...

IF YOU'RE INTERESTED in starting a speaking circle, contact the NSP office for the chapter leader packet. It has an audio tape, a video, and all the printed materials you need...8 to 10 [people] is ideal for a 2 1/2 hour program.

Annie Bradburry, Executive Director of the National Stuttering Project, described her experiences with speaking circles:

There is a big difference between a regular NSP meeting and the speaking circles. I have enjoyed the NSP meeting environment for 16 years now and they can't be replaced.

What the speaking circle does for me is provide the same safe environment as an NSP meeting but the opportunity to work on public speaking. How to speak spontaneous, take control of the room (make it mine) and in doing that, realizing that as the speaker, I set the pace.

We have heard from many who have experienced Toastmasters how much they have grown from getting involved.

I tried Toastmasters years ago, but at that time in my life, found the structure too intimidating for me. The Speaking Circle atmosphere is more informal and again, we have the added support of our fellow NSP members. Don't get me wrong, this is not an "avoidance" of any sort. Actually quite the opposite. Being comfortable with my NSP friends has given me a more "free" environment to really step out of my comfort zone. And, sometimes it is harder doing uncomfortable things in front of peers.

Another difference between the Speaking Circles and a regular NSP meeting are the timed speeches. They are not planned ahead of time, yet for those who have a speech coming up for work or school, planned speeches can be used and a great time to practice and prepare. Not planning in advance helps one-on-one conversations. It has helped me think on my feet.

Out here in California, people sign up (RSVP) for each meeting. This allows the group to set amounts of time for each speech. Everyone gets the same time and opportunities. The speeches are videotaped. Yes, videotaped. The important thing to remember is that you are the only one who watches your tape. I watch mine in the privacy of my own home. John Harrison recommends that we watch it more than once, at least three times. The reason is that the first time, we tend to criticize our physical self...which I did. The second time...I still criticized my physical but also attacked my stuttering. It is amazing what my chin does during a "good" block. By the third time I was so tired of picking on myself that I finally just watched it. I saw that I was not as bad as I thought. In fact, and this is hard to say here....I thought I was okay!

I had the opportunity a few years ago to attend one of the Speaking Circle meetings in San Francisco that John Harrison has been attending for years. Even though I declined to participate in the beginning, I did finally. I knew that If I didn't, I would be kicking myself later that night. I felt the effects of that one experience during the opening of the general session at the San Diego convention. It was the first time I remembered what I had said after I sat down after speaking. Seriously, before then, I would have no idea what I had said when addressing a group of people.

I continue to attend the regular NSP meetings, while attending Speaking Circles as often as possible.

It is important to remember that the Speaking Circles were not added to the NSP program to replace regular NSP meetings. They are not for everyone, though this could be just the thing for some in your group.

Politically-Correct Stuttering Words

It's incorrect to say that someone "stutters badly," or "is a bad stutterer."

What is "bad stuttering"? What is "good stuttering"? If you can stutter on any sound, any word, in any situation, you must be good at stuttering. Long blocks, with great physical struggle, must be excellent stuttering.

The worst stutterers are speech pathology students assigned to stutter for one day to see what stuttering feels like. The students go out and do a little repetition here and there. No laryngeal blocks, no physical struggle. I'd give these students a "D" in stuttering!

"Good stuttering" is when you stutter without fear or anxiety. Voluntary stuttering (a part of stuttering modification therapy) is always "good stuttering."

"Bad stuttering" is when you hide your stuttering, not talking when you want to, or substituting a word you can say for the word you want to say. Bad stuttering makes ruins your life.

If this confuses you, say "severe stuttering" and "mild stuttering."

Some people object to the term "stutterer," preferring "person who stutters" (or PWS), or even "person who occasionally stutters." The idea is that stuttering is something we do, not something we are.

This point is debatable. A person who flies an airplane is a pilot. A person who creates art is an artist.

People are happy to "be" something they are proud of. People don't want to be something that is embarrassing and disrespected. Saying "person who stutters" suggests that you are embarrassed about stuttering. Referring to yourself as a "stutterer" suggests you are not embarrassed.

What about the unfortunate 99% that never learned to stutter? We can't call them "fluent speakers," because they are disfluent about 2% of the time. Calling them "normal speakers" doesn't sound politically-correct. "Person who doesn't stutter" is a mouthful. Call them "non-stutterers."

Some people use the euphemism "speech impediment" instead of "stuttering." If someone has myopia, do you say he has a "vision impediment"? Of course not, you say he's near-sighted, or wears glasses. "Speech impediment" suggests that stuttering is too embarrassing to talk about.

And, lastly, a few "radical" stutterers (all long-time members of the National Stuttering Project) object to the "f-word." The "f-word," if you haven't guessed, is (dare I say it) "fluency"!

Ten Advantages Of Stuttering

1) You can annoy telemarketers by practicing your therapy techniques. Do really long stretched-vowels, bounces, or whatever your speech therapist wants you to practice. Ask really stupid questions and keep them on the phone as long as possible.

2) Museums give handicapped discounts. When you buy a ticket, get into a good block, with eye blinking, head jerks, facial grimaces, etc., and ask for the handicapped price. This works on buses too.

3) On lie detector tests, detectives first ask simple "baseline" questions such as your name. Our stress levels go so high struggling to say our names that any lie after that is undetectable.

4) Substituting words builds vocabulary!

5) Being handicapped is politically-correct. Try saying, "My people are oppressed by a society that judges us by how we speak, not by who we are."

6) If you get a ticket for parking in a handicapped space, stutter to the parking patrol officer. (I doubt this works.) If you want to avoid the draft, try to get a 4-F for stuttering. (That didn't work either.)

7) Oliver Stone's producer, after saying that they "loved" my screenplay "but it's not what Oliver wants to do right now" (the oldest line in Hollywood), added that stuttering was an advantage, because the movie industry likes people who are "brilliant but not perfect."

8) Tell people that stutterers are, on average, 15 IQ points smarter than non-stutterers. It's not true, but they'll never find out. Or say that we're better at math, more artistic, or better drivers. Whatever fits the occasion.

9) Stuttering can be an advantage or a disadvantage in dating. If you're open about it and show that you are working on improving your speech, stuttering can be an attraction. Revealing a minor fault creates emotional intimacy. If you show that stuttering isn't stopping you from doing the things you want, you come across as courageous. In contrast, if you stutter severely but aren't doing anything about it, or if you are afraid to talk and reveal that you stutter, you come across as a having major personality problems. I met one girlfriend by introducing myself and saying that my speech therapist wanted me to work on therapy techniques with strangers. Recently a woman told me that she thinks my stuttering is cute!

10) "Stuttering is frustrating and can feel demeaning, but if understood, and confronted, it need not change the quality of one's life. I would even say, that it can enhance one's life experience. You know the expression, 'What doesn't kill us makes us stronger'? Stuttering is a chronic problem, but it is also a chronic challenge which calls on us to be more than we might normally be." — John Ahlbach, former Executive Director of the National Stuttering Project.

REFERENCES

Ambrose, N., Yairi, E., Cox, N. "Genetic Aspects of Early Childhood Stuttering." *Journal of Speech and Hearing Research, 36,* 701-706, August 1993.

Andrews, G., Cutler, J. "Stuttering Therapy: The relation between changes in symptom level and attitudes." *Journal of Speech and Hearing Disorders, 39,* 312-319, 1974.

Andrews, G., Guitar, B., Howie, P. (1980) "Meta-Analysis of the Effects of Stuttering Treatment." *Journal of Speech and Hearing Disorders.* 45:287-307.

Andrews, *et al.*, "Stuttering: a review of research findings and theories," *Journal of Speech and Hearing Disorders*, 48, 226-246, 1983.

Andrews, G., Craig, A. (1988) "Prediction of Outcome after Treatment for Stuttering." *British Journal of Psychiatry.* 153: 236-240.

APA, *Diagnostic and Statistical Manual of Mental Disorders*, American Psychiatric Association, 1987.

Armson, J., Jenson, S., Gallant, D., Kalinowski, J., Fee, J. "The Relationship Between Degree of Audible Struggle and Judgements of Childhood Disfluencies as Stuttered or Not Stuttered." *American Journal of Speech-Language Pathology*, 6, 42-50, February 1997.

Armson, J., Kalinowski, J., Foote, S., Witt, C., Stuart, A. "Effect of Frequency Altered Feedback and Audience Size on Stuttering." *European Journal of Disorders of Communication* (1997).

Armson, J., Stuart, A. "Effect of Extended Exposure to Frequency-Altered Feedback on Stuttering During Reading and Monologue." *Journal of Speech, Language, and Hearing Research, 41,* 479-490, June 1998.

ASHA Code of Ethics, I-F, 1993.

Bakker, Klaas. "Instrumentation For The Assessment And Treatment Of Stuttering." In *Nature and Treatment of Stuttering: New Directions*, edited by R.F. Curlee and G.M. Siegel. (1996) Needham Heights, MA: Allyn & Bacon.

Bebout, L., Arthur, B. "Cross-Cultural Attitudes Toward Speech Disorders." *Journal of Speech and Hearing Research, 35,* 45-52, February 1992.

Blood, I., Wertz, H., Blood, G., Bennett, S., Simpson, K. "The Effect of Life Stressors and Daily Stressors on Stuttering." *Journal of Speech, Language, and Hearing Research, 40,* 134-143, February 1997.

Bloodstein, Oliver (1993) *Stuttering: The Search For A Cause And Cure.* Boston: Allyn & Bacon.

Bloodstein, Oliver (1995) *A Handbook On Stuttering,* 5th edition, San Diego: Singular Press.

Bloodstein, Oliver (1996) "Stuttering As An Anticipatory Struggle Reaction," in R.F. Curlee & G.M.Siegel, *Nature and Treatment of Stuttering: New Directions.* Boston: Allyn&Bacon.

Bly, Robert. *Iron John* (Georges Borchardt, Inc., 1991).

Bobrick, Benson. *Knotted Tongues.* New York: Simon&Schuster, 1995

Bosshardt, H., Fransen, H. (1996) "Online Sentence Processing in Adults Who Stutter and Adults Who Do Not Stutter." *Journal of Speech and Hearing Research, 39:4,* 785-797.

Bosshardt, H. "Mental Effort and Speech Fluency," in *Speech Production: Motor Control, Brain Research and Fluency Disorders*, edited by W. Hulstijn, H.F.M. Peters, and P.H.H.M. Van Lieshout, Amsterdam: Elsevier, 1997.

Botterill, W., Cook, F. "Personal Construct Theory and the Treatment of Adolescent Dysfluency," in *Progress in the Treatment of Fluency Disorders*, ed. Rustin, L., Pursor, H., Rowley, D. London: Taylor&Francis, 1987.

Brady, J.P., Price, T.R., McAllister, T.W., Dietrich, K. (1989). A trial of verapamil in the treatment of stuttering in adults. *Biological Psychiatry, 25(5)*, 630-633.

Braun, A.R., Varga, M., Stager, S., Schulz, G., Selbie, S., Maisog, J.M., Carsom, R.E., Ludlow, C.L. "Atypical Lateralization of Hemispehral Activity in Developmental Stuttering: An $H_2{}^{15}O$ Positron Emission Tomography Study," in *Speech Production: Motor Control, Brain Research and Fluency Disorders*, edited by W. Hulstijn, H.F.M. Peters, and P.H.H.M. Van Lieshout, Amsterdam: Elsevier, 1997.

Brenaut, L., Morrison, S., Kainowski, J., Armson, J., Stuart, A. "Effect of Altered Auditory Feedback on Stuttering During

Telephone Use." Dalhousie University, Halifax, Nova Scotia, Canada. 1995.

Brenner, Marie. "I Never Sang For My Mother." *Vanity Fair, 58*, August 1995, p.128.

Brutten, G., Dancer, J. "Stuttering adapation under distributed and massed conditions." Journal of Fluency Disorders, 5, 1-10.

Brown, Walter A. "The Placebo Effect." *Scientific American*, January 1998, 90-96.

Butcher, S. Stut-hlp posting, January 27, 1998. Reprinted with permission.

Carlin, Peter Ames. "Even Clinton wigged out." *People Weekly*, November 3, 1997, v48, n18, p28.

Carlisle, J., *Tangled Tongue*, University of Toronto Press, 1985.

Carlson, T. "Peaks pique viewers interest; Series is Lipton's cup of tea." *TV Guide*, 38:16, p.41, April 27, 1990.

Carlton, Jim. *Apple: The Inside Story of Intrigue, Egomania, and Business Blunders*. (New York: Random House, 1997).

Carpenter, Andrew. E-mail discussion on stutt-x, 1996.

Caruso, A., *et al.* "Adults Who Stutter: Responses to Cognitive Stress." *Journal of Speech and Hearing Research, 37,* 746-754, August 1994.

Caruso, A., Max, L. "Applications of Motor Learning Theory To Stuttering Research," in *Speech Production: Motor Control, Brain Research and Fluency Disorders*, edited by W. Hulstijn, H.F.M. Peters, and P.H.H.M. Van Lieshout, Amsterdam: Elsevier, 1997.

Chadwick, E.F.K. "Readers' Letters: Stuttering Aid Dogs." *Speaking Out*, 18:2, Summer 1997.

Comings, D., et al., "Polygenic Inheritance of Tourette Syndrome, Stuttering, Attention Deficit Hyperactivity, Conduct, and Oppositional Defiant Disorder," *American Journal of Medical Genetics 67*:264-288 (1996).

Cook, Lynn E. "Textbook on Masking for Student Clinicians," *ADVANCE For SLPs*, September 9, 1996, p.11.

Cooper, E., "The Mentally Retarded Stutterer," in *The Atypical*

Stutterer, ed. Kenneth St. Louis, New York: Academic Press, 1986.

Cooper, E.B., and Cooper, C.S. "A fluency disorders prevention program for preschoolers and children in the primary grades." *American Journal of Speech-Language Pathology*, 1, 28-32 (1991).

Cooper, E.B, Cooper, C.S. "Clinician Attitudes Towards Stuttering"

Craig, A., Cleary, P. "Reduction of Stuttering by Young Male Stutterers Using EMG Feedback." *Biofeedback and Self-Regulation*, Vol. 7, No. 3, 1982.

Craig, A., Calver, P. "Following Up on Treated Stutterers: Studies of Perceptions of Fluency and Job Status." *Journal of Speech and Hearing Research, 34,* 279-284, April 1991.

Craig and Kearns. June 1995 *Journal of Speech and Hearing Disorders* ("Results of a Traditional Acupuncture Intervention for Stuttering")

Craig, A., et al. "A Controlled Clinical Trial for Stuttering in Persons Aged 9 to 14 Years" *Journal of Speech and Hearing Research, 39:4,* 808-826, August 1996.

Csikszentmihaly, Mihaly. *Creativity.* 1996, New York: HarperCollins.

Culatta, R., Bader, J., McCaslin, A., Thomason, N. "Primary School Stutterers: Have Attitudes Changed?" *Journal of Fluency Disorders, 10.* 87-91, 1985.

Culatta, R., Goldberg, S. *Stuttering Therapy: An Integrated Approach to Theory and Practice.* Boston: Allyn and Bacon, 1995.

Daily Mail, "A Pill To End The Agony Of Stammering" 20 January 1998.

Daly, David. "Cluttering," in *Stuttering and Related Disorders of Fluency,* edited by Richard F. Curlee, Ph.D., New York: Thieme Medical Publishers, 1993.

De Nil, L., Brutten, G. "Speech-Associated Attitudes of Stuttering and Nonstuttering Children," *Journal of Speech and Hearing Research, 34,* 60-66, February 1991.

De Nil, L., & Kroll, R. "The Relationship Between Locus of Control and Long-Term Stuttering Treatment Outcome in Adult Stutterers," *Journal of Fluency Disorders*, 20:4, December 1995.

De Nil, L., Kroll, R., Houle, S., Ludlow, C., Braun, A., Ingham, R.J.

(1995). "Advances in stuttering research using positron emission tomography brain imaging." *ASHA, 37,* 89.

De Nil, L., Kroll, R., & Ham, R. "Therapy Review," *Journal of Fluency Disorders*, 21, 1996 61-67.

Dewar, A., Dewar, A.D., Austin, W.T.S., Brash, H.M. (1979) "The Long Term Use of an Automatically Triggered Auditory Feedback Masking Device in the Treatment of Stammering," *British Journal of Disorders of Communication*, vol. 14, no. 3.

Doman, Glenn, *What To Do About Your Brain-Injured Child*, 1974.

Douglas, John. *Mindhunter: Inside the FBI's Elite Serial Crime Unit.* New York: Scribner, 1995.

Drew, Polly. "A Stutter Won't Stop You," *Milwaukee Journal-Sentinal*, July 27, 1997, p.4L.

Druce, T., Debney, S., Byrt, T. "Evaluation of an Intensive Treatment Program for Stuttering in Young Children." *Journal of Fluency Disorders, 22,* August 1997, 169-186.

EEOC, 1990. Equal Employment Opportunity Commission Technical Assistance Manual, page II-10.

Felsenfeld, S. (1996) "Epidemiology and Genetics of Stuttering" in R.F. Curlee & G.M. Siegel, *Nature & Treatment of Stuttering: New Directions.* Boston: Allyn&Bacon.

Finn, Patrick. "Establishing the Validity of Recovery From Stuttering Without Formal Treatment," *Journal of Speech & Hearing Research, 39,* 1171-1181, December 1996.

Finn, Patrick. "Adults Recovered From Stuttering Without Formal Treatment: Perceptual Assessment of Speech Normalcy," *Journal of Speech, Language, and Hearing Research, 40*, 821-831, August 1997.

Finn, Patrick. "Children Recovered From Stuttering Without Formal Treatment: Perceptual Assessment of Speech Normalcy," *Journal of Speech, Language, and Hearing Research, 40*, 867-876, August 1997.

Fonzi, Gaeton. *Annenberg.* New York: Weybright & Talley, 1969.

Fosnot, S. (1993). "Research design for examining treatment efficacy in fluency disorders." *Journal of Fluency Disorders, 18,* 221-251.

Fox, PT, Ingham, RJ, Ingham, JC, et al., "A PET study of the neural systems of stuttering," *Nature*, vol. 382, July 11 1996, 158-162.

Fraser, Antonia. *King James VI of Scotland, I of England.* (London: Weidenfeld and Nicolson; 1974) p. 163.

Fraser, Jane (1996). Personal correspondance.

Freeman, Frances. 1993. University of Texas, personal correspondence.

Gathman, Bob. "Tommy John," *The Speak Easy Newsletter*, 18:1 (Spring 1998).

Ghostwriter, 1993 PBS drama series focused on illiteracy.

Giret, Karen. *Letting GO*, National Stuttering Project newsletter, July/August 1996.

Gladwell, Malcolm. "Do Parents Matter?" *The New Yorker*, August, 17, 1998.

Glenn, Larry A., alt.support.stuttering (June 19, 1996).

Glover, Helen, Kalinowski, J., Rastatter, M., Stuart, A. "Effect of Instruction To Sing On Stuttering Frequency At Normal and Fast Rates", *Perceptual and Motor Skills*, 1996, 83, 511-522.

Goldberg, G. (1985). "Supplementary motor area structure and function: Review and hypothesis." *The Behavioral and Brain Sciences, 8,* 567-616.

Goldberg, H., 1994 Personal correspondence. Foundation For Fluency, 9242 Gross Point Road #305, Skokie, IL 60077.

Goleman, Daniel, and Joel Gurin *Mind/Body Medicine*, by , Consumer Reports Books, 1993.

Goleman, Daniel, *Emotional Intelligence*, 1995. New York: Bantam Books, page 43.

Gottwald, S., Starkweather, W., "Fluency Intervention for Preschoolers and Their Families in the Public Schools," *Language, Speech, and Hearing Services in Schools*, Vol. 26, April 1995.

Guitar, B., Bass, C. "Stuttering Therapy: The relation between attitude change and long-term outcome." *Journal of Speech and Hearing Disorders, 43,* 392-400.

Häge, A., Rommel, D., Johannsem, H., Schulze, H. "Cognitive and

Linguistic Abilities of Stuttering Children," in *Speech Production: Motor Control, Brain Research and Fluency Disorders*, edited by W. Hulstijn, H.F.M. Peters, and P.H.H.M. Van Lieshout, Amsterdam: Elsevier, 1997.

Ham, R., *Techniques of Stuttering Therapy*, Englewood Cliffs: Prentice-Hall, 1986.

Hancock, K., Craig, A., McCready, C., McCaul, A., Costello, D., Campbell, K., Gilmore, G. "Two- to Six-Year Controlled-Trial Stuttering Outcomes for Children and Adolescents," *Journal of Speech, Language, and Hearing Research*, *41*:1242-1252, December 1998.

Hansen, Barry. Personal correspondence, 1999.

Hargrave, S., Kalinowski, J., Stuart, A., Armson, J., Jones, K. (1994) "Stuttering reduction under frequency-altered feedback at two speech rates." *Journal of Speech and Hearing Research, 37,* 1313-1320.

Harkness, Richard, 1996. Internet discussion group.

Helm-Estabrooks, Nancy. "Stuttering Associated With Acquired Neurological Disorders," in *Stuttering and Related Disorders of Fluency*, edited by Richard F. Curlee, Ph.D., New York: Thieme Medical Publishers, 1993.

Hollins Communications Research Institute, July 26, 1993.

Howell, P., Sackin, S., Glenn, K. "Development of a Two-Stage Procedure for the Automatic Recognition of Dysfluencies in the Speech of Children Who Stutter." *Journal of Speech, Language, and Hearing Research, 40*, 1073-1096, October 1997.

Howell, P., Kapoor, A, Rustin, L. "The Effects of Formal and Casual Interview Styles on Stuttering Incidence," in *Speech Production: Motor Control, Brain Research and Fluency Disorders*, edited by W. Hulstijn, H.F.M. Peters, and P.H.H.M. Van Lieshout, Amsterdam: Elsevier, 1997.

Howell, P., Sackin, S., Williams, R. "Differential Effects of Frequency-Shifted Feedback Between Child and Adult Stutterers." Journal of Fluency Disorders, 24 (1999) 127-136.

Howie, P.M., Tanner, S., Andrews, G. "Short- and Long-Term Outcomes in an Intensive Treatment Program for Adult Stutterers." Journal of Speech and Hearing Disorders, 46: 104-109, 1981.

Hurwitz, Michael, Stutt-L listserv, December 12, 1997.

Hutchings, D. "Can You Dig It? *The Mod Squad's* Peggy Lipton, One Marriage and 15 Years Later, Returns To Acting." *People Weekly*, 29:13, April 4, 1988.

Ingham, R.J., Fox, P.T., et al. "Functional-Lesion Investigation of Developmental Stuttering With Positron Emission Tomography." *Journal of Speech & Hearing Research, 39,* 1208-1227, December 1996.

Ingham, R., Moglia, R., Frank, P., Ingham, J., Cordes, A. "Experimental Investigation of the Effects of Frequency-Altered Auditory Feedback on the Speech of Adults who Stutter." *Journal of Speech and Hearing Research*, 40:2, 361-373, April 1997.

Ingham R.J., Fox, P.T., Ingham, J.C.. "A $H_2{}^{15}O$ Positron Emission Tomography (PET) Study On Adults Who Stutter: Findings and Implications," in *Speech Production: Motor Control, Brain Research and Fluency Disorders*, edited by W. Hulstijn, H.F.M. Peters, and P.H.H.M. Van Lieshout, Amsterdam: Elsevier, 1997.

James, J.E. "Punishment of stuttering: Contingency and stimulus parameters." *Journal of Communication Disorders*, 1981, 14, 375-386.

Jäncke, L., Bauer, A., Kalveram, K. "Prosodic Disturbances in Stuttering Adults," in *Speech Production: Motor Control, Brain Research and Fluency Disorders*, edited by W. Hulstijn, H.F.M. Peters, and P.H.H.M. Van Lieshout, Amsterdam: Elsevier, 1997.

Janssen, P., Kloth, S., Kraaimat, F., Brutten, G. "Genetic Factors In Stuttering: A Replication of Ambrose, Yairi, and Cox's (1993) Study With Adult Probands," *Journal of Fluency Disorders,* 21(June 1996), 105-106.

Johnson, B. "Bruce Oldfield Makes Clothes Fit For A (Future) Queen." *People Weekly*, April 13, 1987, p.137.

Johnson, W., Rosen, L. "Studies in the psychology of stuttering," *Journal of Speech Disorders, 2,* 1937, 105-110.

Johnson, W. *Stuttering and what you can do about it.* Garden 'City, NY: Doubleday, 1961.

Jones, James Earl. *Voices and Silences.* New York: Scribners, 1993.

Kalinowski, J., Armson, J., Stuart, A., Graco, V., and Roland-Mieskowski, M. "Effects of alterations in auditory feedback and speech rate on stuttering frequency," *Language and Speech*, 1993, 36, 1-16.

Kalinowski, Joseph, Joy Armson, *et al.*, "Effect of Frequency-Altered Feedback on Stuttering Frequency at Normal and Fast Speech Rates," *Journal of Speech and Hearing Research*, 37:6, December 1994.

Kalinowski, J., Rastatter, M., Cranford, J., Stuart, A. "Topographic EEG Mapping Of Stuttering Subjects During Speech Tasks Under Normal and Altered Feedback Conditions." 1997. East Carolina University, unpublished.

Kaylin, L. "Big Bad Bruce." *Gentleman's Quarterly,* v66, n6, June 1996, p.159.

Kehoe, Alice. *North American Indians: A Comprehansive Account*, 2nd Edition, p.245. Prentice-Hall, Inc. (Englewood Cliffs, NJ), 1992. See also *Hiawatha and the Iroquois Confederation* and *Proc. of the American Association for the Advancement of Science* 30:324-341, both by Horatio E. Hale, 1882; and "Hi-a-wat-ha," by William M. Beauchamp, *Journal of American Folklore* 4(15):295-306, 1891.

Kelly, E.M. & Conture, E.G. (1992) "Speaking rates, response time latencies, and interrupting behaviors of young stutterers, non-stutterers, and their mothers." *Journal of Speech and Hearing Research, 37,* 1256-1267.

Kelly, E.M. (1994) "Speech rates and turn-taking behaviors of children who stutter and their fathers." *Journal of Speech and Hearing Research, 37,* 1284-1294.

Kelly, Ellen. "Orofacial Muscle Activity of Children Who Stutter," *et al.*, *Journal of Speech and Hearing Research*, 38:5, October 1995.

Kelly, G., *The Psychology of Personal Constructs*, New York: Norton, 1955.

Kinsbourne, Marcel. "Single-Channel Theory," in *Human Skills*, edited by Dennis Holding, New York: John Wiley, 1981.

Kloth, S.A.M., Jannsen, P., Kraaimaat, F.W., Brutten, G.J. (1995) "Communicative Behavior of Mothers of Stuttering and Nonstuttering High-Risk Children Prior to the Onset of Stuttering," *Journal of Fluency Disorders, 20,* 365-377.

Kottke, F.J., Halpern, D., Easton, J.K.M., Ozel, A.T., Burrill, C.A. "The Training of Coordination." *Archives of Physical Medicine and*

Rehabilitation, Vol 59, December 1978, 567-572.

Kram, Mark. "Ben Still Needs To Run," Outside, Vol. 23, no. 12, December 1998.

Kroll, R.M., De Nil, L.F., Kapur, S., Houle, S. "A Positron Emission Tomography Investigation of Post-Treatment Brain Activation in Stutterers," in *Speech Production: Motor Control, Brain Research and Fluency Disorders*, edited by W. Hulstijn, H.F.M. Peters, and P.H.H.M. Van Lieshout, Amsterdam: Elsevier, 1997.

Kottke, F.J., Halpern, D., Easton, J.K.M., Ozel, A.T., & Burrill, C.A. (1978). The training of coordination. *Archives of Physical Medicine and Rehabilitation*, 59, 567-572.

Kuehn, Donald (1994). Official correspondence from the National Institute of Deafness and Communication Disorders.

Kuhr, Armin "The Rise and Fall of Operant Programs for the Treatment of Stuttering," *Folia Phoniatrica et Logopaedica*, September 1994.

Laboy, Julio. *Newsday*, September 12, 1993.

Langlois, A., Hanrahan, L.L., & Inouye, L.L. (1986) A comparison of interactions between stuttering children, nonstuttering children, and their mothers." *Journal of Fluency Disorders, 11*, 263-273.

Lawrence, M. "A Man of Many Words." *Sports Illustrated*, v79, n18, November 1, 1993, p.91.

Lee TD, Swanson LR, Hall AL. "What is repeated in repetition? Effects of practice conditions on motor skill acquisition." *Physical Therapy*, 1991;71:150-156.

Leith, W. "Treating the Stutterer With Atypical Cultural Influences," in *The Atypical Stutterer*, ed. Kenneth St. Louis, New York: Academic Press, 1986.

Lincoln, A., Onslow, M. "Long-Term Outcome of Early Intervention for Stuttering." *American Journal of Speech-Language Pathology, 6,* 51-58, February 1997.

Logan, K., Conture, E. "Selected Temporal, Grammatical, and Phonological Characteristics of Conversational Utterances Produced by Children Who Stutter." *Journal of Speech, Language, and Hearing Research, 40.* 107-120. February 1997.

Louganis, G., Marcus, E. *Breaking The Surface.* New York: Random

House, 1995.

Ludlow, C., Siren, K, Zikria, M. "Speech Production Learning In Adults With Chronic Developmental Stuttering," in *Speech Production: Motor Control, Brain Research and Fluency Disorders*, edited by W. Hulstijn, H.F.M. Peters, and P.H.H.M. Van Lieshout, Amsterdam: Elsevier, 1997.

Maccoby, Eleanor E. "Gender and Relationships: A Developmental Account." *American Psychologist*, vol. 45, no. 4, April 1990, pages 513-520.

MacLeod, J., Kalinowski, J., Stuart, A., and Armson, J. (1995). Effect of single and combined altered auditory feedback on stuttering frequency at two speech rates. *Journal of Communication Disorders*. 28 218-226).

Maguire, Gerald. "Nimodipine in the Treatment of Stuttering," , *et al.*, *UCI Psychiatry* Journal, 2:1, 1995.

Maguire, Gerald. Lecture at National Stuttering Project convention, 1996.

Maguire, G., Riley, G.D., Wu, J.C., Franklin, D.L., Potkin, S. "Effects of risperidone in the treatment of stuttering," in *Speech Production: Motor Control, Brain Research and Fluency Disorders*, edited by W. Hulstijn, H.F.M. Peters, and P.H.H.M. Van Lieshout, Amsterdam: Elsevier, 1997.

Mahr, G., Leith, W., "Psychogenic Stuttering of Adult Onset." *Journal of Speech and Hearing Research*, 35:283-286, April 1992.

Manschreck, T., Kalotkin, M., Jacobson, A. "Utility of Electromyographic Biological Feedback in Chronic Stuttering: A Clinical Study With Follow-Up." *Perceptual and Motor Skills*, 1980, 51, 535-540.

Marsh, Dave. *Before I Get Old* (St. Martin's Press, 1983).

Max, L., Caruso, A. "Adaptation of Stuttering Frequency During Repeated Readings: Associated Changes in Acoustic Parameters of Perceptually Fluent Speech." *Journal of Speech, Language, and Hearing Research, 41*, 1265-1281, December 1998.

McInerney, J. "Bruce Willis In The Hot Zone." *Esquire*, 123:5, p.62, May 1995.

Merzenich, M., Jenkins, W., Johnston, P., Schreiner, C., Miller, S., and Tallal, P. "Temporal Processing Deficits of Language-Learning

Impaired Children Ameliorated by Training," *Science* vol. 271, January 5 1996, p.77-80.

Meyers, S.C., & Freeman, F.J. (1985a) "Are mothers of stutterers different? An investigation of social-communicative interaction." *Journal of Fluency Disorders, 10,* 193-209.

Meyers, S.C., & Freeman, F.J. (1985b) "Interruptions as a variable in stuttering and disfluency." *Journal of Speech and Hearing Research, 28,* 428-435.

Meyers, S.C., & Freeman, F.J. (1985c) "Mother and child speech rates as a variable in stuttering and disfluency." *Journal of Speech and Hearing Research, 28,* 436-444.

Meyers, S.C. (1986) "Qualitative and quantitative differences and patterns of variability in disfluencies emitted by preschool stutterers and non-stutterers during dyadic conversation." *Journal of Fluency Disorders, 11,* 293-306.

Meyers, S.C. (1990) "Verbal behaviors of preschool stutterers and conversational partners: Observing reciprocal relationships." *Journal of Speech and Hearing Disorders, 54,* 706-712.

Miller, S., Watson, B. "The Relationship Between Communication Attitude, Anxiety, and Depression in Stutterers and Non-stutterers." *Journal of Speech and Hearing Research, 35,* 789-798, August 1992.

Moore, W.E. "Hypnosis in a system of therapy for stutterers." *Journal of Speech Disorders, 11,* 117-22 (1946).

Morthland, John. "Guitar Rock 1974-1975." Time/Life Music, 1993.

Nefsky, Art. Letter from Mel Tillis, Sept. 30, 1997, http://www.nefsky.com/tillis.htm

Neiders, Gunars. Stutt-x e-mail correspondance, December 18, 1997.

Newman-Tancredi, Adrian. "Noradrenaline and adrenaline are high affinity agonists at dopamine D4 receptors." European Journal of Pharmacology 319 (1997) 379-383. 101511,274@compuserve@com. Valerie Audinot-Bouchez, Alain Gobert, Mark J. Millan, Department pf Psychopharmacology, Institut de Recherches, 125 Chemin de Ronde, 78290 Croissy-sur-Seine (Paris), France.

Nippold, M., Rudzinski, M. "Parents' Speech and Children's

Stuttering: A Critique of the Literature," *Journal of Speech and Hearing Research*, 38:5, October 1995.

Onslow, M. "Choosing a Treatment Procedure for Early Stuttering: Issues and Future Directions." *Journal of Speech and Hearing Research, 35,* 983-993, October 1992.

Onslow, Mark. et al. "A Control/Experimental Trial of an Operant Treatment for Early Stuttering," *Journal of Speech and Hearing Research*, 37:6, December 1994.

Onslow, Mark. et al. (1996) "Speech Outcomes of a Prolonged-Speech Treatment for Stuttering," *Journal of Speech and Hearing Research, 39:4*, August 1996.

Onslow, M., Packman, A., Stocker, S., van Doorn, J., Siegel, G. "Control of Children's Stuttering With Response-Contingent Time-Out: Behavioral, Perceptual, and Acoustic Data." *Journal of Speech, Language, and Hearing Research, 40.* 121-133, February 1997.

Oxendine, Jospeh B. Psychology of Motor Learning, 2nd edition. Englewood Cliffs: Prentice-Hall, 1984.

Perkins, W., Dabul, B. "The Effects of Stuttering on Systolic Blood Pressure." *Journal of Speech & Hearing Research*, Vol. 16, No. 4, December 1973.

Perkins, W., Rudas, J., Johnson, L., Bell, J. "Stuttering: Discoordination of Phonation with Articulation and Respiration." *Journal of Speech & Hearing Research*, Vol. 19, No. 3, September 1976.

Perkins, W., Kent, R., Curlee, R. "A Theory of Neuropsycholinguistic Function in Stuttering," *Journal of Speech and Hearing Research*, 34:734-752, August 1991.

Perkins, William. "Fluency Controls And Automatic Fluency," *American Journal of Speech-Language Pathology,* January, 1992.

Perkins, William. *Stuttering And Science*, Singular Publishing Group, San Diego, 1996

Peters, T., Guitar, B. *Stuttering: An Integrated Approach To Its Nature and Treatment*, Baltimore: Williams&Wilkins, 1991. (800) 577-5730

Porterfield, K. "British Researchers Identify Genetic Area Affecting Speech." *ASHA Leader*, Vol. 3, No. 4, March 3, 1998, p.1. Refers to the February, 1998, issue of *Nature Genetics*.

Postma, A., Kolk, H. "Error Monitoring in People Who Stutter: Evidence Against Auditory Feedback Defect Theories." *Journal of Speech and Hearing Research, 35*, 1024-1032, October 1992.

Prins, D., Madelkorn, T., Cerf, A. "Principal and Differential Effects of Haloperidol and Placebo Treatments Upon Speech Disfluencies in Stutterers." *Journal of Speech & Hearing Research, 23,* 614-629, September 1980.

Ramig, L. "Comparison of Two Forms of Intensive Speech Treatment for Parkinson Disease," Lorraine Olson Ramig, et al., *Journal of Speech and Hearing Research*, 38:6, December 1995.) The LSVT treatmnet is also described in the February 26, 1996 issue of the weekly newspaper *ADVANCE For Speech-Language Pathologists* .

Ramig, P., Adams, M. "Vocal Changes in Stutterers and Non-stutterers During High- and Low-Pitched Speech," *Journal of Fluency Disorders, 6* (1981), 15-33.

Ramig, P., Bennett, E. "Working With 7- to 12-Year-Old Children Who Stutter: ideas for Intervention in the Public Schools." *Language, Speech, And Hearing In Schools*, 26:2, April 1995, p.138-150.

Riley, G.D., Wu, J.C., Maguire, G. "PET Scan Evidence of Parallel Cerebral Systems Related To Treatment Effects," in *Speech Production: Motor Control, Brain Research and Fluency Disorders*, edited by W. Hulstijn, H.F.M. Peters, and P.H.H.M. Van Lieshout, Amsterdam: Elsevier, 1997.

Riley, G.D., Maguire, G. "National Enquirer Article" memo, 1998.

Rommel, D., Häge, A., Johannsen, H., Schulze, H. "Linguistic Aspects of Stuttering In Childhood," in *Speech Production: Motor Control, Brain Research and Fluency Disorders*, edited by W. Hulstijn, H.F.M. Peters, and P.H.H.M. Van Lieshout, Amsterdam: Elsevier, 1997.

Rothenberger, A., Johannsem, H., Schulze, H., Amorosa, H., Rommel, D. "Use of Tiapride on Stuttering in Children and Adolescents," *Perceptual and Motor Skills*, 1994, 79, 1163-1170.

Ryan, B.P., Van Kirk, B. "The Establishment, Transfer and Maintenance of Fluent Speech in 50 Stutterers Using Delayed Auditory Feedback and Operant Procedures." *Journal of Speech and Hearing Disorders*, 39:1, February, 1974.

Ryan, Bruce and Barbara Van Kirk Ryan. "Programmed Stuttering Treatment for Children: Comparison of Two Establishment Programs

Through Transfer, Maintenance, and Follow-Up," *Journal of Speech and Hearing Research*, 38:1, February 1995.

St. Louis, Kenneth and Florence Myers. "Clinical Management of Cluttering," , *Language, Speech, and Hearing Services in Schools*, Vol. 26, April 1995

Salmelin R, Schnitzler A, Schmitz F, Jancke L, Witte OW, Freund HJ. "Functional organization of the auditory cortex is different in stutterers and fluent speakers." *Neuroreport* 1998 Jul 13;9(10):2225-2229

Sark, S., Kalinowski, J., Stuart, A., Armson, J. "Stuttering amelioration at various auditory feedback delays and speech rates," European Journal of Disorders of Communication, 31, 259-269, 1996.

Schwartz, Martin *Stutter No More* (New York: Simon & Schuster, 1991, p.21).

Schwartz, Martin, 1996a. Personal correspondance.

Schwartz, Martin, 1996b. National Center for Stuttering World Wide Web site.

Scott, Abigail. "Visualizing Fluency." *ADVANCE For Speech-Language Pathologists & Audiologists*, February 2, 1998, page 10.

Sculley, John. *Odyssey* (1987). p.111.

Shapiro, Francine. *Eye Movement Desensitization & Reprocessing*, 1995.

Shea, C.H., Shebilske, W.L., Worchel, S. *Motor Learning and Control.* Englewood Cliffs: Prentice-Hall, 1993.

Sheehan, J.G. *Stuttering: Research and Therapy*, New York: 1970, p.4.

Shoemaker, Abigail. "Consumers Are Focus of World Fluency Congress." *ADVANCE For SLPs*, July 7, 1997.

Silverman, S., Bernstein Ratner, N. "Syntactic Complexity, Fluency, and Accuracy of Sentence Imitation in Adolescents." *Journal of Speech, Language, and Hearing Research, 40.* 95-106. February 1997.

Singer, Harvey. "In Search of a Trigger." *ADVANCE For Speech-Language Pathologists and Audiologists*, July 6, 1998, page 22.

Smith, A. "Commentary on 'A Theory of Neuropsycholingusitic Function in Stuttering'," *Journal of Speech and Hearing Research*, 35:805-809, August 1992.

Smith, Denny, Shaffer, Kelly and Hirano, "Activity of Intrinsic Laryngeal Muscles in Fluent and Disfluent Speech," *Journal of Speech and Hearing Research, 39,* 329-348, April 1996.

Somer, Elizabeth, *Food and Mood.* New York: Holt, 1995.

Spivey, K. "The Superstar Who Couldn't Speak." *Reader's Digest*, 141:847, November 1992, p.49.

Stager, Ludlow, Gordon, Cotelingam, and Rapoport. "Fluency Changes in Persons Who Stutter Following a Double Blind Trial of Clomipramine and Desipramine," June 1995 *Journal of Speech and Hearing Research.*

Stager, S., Denman, D., Ludlow, C. "Modifications in Aerodynamic Variables by Persons Who Stutter Under Fluency-Evoking Conditions." *Journal of Speech, Language, and Hearing Research*, Volume 40, 832-847, August 1997.

Stager, S., Calis, K., Grothe, D., Bloch, M., Turcasso, N., Ludlow, C., Braun, A. "A Double-Blind Trial of Pimozide and Paroxetine For Stuttering," in *Speech Production: Motor Control, Brain Research and Fluency Disorders*, edited by W. Hulstijn, H.F.M. Peters, and P.H.H.M. Van Lieshout, Amsterdam: Elsevier, 1997.

Starkweather, C.W. *Fluency and Stuttering.* Englewood Cliffs: Prentice-Hall (1987).

Starkweather, Woodruff. 1993. *Letting GO,* National Stuttering Project newsletter.

Starkweather, Woodruff, "A Simple Theory of Stuttering," *Journal of Fluency Disorders*, Vol. 20, No. 2, June 1995.

Starkweather, Woodruff. "The Importance of Being Aware," *Letting GO*, March/April 1996.

Starkweather, Woodruff. "Therapy For Younger Children," in *Nature and Treatment of Stuttering: New Directions, 2nd edition*, edited by Richard Curlee and Gerald Siegel. Needham Heights: Allyn & Bacon, 1997.

Stephenson-Opsal, D., & Bernstein Ratner, N. (1988) "Maternal speech rate modification and childhood stuttering." *Journal of Fluency Disorders, 13,* 49-56.

Stewart, T. (1996) "Good Maintainers and Poor Maintainers: A Personal Construct Approach To An Old Problem," *Journal of Fluency Disorders, 21*, 33-48.

Stewart, T., Brosh, H. (1997) "Use of Drawings With Adult Stammerers," *Journal of Fluency Disorders, 22*, 35-50.

Stossel, J. "Stossel's Biggest Story: Overcoming the Fear of Stuttering." *ADVANCE For Speech-Language Pathologists and Audiologists*, May 12, 1997.

Stuart, A., Kalinowski, J., Armson, J., Stenstrom, R., and Jones, K. (1996). Stuttering reduction under frequency-altered feedback of plus and minus one-half and one-quarter octaves at two speech rates. *Journal of Speech and Hearing Research*, 39, 396-401.

Stuart, A., Kalinowski, J., and Rastatter, M. (in press). Effect of monaural and binaural altered auditory feedback on stuttering frequency, *Journal of the Acoustical Society of America.*

Stuttering Foundation of America, "Complete Set of Books On Stuttering", 1994. P.O. Box 11749, Memphis, TN 38111.

Toch, Thomas, "One man's gift to public education." *U.S. News & World Report*, November 1, 1993, v115, n17, p20.

van Lieshout, Hulstijn, and Peters, "Speech Production in People Who Stutter: Testing the Motor Plan Assembly Hypothesis," *Journal of Speech and Hearing Research*, vol. 39, No. 1, February 1996a, pages 76-92.

van Lieshout, P., Hulstijn, W., Peters, H. "From Planning to Articulation in Speech Production," *Journal of Speech and Hearing Research, 39*, 546-564, June 1996b.

Van Riper, C. *The Nature of Stuttering*, Englewood Cliffs, NJ: Prentice-Hall, 1971.

Van Riper, C. "Stuttering: Where and Whither?," *Asha*, September 1974.

Venkatagiri, H.S. Review of *Stuttering: Science, Therapy & Practice. Journal of Fluency Disorders*, in press 1998.

Venturi, Ken. Stuttering Foundation of America newsletter, 1994.

Wallichenski, David. *Book of Lists* (Boston: Little, Brown, 1995)

Walton, Bill. Stuttering Foundation of America newsletter, Vol. V, No.

1, Spring/Summer 1996

Watkins, R., Yairi, E. "Language Production Abilities of Children Whose Stuttering Persisted or Recovered." *Journal of Speech, Language & Hearing Research, 40,* 385-399, April 1997.

Watson, B.C., Freeman, F.J., Devous, M.D., Chapman, S.B., Finitzo, T., Pool, K.D. "Linguistic Performance and Regional Cerebral Blood Flow in Persons Who Stutter." Journal of Speech and Hearing Research, 37:6, December 1994, 1221-1228.

Watson, B., Freeman, F. (1996) "Brain Imaging Contributions," in R.F. Curlee & G.M. Siegel (eds.) *Nature and Treatment of Stuttering: New Directions*, Boston: Allyn&Bacon.

Webster, Ronald. "Manipulation of Vocal Tone: Implications For Stuttering," in *Speech Motor Controls and Stuttering*, ed. Peters, Hulstijn, and Starkweather, New York: Elsevier, 1991.

Weil, Andrew. New Dimensions Radio , fall 1995.

Weiner, Tim. "Sidney Gottlieb, 80, Dies; Took LSD to C.I.A." *New York Times*, March 10, 1999.

Weiss, A.L., & Zebrowski, P.M. (1992) "Disfluencies in the conversations of young children who stutter: Some answers about questions." Journal of Speech and Hearing Research, 35, 1230-1238.

Weliky, Berta . White Memorial Medical Center, 1720 E. Cesar Chavez Ave., Los Angeles, CA 90033. 1994. Paper presented at ASHA convention poster session.

Wilson, Robert. *ArtNews*, December 1996, p.98

Wingate, M.E. "Recovery From Stuttering." *Journal of Speech & Hearing Disorders, 29,* 312-21 (1964).

Wingate, M. (1986) "Physiological and genetic factors." In G.H. Shames & H. Rubin, Eds.), *Stuttering Then And Now* (pp.49-69). Columbus: Charles E. Merrill Publishing Co.

Winslow, M. & Guitar, B. (1994) "The effects of structured turntaking on disfluencies: A case study." *Language, Speech, and Hearing Services in Schools, 25,* 251-257.

Wu, Joseph, Gerald Maguire, Glyndon Riley, "A positron emission tomography [18-F]deoxyglucose study of developmental stuttering," in *Cognitive Neuroscience and Neuropsychology*, Vol. 6 No. 3,

February 1995, p.501-503.

Wu, J.C., Maguire, G., Riley, G., Fallon, J., LaCasse, L., Chin, S., Klein, E., Tang, C., Cadwell, S., Lottenberg, S. (1995). "A positron emission tomography [18F]deoxyglucose study of developmental stuttering." *Neuroreport*, 6, 501-505.

Wu, J.C., Maguire, G., Riley, G.D., in *Speech Production: Motor Control, Brain Research and Fluency Disorders*, edited by W. Hulstijn, H.F.M. Peters, and P.H.H.M. Van Lieshout, Amsterdam: Elsevier, 1997.

Wurtman, Judith, *Managing Your Mind And Mood Through Food*. New York: Harper & Row, 1986.

Yairi, E. (1983) "The onset of stuttering in two- and three-year-old children," *Journal of Speech and Hearing Research*, *25* 155-160.

Yairi, E., Ambrose, N. "Onset of stuttering in preschool children: Selected factors," *Journal of Speech and Hearing Research, 35*, 1992, 782-788.

Yairi, E., Ambrose, N. "The early months of stuttering: A developmental study," *Journal of Speech and Hearing Research, 36*, 1993, 521-528.

Yairi, E. (1993) "Epidemiologic and other considerations in treatment efficacy research with preschool-age children who stutter," *Journal of Fluency Disorders*, *18*, 197-220.

Yairi, E. Ambrose, N., Cox, N. (1996) "Genetics of Stuttering: A Critical Review," *Journal of Speech and Hearing Research*, 39 771-784.

Yairi, E. (1996) "Home Environment and Parent-Child Interaction in Childhood Stuttering," in R.F. Curlee & G.M. Siegal (eds.) *Nature and Treatment of Stuttering: New Directions, 2nd ed.*, Boston: Allyn&Bacon.

Yaruss, J.S., Conture, E.G. (1995) "Mother and Child Speaking Rates and Utterance Lengths in Adjacent Fluent Utterances: Preliminary Observations," *Journal of Fluency Disorders*, 20, 257-278.

Yaruss, J.S. (1997) "Utterance Timing and Childhood Stuttering," *Journal of Fluency Disorders*, 22, 263-286.

Zimmerman, I. "For $500, Who is Ira Zimmerman?" *ADVANCE For Speech-Language Pathologists and Audiologists*, December 15,

1997, page 4.

Zimmerman, I. "Photography That Speaks Volumes"" *ADVANCE For Speech-Language Pathologists and Audiologists*, 7:50, March 23, 1998, page 22.

Zimmerman, S., Kalinowski, J., Stuart, A., Rastatter, M. "Effect of Altered Auditory Feedback on People Who Stutter During Scripted Telephone Conversations." *Journal of Speech, Language, and Hearing Research*, Vol. 40, 1130-1134, October 1997.

INDEX

C

D

I

J

K

L

M

N

O

P

R

S

T